Pediatric Otolaryngology

Scott R. Schoem, MD, FAAP
David H. Darrow, MD, DDS, FAAP
Editors

American Academy of Pediatrics
DEDICATED TO THE HEALTH OF ALL CHILDREN™

American Academy of Pediatrics Department of Marketing and Publications Staff
Maureen DeRosa, MPA, Director, Department of Marketing and Publications
Mark Grimes, Director, Division of Product Development
Diane E. Lundquist, MS, Senior Product Development Editor
Carrie Peters, Editorial Assistant
Sandi King, MS, Director, Division of Publishing and Production Services
Theresa Wiener, Manager, Publications Production and Manufacturing
Jason Crase, Editorial Specialist
Peg Mulcahy, Manager, Graphic Design and Production
Kevin Tuley, Director, Division of Marketing and Sales
Linda Smessaert, Manager, Clinical and Professional Publications Marketing

Library of Congress Control Number: 2011903232
ISBN: 978-1-58110-604-6
eISBN: 978-1-58110-727-2
MA0596

Cover illustration: Brian Evans/Photo Researchers, Inc.
Book design: Peg Mulcahy

The recommendations in this publication do not indicate an exclusive course of treatment or serve as a standard of medical care. Variations, taking into account individual circumstances, may be appropriate.

The mention of product names in this publication is for informational purposes only and does not imply endorsement by the American Academy of Pediatrics.

Every effort has been made to ensure that the drug selection and dosages set forth in this text are in accordance with the current recommendations and practice at the time of publication. It is the responsibility of the health care provider to check the package insert of each drug for any change in indications and dosage and for added warnings and precautions.

The publishers have made every effort to trace the copyright holders for borrowed material. If they have inadvertently overlooked any, they will be pleased to make the necessary arrangements at the first opportunity.

9-299/0512

1 2 3 4 5 6 7 8 9 10

AMERICAN ACADEMY OF PEDIATRICS
SECTION ON OTOLARYNGOLOGY–HEAD AND NECK SURGERY
EXECUTIVE COMMITTEE
2011–2012

Scott R. Schoem, MD, FAAP
Chairperson

Charles M. Bower, MD, FAAP
Joshua A. Gottschall, MD, FAAP
Diego Preciado, MD, PhD, FAAP
Kristina W. Rosbe, MD, FACS, FAAP
Sally R. Shott, MD, FACS, FAAP
Steven E. Sobol, MD, FAAP

David H. Darrow, MD, DDS, FAAP
Immediate Past Chairperson

To the pioneers of pediatric otolaryngology who developed our subspecialty and dedicated their lives to the art and craft of caring for children with head and neck disorders.

We also recognize the sacrifices of David's wife, Beth, and his children, Evan, Julia, Joshua, and Gwendolyn, and Scott's wife, Rachel, and his son, Noah, whose patience and support made this book possible.

CONTRIBUTORS

Tiffiny Ainsworth, MA, MD
Division of Otolaryngology
Connecticut Children's Medical
   Center
Hartford, CT

Randall A. Bly, MD, FAAP
Department of Otolaryngology-Head
   and Neck Surgery
University of Washington School
   of Medicine
Seattle, WA

Charles M. Bower, MD, FAAP
Division of Otolaryngology
Arkansas Children's Hospital
Little Rock, AR

David H. Chi, MD, FAAP
Children's Hospital of Pittsburgh
Pittsburgh, PA

Sukgi S. Choi, MD, FAAP
Department of Otolaryngology
Children's National Medical Center
Washington, DC

David H. Darrow, MD, DDS, FAAP
Professor of Otolaryngology
   and Pediatrics
Director, Center for Hemangiomas
   and Vascular Birthmarks
Children's Hospital of The
   King's Daughters
Eastern Virginia Medical School
Norfolk, VA

Carrie L. Francis, MD, FAAP
Assistant Professor, Pediatric
   Otolaryngology
Department of Otolaryngology,
   Head & Neck Surgery
Kansas University Medical Center
Kansas City, KS

John Gavin, MD, FAAP
Assistant Professor, Pediatric
   Otolaryngology
Department of Surgery
Albany Medical College
Albany, NY

Christopher Hartnick, MD, FAAP
Massachusetts Eye and Ear Infirmary
Boston, MA

Dorsey Heithaus, MA
Cincinnati Children's Hospital
   Medical Center
Cincinnati, OH

Ian N. Jacobs, MD, FAAP
Department of Otolaryngology
Children's Hospital of Philadelphia
Philadelphia, PA

Eric M. Jaryszak, MD, PhD, FAAP
Department of Otolaryngology
Children's National Medical Center
Washington, DC

Raymond Maguire, DO, FAAP
Children's Hospital of Pittsburgh
Pittsburgh, PA

David L. Mandell, MD, FAAP
Volunteer Associate Professor
Department of Otolaryngology
University of Miami
Miami, FL
Clinical Associate Professor
Division of Otolaryngology
NOVA Southeastern University
Ft. Lauderdale, FL

Steve Maturo, MD, FAAP
Massachusetts Eye and Ear Infirmary
Boston, MA

Anna K. Meyer, MD, FAAP
Lucille Packard Children's Hospital
Stanford, CA

Patrick D. Munson, MD, FAAP
Division of Otolaryngology
Arkansas Children's Hospital
Little Rock, AR

T.J. O-Lee, MD, FAAP
Division of Otolaryngology
University of Nevada School
   of Medicine
Las Vegas, NV

Blake Papsin, MD, FAAP
Department of Otolaryngology-Head
   and Neck Surgery
Hospital for Sick Children
Toronto, ON

Sanjay R. Parikh, MD, FACS
Seattle Children's Hospital
Seattle, WA

Maria T. Peña, MD, FAAP
Department of Otolaryngology
Children's National Medical Center
Washington, DC

Seth M. Pransky, MD, FAAP
Clinical Professor of Surgery
Division of Otolaryngology
University of California, San Diego
San Diego, CA
Director, Pediatric Otolaryngology
Rady Children's Specialist Medical
   Foundation
San Diego, CA

Eileen M. Raynor, MD, FACS, FAAP
Assistant Professor, Otolaryngology-
   Head and Neck Surgery and
   Pediatrics
Duke University Department
   of Surgery
Chapel Hill, NC

Corrie E. Roehm, MD
Division of Otolaryngology
Connecticut Children's Medical
   Center
Hartford , CT

Kristina W. Rosbe, MD, FACS, FAAP
Division of Otolaryngology
University of California,
   San Francisco
San Francisco, CA

Scott R. Schoem, MD, FAAP
Division of Otolaryngology
Connecticut Children's Medical
   Center
Hartford, CT

Anthony Sheyn, BS
Cincinnati Children's Hospital
   Medical Center
Cincinnati, OH

Sally R. Shott, MD, FACS, FAAP
Cincinnati Children's Hospital
   Medical Center
Department of Otolaryngology-Head
   Neck Surgery
University of Cincinnati
Cincinnati, OH

Yamilet Tirado, MD, FAAP
Department of Otolaryngology
Hospital for Sick Children
Toronto, ON

Tulio A. Valdez, MD, FAAP
Division of Otolaryngology, 2L
Connecticut Children's Medical
  Center
Hartford, CT

Mark S. Volk, MD, DMD, FAAP
Department of Otolaryngology
Boston Children's Hospital
Boston, MA

Amy S. Whigham, MD
Department of Otolaryngology
Children's National Medical Center
Washington, DC

J. Paul Willging, MD, FAAP
Department of Otolaryngology
Cincinnati Children's Hospital
  Medical Center
Cincinnati, OH

Daniel L. Wohl, MD, FACS, FAAP
Pediatric and Adolescent
  Otolaryngology
Department of Surgery
University of Florida-Jacksonville
Jacksonville, FL

Robert F. Yellon, MD, FACS, FAAP
Children's Hospital of Pittsburgh
Pittsburgh, PA

FOREWORD

As a busy community pediatrician serving a large rural population for the last 35 years, I have encountered numerous pediatric head and neck dilemmas. I have intubated more babies than I can count, clipped more tongues than most doctors, put needles in peritonsillar abscesses in the office, done incision and drainage procedures on children with lymphadenitis/abscesses in the head and neck region, performed myringotomies on complicated children with otitis media, and sweated through the management of really sick young children with croup and impending respiratory failure. I have been fortunate in my rural hospital to have the support of otolaryngologists and anesthesiologists, such that most of my patients have achieved good outcomes and most have completed courses of therapy in our hospital or as outpatients in our practice. I have never owned a book that was specifically written to assist pediatricians in the day-to-day management of pediatric head and neck problems. I see the American Academy of Pediatrics Section on Otolaryngology–Head and Neck Surgery *Pediatric Otolaryngology* as an essential reference text for busy pediatricians.

Head and neck problems are pervasive in community pediatrics. Pediatricians need a user-friendly resource to help them quickly address puzzling head and neck problems they encounter every day in their practices. This book is the ideal head and neck resource for busy pediatricians.

In the newborn nursery, pediatricians frequently need to know what to do about babies with cleft lip and palate, stridor, choanal atresia, outer ear anomalies, and vascular malformations of the head and neck. Can the baby be managed conservatively without consultation, or should the baby be evaluated by a subspecialist skilled in the care of newborns, infants, and children with head and neck problems? What syndromes should be considered in these situations? There are specific chapters in this book that will assist pediatricians in making these big decisions.

Most babies undergo hearing screening as newborns. Sometimes the results of these screening procedures are confusing. Even if the newborn hearing screening turns out to be normal, only 50% of pediatric hearing loss is congenital. The other half is acquired. Pediatricians need expertise in screening babies and young children for speech and hearing problems. Pediatricians need to have appropriate equipment in their offices to evaluate children for hearing loss. Many babies and young children have speech development delay and need to be carefully assessed by an otolaryngologist. This handy resource explains audiologic, speech, and language problems in a practical format for pediatricians.

In the outpatient practice setting, babies and children often present with feeding problems ranging from ankyloglossia (tongue-tie), to gastroesophageal reflux, to excessive drooling. Usually, the pediatrician can manage a wide range of feeding problems without the consultation services of a subspecialist. This book provides valuable information to support the busy pediatrician in addressing feeding problems in newborns, infants, and children.

Children often present with problems related to the upper airway, including acute and chronic illness. When do children need adenoidectomy or tonsillectomy? Which children need sleep studies? When do they need bronchoscopy? What are the life-threatening airway emergencies of children? What are criteria for putting tubes in children's ears? All of these issues are addressed in the book.

Head and neck masses in children range from vascular malformation, to lymph node enlargement, to salivary gland inflammatory disease, to thyroid enlargement and cancer. Making the right diagnosis and prescribing the right course of treatment are often challenging exercises for the pediatrician. Plain radiographs, ultrasound, computed tomography, and magnetic resonance imaging modalities are often helpful, but pediatricians need to know when to order which imaging study. This resource provides helpful information and guidance.

Parents frequently bring their children to the pediatrician because of head and neck emergencies. How should physicians evaluate children suspected of having nasal bone fractures? When does the child with epistaxis (nosebleed) need to be evaluated for a coagulation problem? When does the child need to see the otolaryngologist? This reference has answers for these questions.

And what about facial nerve paresis or paralysis? Pediatricians need an evidence-based approach to this situation because most parents are very upset when they see that their children may be having a stroke. This resource provides a logical approach to facial nerve problems in children.

The authors have done an excellent job reviewing common head and neck dilemmas in pediatrics. I consider this reference a must for the busy community pediatrician and a most helpful resource for all physicians who are expected to address head and neck problems in children.

David Tayloe, MD, FAAP
Goldsboro, NC

INTRODUCTION

Otolaryngologic disorders comprise more than 25% of a pediatrician's daily practice. As new research, pharmaceuticals, and technologies emerge, it is increasingly difficult for the pediatric primary care practitioner to maintain proficiency in the management of these problems. At the same time, the scope of otolaryngology–head and neck surgery has expanded widely over the past 30 years. In addition to continued advances in traditional disorders of the ear, nose, and aerodigestive tract, the field of pediatric otolaryngology incorporates diagnosis and management of congenital and neoplastic masses of the head and neck, craniofacial anomalies, vascular malformations, and diseases of the thyroid gland. Refinement and miniaturization in surgical instrumentation has revolutionized management of sinus disease and skull base tumors, and technologic advancements in cochlear implantation have enabled children who are deaf to develop excellent speech and integrate into mainstream society.

Through our experience with the American Academy of Pediatrics Section on Otolaryngology–Head and Neck Surgery, we have identified a need for a resource to which the pediatric primary care practitioner can turn for practical, current approaches to the many ear, nose, and throat disorders encountered on a daily basis. Although there are several all-encompassing tomes for pediatric otolaryngologists and a few rudimentary publications for primary care, there are no otolaryngology texts that seem just right for pediatric primary care practitioners. In *Pediatric Otolaryngology,* we have endeavored to create a readable reference designed just for our colleagues in pediatric medicine, with the right level of detailed, practical information for everyday use, and clinical pearls to help guide diagnosis and treatment.

Our sincere wish is that you find this book helpful in your daily practice to better manage our mutual patients. We invite your comments and suggestions to improve this text for future editions.

Scott R. Schoem, MD, FAAP
David H. Darrow, MD, DDS, FAAP

SECTION 1

Ear and Temporal Bone

CHAPTER 1

Neonatal Hearing Screening, Hearing Loss, and Treatment for Hearing Loss

Anna K. Meyer, MD

■ Introduction

Hearing impairment in infants and children is a common and serious disability that can have far-reaching implications in cognitive, psychosocial, and academic development. Hearing in the earliest years of life is an essential aspect of the development of speech and language, and even mild impairment can impede this process. Unfortunately, primary care residencies and medical schools provide little education about the diagnosis of hearing loss, the counseling of families, and the interventions that are available. The most important aspect of pediatric hearing loss is early identification and intervention. Universal newborn hearing screening (UNHS) programs have markedly improved the ability of health care professionals to diagnose congenital hearing loss at an earlier age. However, children who have late-onset or progressive loss are still at risk for delays in diagnosis. Recognizing children who have problems with speech acquisition and hearing impairment is essential to ensure early referral to audiologists and otolaryngologists.

Once a hearing loss is identified, the next key step is identifying the best intervention strategy for each individual child and family. Interventions can range from sign language to cochlear implantation. Many of the interventions depend on the type and cause of hearing loss. Pediatricians should have an understanding of the common causes of hearing loss and the equipment and resources that will assist a hearing-impaired child in developing the best possible auditory perception and speech, as well as maximizing social and academic performance.

> **Pearl:** Early identification and intervention for childhood hearing loss are essential for the best outcomes in speech and language as well as cognitive, social, and academic functioning.

■ Epidemiology

The estimated incidence of permanent childhood hearing loss identified in the newborn period is 1 to 3 per 1,000 screened neonates. The prevalence of hearing loss in older children and adolescents is as high as 3.1%. Hearing loss is slightly more common among boys with a ratio of 1.2 to 1. Ethnic and socioeconomic variation exists with a higher prevalence of hearing loss among Mexican Americans, African Americans, and children living in lower income households.

A tremendous shift in the common etiologies of pediatric hearing impairment has occurred since the advent of antibiotics and immunizations. While the early 20th century was dominated by hearing loss caused by childhood infection, the last 50 years have seen a relative increase in the proportion of hearing loss due to inherited causes. In developed countries it is estimated that 20% of all pediatric hearing loss and 50% of congenital loss is genetic. Approximately 25% to 50% of hearing loss is acquired. However, 25% to 50% of children will never have a cause identified.

Causes of acquired congenital pediatric hearing loss include maternal infections or toxins taken during pregnancy, maternal diabetes, and birth-related problems. Acquired causes of childhood hearing loss include ear infections, ototoxic medications, meningitis, viral illnesses, trauma, and noise exposure. An ever-growing number of gene mutations have been linked to hearing loss; approximately 80% of hereditary hearing loss is autosomal recessive and 15% autosomal dominant. Many syndromes are associated with hearing loss, the most common of which is Down syndrome.

> **Pearl:** Hearing impairment is more common than all other diseases screened for in the newborn period combined.

■ Presenting Symptoms

One of the greatest challenges in infants is recognizing symptoms of hearing loss. Nearly two-thirds of children identified were initially suspected to have hearing loss by their parents. While audiologic evaluation should be initiated whenever a parent or caregiver has concerns about hearing or speech development, a lack of parental concern is not a reliable indicator of intact hearing in an infant or child. For example, children with moderate hearing loss may respond when their parent yells or may startle at a loud noise, and parents may interpret this as normal hearing, although careful questioning will reveal that the children struggle with quieter speech and sounds. On average the time between suspicion and diagnosis of hearing loss is 9 months. Table 1-1 lists expected hearing, speech, and language milestones for young children. Those who do no meet the milestones should be evaluated for hearing loss.

Preschoolers and older children are somewhat easier to assess for symptoms of hearing loss, but subtle indicators can still be overlooked.

Table 1-1. Normal Hearing, Speech, and Language Development

	Birth to 3 mo	4 to 6 mo	7 to 12 mo	12 to 24 mo
Expressive language	◆ Smiles or coos[a] ◆ Cries differently for different needs[a]	◆ Makes vowel babbling sounds[a] ◆ May begin consonant sounds p, b, m ◆ Laughs ◆ Vocalizes excitement or displeasure ◆ Entertains oneself with gurgling sounds	◆ Babbles many consonants and vowels ◆ Says "mama" or "dada" or other words by first birthday ◆ Repeats some sounds made by others ◆ Uses voice to get attention	◆ Uses more words each month ◆ Names common objects ◆ Puts 2 words together
Receptive language	◆ Startles or awakens to loud noises ◆ May turn head in direction of sound ◆ Changes sucking behavior in response to sound ◆ May seem to recognize parent voice	◆ Turns toward familiar sounds ◆ Responds to tone of voice ◆ Smiles when spoken to[a] ◆ Notices sound-making toys[a] ◆ Pays attention to music	◆ Responds to name ◆ Listens when spoken to ◆ Turns and looks in direction of sounds ◆ Understands simple requests	◆ Points to familiar objects when named ◆ Listens to stories, songs, and rhymes ◆ Follows simple commands ◆ Points to body parts when asked ◆ Points to pictures in book when named

[a] Hearing-impaired children can be very responsive to facial expressions and visual stimuli and will also make sounds, which can fool parents and providers into believing hearing is intact.

Often, not hearing can be interpreted as ignoring or not listening. Children should be observed for the following symptoms of possible hearing loss:

- Turning up the volume of the radio or television
- Responding inappropriately to questions
- Having difficulty understanding what people are saying
- Not replying when called
- Problems with articulation or difficulty for others to understand the child's speech
- Speech/language delays
- Decline in previous language skills
- Ear pain/aches or head noise complaints
- School performance problems
- Behavioral problems

In addition, clinicians should be aware of high-risk indicators for hearing loss in children (Table 1-2) and should ensure that these children have been appropriately evaluated.

A family history of hearing loss including first- and second-degree relatives should be elicited as well as determination of common origin from ethnically isolated locations or consanguinity.

> **Pearl:** All children who have a speech delay should undergo evaluation for hearing loss.

■ Physical Examination

A complete physical examination should be performed in all children who present with hearing loss because nearly every organ system can have abnormalities associated with hearing loss. The head and face should be evaluated for any features that could be consistent with a craniofacial syndrome associated with hearing loss (Table 1-3). For example, the hair should be examined for a white forelock, which suggests Waardenburg syndrome. The external ear should be thoroughly inspected for abnormalities including low-set ears, abnormal shape, preauricular pits and tags, and branchial cleft anomalies. The canal should be evaluated for infection, stenosis, or atresia, and the presence of obstructing foreign bodies or cerumen. The tympanic membrane should be visualized in its entirety to examine for perforations, areas of retraction, tympanosclerosis (scar of the tympanic membrane), and squamous debris that

Table 1-2. Acquired Causes of Pediatric Hearing Loss		
Prenatal	**Perinatal**	**Postnatal**
◆ Congenital infection — Cytomegalovirus — Rubella — Toxoplasmosis — Herpes — Syphilis — Varicella ◆ Teratogens — Alcohol — Cocaine — Methyl mercury — Thalidomide ◆ Ototoxic medications — Aminoglycosides — Loop diuretics — Quinine, chloroquine ◆ Gestational diabetes or diabetes mellitus	◆ Prematurity ◆ Low birth weight ◆ Birth hypoxia/low Apgar ◆ Hyperbilirubinemia ◆ Sepsis ◆ NICU admission ◆ Ototoxic medications	◆ Infection — Mumps — Measles — Varicella — Lyme disease — Meningitis ◆ Recurrent acute otitis media or persistent OME ◆ Head trauma ◆ Noise exposure ◆ Ototoxic medications ◆ Neurodegenerative disorders

Abbreviations: NICU, neonatal intensive care unit; OME, otitis media with effusion.

could be consistent with cholesteatoma. This is especially important because many clinicians rely on the "light reflex," which is an unreliable indicator of disease of the tympanic membrane and middle ear. Reliance on the light reflex may mislead providers to examine only the anterior-inferior portion of the eardrum. Pneumatic otoscopy should always be performed to assess for the presence of middle-ear effusion, as well as the integrity of the tympanic membrane. The eyes should be evaluated for the presence of colobomas of the lids, iris, or retina and for heterochromia of the irises. The maxilla and mandible should be assessed for hypoplastic or dysmorphic growth. The nose should be evaluated for bilateral nasal patency and if obstruction is suspected, endoscopic evaluation for choanal atresia should be performed. The neck should be examined for any pits that could be consistent with branchial cleft anomalies. A complete cranial nerve examination should be performed. In children who are old enough to cooperate, vestibular testing may be performed because hearing loss and balance problems may be associated.

> **Pearl:** The light reflex is not a reliable indicator of middle-ear or tympanic membrane disease.

Table 1-3. Common Syndromes Associated With Hearing Loss

Name	Inheritance	Gene	Phenotype
Down	Sporadic	Trisomy 21	SNHL, CHL, or MHL; classic facies, mental retardation, congenital heart disease; intestinal, thyroid, and skeletal problems
Stickler	Autosomal dominant and autosomal recessive	COL2A, COL9A1 COL11A, COL11A2	Congenital high frequency SNHL, Pierre Robin syndrome (micrognathia and cleft palate), myopia
Treacher Collins	Autosomal dominant	TCOF1	CHL, microtia, external auditory canal atresia, ossicular malformation, cleft palate, micrognathia, hypoplastic zygomas, cleft palate, coloboma
Crouzon	Autosomal dominant	FGFR2	CHL or MHL; ear malformations, craniosynostosis
Waardenburg	Autosomal dominant	EDN3, EDNRB MITF, PAX3, SNAI2, SOX10	Dystopia canthorum, congenital SNHL, heterochromia irises, white forelock
Branchio-oto-renal	Autosomal dominant	EYA1	SNHL, MHL, or CHL; external ear abnormalities, preauricular pits, branchial cleft anomalies, renal abnormalities
Pendred	Autosomal recessive	SLC26A4	SNHL stable or progressive, enlarged vestibular aqueduct ± cochlear aplasia, goiter
Usher	Autosomal recessive	CDH23, CLRN, GPR98, MYO7A, PCDH15, USH1, USH1G, USH2A	Type 1: congenital or progressive SNHL, progressive vision loss, ± vestibular dysfunction
Alport	X-linked 80% Autosomal recessive 15% Autosomal dominant 5%	COL4A, COL4A4, COL4A5	Progressive SNHL, progressive renal failure, anterior lenticonus and perimacular flecks

Abbreviations: CHL, conductive hearing loss; MHL, mixed hearing loss; SNHL, sensorineural hearing loss.

■ Diagnosis

UNIVERSAL NEWBORN HEARING SCREENING

In 1993, an expert panel at the National Institutes of Health recommended that all babies be screened for hearing loss. A great improvement in the early detection and intervention of congenital hearing loss subsequently occurred with the advent of the UNHS program, and currently 95% of newborns are screened in the United States. In addition, agencies such as the National Center for Hearing Assessment and Management and state-based early hearing detection and intervention (EHDI) programs have markedly improved identification of and education about pediatric hearing loss. Prior to the advent of UNHS, the average age of identification of congenital hearing loss was 2.5 to 3 years of age; that has now dropped to 14 months. The goal of UNHS is not only to have all neonates screened for hearing loss before discharge or by 1 month of age but also to ensure appropriate follow-up is obtained. Newborns who fail newborn hearing screening should have follow-up evaluation by 3 months of age, and those with identified hearing loss should have appropriate hearing rehabilitation and services by 6 months of age. Despite the great success that has occurred with initial newborn hearing screening, half of those who fail screening do not receive follow-up testing. Children who are identified with hearing loss and receive intervention by 6 months of age usually have normal language development by 5 years; children who have delays in identification and intervention have difficulty catching up to their hearing peers.

Universal newborn hearing screening cannot identify all children with hearing loss because many with mild hearing loss will be missed and a proportion of children who pass UNHS will go on to develop hearing loss later in life. Those children often are not identified until the preschool or school years. Because of the risk of delayed diagnosis in these children, in 2007, the Joint Committee on Infant Hearing updated its guidelines to improve identification of newborns at risk for late-onset hearing impairment (Box 1-1).

The pediatrician plays an essential role in the ongoing screening for hearing loss. After UNHS, the next formalized hearing evaluation does not occur until the beginning of school. Pediatricians should be vigilant in screening for signs of developing hearing loss. They should provide parents with information on hearing, speech, and language milestones; identify and treat middle-ear disease; and provide ongoing developmental surveillance. Pediatricians should also be aware of and assess neonates for any of the risk factors for late-onset hearing loss.

> ## Box 1-1. 2007 Joint Committee on Infant Hearing Risk Indicators Associated With Permanent Congenital, Delayed Onset, or Progressive Hearing Loss
>
> ♦ Caregiver concern about hearing, speech, language, or developmental delay.
> ♦ Family history of permanent childhood hearing loss.
> ♦ Neonatal intensive care of more than 5 days or any of the following regardless of length of stay: extracorporeal membrane oxygenation, assisted ventilation, exposure to ototoxic medications (gentamicin, tobramycin) or loop diuretics (furosemide/Lasix), and hyperbilirubinemia that requires exchange transfusion.
> ♦ In utero infections, such as cytomegalovirus, herpes, rubella, syphilis, and toxoplasmosis.
> ♦ Craniofacial anomalies, including those that involve the pinna, ear canal, ear tags, ear pits, and temporal bone anomalies.
> ♦ Physical findings, such as white forelock, that are associated with a syndrome known to include a sensorineural or permanent conductive hearing loss.
> ♦ Syndromes associated with hearing loss or progressive or late-onset hearing loss, such as neurofibromatosis, osteopetrosis, and Usher syndrome; other frequently identified syndromes include Waardenburg, Alport, Pendred, and Jervell and Lange-Nielson.
> ♦ Neurodegenerative disorders, such as Hunter syndrome, or sensory motor neuropathies, such as Friedreich ataxia and Charcot-Marie-Tooth syndrome.
> ♦ Culture-positive postnatal infections associated with sensorineural hearing loss, including confirmed bacterial and viral (especially herpesviruses and varicella) meningitis.
> ♦ Head trauma, especially basal skull/temporal bone fracture that requires hospitalization.
> ♦ Chemotherapy.

Hospitals and clinics use 2 types of newborn hearing screening. Many use otoacoustic emissions (OAE) testing. This test measures the function of the external auditory canal, tympanic membrane, middle ear, and outer hair cells of the cochlea but does not assess the inner hair cells of the cochlear or cochlear nerve. Other hospitals use automated auditory brain stem response (ABR) testing. This assesses the entire hearing pathway with a sensitivity down to 30 dB (normal hearing is considered ≤20 dB). Screening OAEs and automated ABR provide only a pass or fail report and do not require the interpretation of an audiologist. False positives can occur because of amniotic fluid present in the middle ear. Neither determine the degree of hearing loss and both can miss mild hearing loss (<30 dB). One type of hearing loss, auditory neuropathy/dyssynchrony, may not be detected by UNHS programs using OAEs. Auditory neuropathy/dyssynchrony is a disorder in which sound enters the inner ear normally, but the transmission of sound via the cochlear nerve to the brain is abnormal. Children who are admitted to the neonatal intensive care unit (NICU) are at higher risk for auditory neuropathy/dyssynchrony and thus should always be screened with automated ABR and not OAEs alone. In addition, children who are readmitted in the newborn period for conditions associated with hearing loss, such as hyperbilirubinemia requiring exchange transfusion or sepsis, should undergo repeat hearing screening by automated ABR.

> **Pearl:** All newborns should be screened for hearing loss by discharge or 1 month of age; those who fail newborn hearing screening should have follow-up evaluation by 3 months of age; and those with identified hearing loss should have appropriate hearing rehabilitation and services by 6 months of age.

AUDIOLOGIC EVALUATION

Neonates who fail UNHS should undergo timely formal audiologic evaluation. This includes an otoscopic inspection, child and family history, assessment of middle-ear function, and OAE and diagnostic ABR testing. Every child with identified permanent hearing loss should be referred to the state EHDI program and requires evaluation by an otolaryngologist.

AUDITORY BRAIN STEM RESPONSE TESTING

The automated ABR used in UNHS gives only a pass or fail reading and does not assess the degree of hearing loss. Diagnostic ABR is used to assess newborn hearing after the neonate has failed UNHS. Auditory brain stem response is an electrophysiologic measurement of the function of the entire hearing pathway, including the brain stem. It is performed by placing earphones or probes in the ears, which give clicks and tones, and electrodes on the head that measure the waveform response to the sounds given. Results can give frequency range and decibel response level information. It requires a quiet room for testing. Auditory brain stem response can be performed in sleeping babies or with sedation. Generally, children younger than 6 months do not require sedation.

OTOACOUSTIC EMISSIONS

Whether the initial hearing screening was OAEs or automated ABR, OAEs will be performed at the audiologic evaluation. Otoacoustic emissions are performed with an ear probe that, like ABR, delivers clicks and tone bursts. The probe also contains a microphone that detects acoustic signals generated by the cochlea in response to sound. The advantages of OAEs are that they can be performed quickly, in children of any age who are awake or asleep. Otoacoustic emissions do not quantify the degree of hearing loss and do not assess the function of the auditory nerve or brain stem. In addition, middle ear or tympanic pathology will affect the accuracy of this test.

Both ABR and OAEs measure only the integrity of the auditory pathway and are not a direct measure of the ability to hear. Hearing cannot be confirmed until the child is old enough to undergo audiometric testing.

AUDIOMETRY

Audiometry is ideally performed in a sound booth in which extraneous noise is eliminated. Children vary in their ability to cooperate with behavioral audiometric testing, and various tests exist for different ages. Audiometry measures the hearing in several ways. Bone conduction transmits sound through the skull directly to the cochlea. Air conduction transmits sound through the ear canal to the tympanic membrane, ossicles, and cochlea. Measurements of these allows the audiologist to determine if hearing loss is *conductive* (caused by pathology in the ear canal, tympanic membrane, middle ear, or ossicles) or *sensorineural* (caused by pathology of the cochlea or eighth nerve). Hearing thresholds greater than 20 dB are considered hearing impairment.

Visual Reinforcement Audiometry

Infants as young as 6 months may be able to provide behavioral hearing responses. For visual reinforcement audiometry, the infant is seated in the caregiver's lap and is trained to turn toward a toy or light when he hears a sound. Some children may tolerate wearing earphones and individual ear hearing data can be obtained. Most young children will not wear earphones and the hearing is assessed in "the sound field," meaning that only the hearing of both ears together can be measured. This allows for accurate measurement of hearing in only the ear that hears better, so unilateral hearing loss cannot be ruled out.

Play Audiometry

Once children are 2 years of age, they may be tested by training them to respond to auditory stimuli by play activities (eg, dropping a block in a box when a sound is heard). Children of this age can usually wear headphones and individual ear hearing levels can be obtained.

Conventional Audiometry

Children older than 4 years can undergo audiometry testing in the same way as adults—by wearing headphones and raising their hand when they hear auditory stimuli.

Tympanometry

Tympanometry assesses the mobility of the tympanic membrane by creating positive and negative pressure in the ear canal. Tympanometry results can provide information about the integrity of the tympanic membrane and the condition of the middle ear and ossicles.

> **Pearl:** Testing of hearing is individualized to the age of the child.

■ Medical Evaluation

OTOLARYNGOLOGY EVALUATION

All children with confirmed hearing loss should be referred to an otolaryngologist as soon as possible. The otolaryngologist will review the history and perform a thorough physical examination, as outlined previously. In addition, the specialist will counsel the family on the consequences of hearing loss and will pursue diagnostic evaluations to potentially determine the cause. The most suitable type of treatment for the hearing loss will then be determined. Hearing aids cannot be distributed without clearance from an otolaryngologist.

LABORATORY TESTS

Historically, a large array of laboratory tests were obtained to look for rare causes of hearing loss. These have included complete blood cell count; serum chemistry; blood glucose; thyroid function test; toxoplasmosis, other agents, rubella, cytomegalovirus (CMV), herpes simplex (TORCH) syndrome antibody tests; autoimmune serologies; and urinalysis. Cost-benefit analyses have suggested that these studies should be limited to selective ordering based on a thorough history and physical examination and perhaps only after other high-yield tests have been performed.

RADIOGRAPHIC EVALUATION

Radiographic imaging is among the highest yield studies in the investigation of the cause of a hearing loss. As many as 40% of children with hearing loss will have an identifiable reason on computed tomography (CT) or magnetic resonance imaging (MRI). Computed tomography is most helpful at identifying middle- and inner-ear abnormalities, while MRI is most often used to identify the cochlear nerve, the patency of the cochlea in children with a history of meningitis, and intracranial masses that could lead to hearing loss. Emerging evidence indicates that there may be long-term risks of malignancy from CT scans performed in young children. Therefore, some otolaryngologists are opting to limit these examinations or use a sequential approach to testing in which other high-yield tests (eg, genetic testing) are performed prior to obtaining a CT scan. Because progressive sensorineural hearing loss (SNHL) is associated with the anatomic abnormality of wide or enlarged vestibular aqueduct (EVA), children with worsening of their baseline hearing loss should undergo CT scanning to assess for EVA if prior imaging was not performed. Almost certainly, the best approach to testing is to engage in an informed discussion with parents or caregivers to come to a mutually acceptable decision about which tests to perform.

Children who have ear anomalies (including those with just preauricular pits or cup ears) and also have hearing loss, dysmorphic features, a family history of deafness, or a maternal history of gestational diabetes or diabetes mellitus, should undergo a renal ultrasound. The ultrasound may aid in the diagnosis of syndromic hearing loss, such as branchio-oto-renal syndrome; coloboma of the eye, heart anomaly, choanal atresia, retardation, and genital and ear anomalies (CHARGE) association; and diabetic embryopathy.

GENETIC TESTING

While imaging remains the highest yield modality for investigating the cause of hearing loss, the number of genes associated with hearing loss is rapidly expanding. Many otolaryngologists are using testing for mutations in GJB2 as their first evaluation of patients with SNHL and proceeding with imaging or laboratory testing only if the genetic test result is negative. In addition, there are many other gene mutations associated with syndromic and non-syndromic hearing loss, the clinical availability of which is constantly evolving.

The interpretation of genetic tests and the understanding of the ramifications of the diagnosis of a syndrome are complex and require the expertise of genetic counselors. A genetics team should always be engaged when evaluating for the presence of a syndrome and are also highly useful for pretest and posttest counseling about genetic testing results.

OPHTHALMOLOGIC EVALUATION

While hearing loss can be associated with abnormalities in every system of the body, the highest association is with ophthalmologic disorders. Syndromic children are especially likely to have ocular anomalies, and all should undergo evaluation by an ophthalmologist. In addition, non-syndromic children with hearing loss are at particular risk for decreased learning and function if they also have visual impairment; thus, it would be wise to ensure that their vision is fully intact.

> **Pearl:** Many otolaryngologists are opting for sequential testing of the highest yield tests to limit radiation and reduce unnecessary evaluations.

CARDIOLOGIC EVALUATION

Electrocardiogram is used to assess the presence of prolonged QT syndrome, a life-threatening cardiac arrhythmia that can lead to sudden death. This is associated with a very rare syndrome with congenital SNHL called Jervell and Lange-Nielsen syndrome. Electrocardiogram should be obtained in all children with profound SNHL, especially those who have a personal history of syncope or a family history of sudden death in childhood.

■ Types of Hearing Loss

Several different types of hearing loss exist. Conductive hearing loss (CHL) occurs whenever there is a disruption of function of the external ear, external auditory canal, tympanic membrane, middle ear, or ossicles. In children, the most common causes of CHL are otitis media with effusion (OME), foreign body in the external auditory canal, and cerumen impaction. Several syndromes are also associated with CHL, particularly those with external auditory canal atresia such as Treacher Collins syndrome. Disruptions in the function of the cochlea, cranial nerve VII, or brain stem can all cause SNHL. The level and quality of sound heard may be diminished. Mixed hearing loss (MHL) is a combination of CHL and SNHL and often occurs in syndromic children. Hearing loss can also be defined as stable or progressive, congenital or delayed onset, and genetic or nongenetic. Auditory neuropathy/dyssynchrony is a special type of nerve hearing loss in which the number of neurons in cranial nerve VII and the coordination of their firing can be affected. Children with this type of hearing loss may have a range of hearing from normal to profound SNHL on audiometric testing and can have particular difficulty understanding speech because of the uncoordinated firing of neurons.

Table 1-4 defines the degrees of hearing loss in terms of decibels (dB) lost. Figure 1-1 gives a pictorial account of the types of sounds that are missed at different levels of hearing loss.

| Table 1-4. Levels of Hearing Loss ||
Degree of Hearing	Hearing Loss Range (dB)
Normal	-10 to 15
Slight	16 to 25
Mild	26 to 40
Moderate	41 to 55
Moderately severe	56 to 70
Severe	71 to 90
Profound	91+

■ Causes of Hearing Loss

GENETIC

Genetic causes account for at least 50% of congenital SNHL and approximately 20% of all pediatric hearing loss. Genetic causes can be divided into non-syndromic (80%) and syndromic (20%). More than 300 genes have been associated with pediatric hearing loss. Seventy-five percent to 80% of non-syndromic hearing loss is autosomal recessive. Therefore, most children with genetic loss are born to parents with normal hearing. The remaining distribution of non-syndromic hereditary hearing loss is 20% autosomal dominant, 2% to 5% X-linked, and 1% mitochondrial. Remarkably, mutations in a single gene, *GJB2*, account for

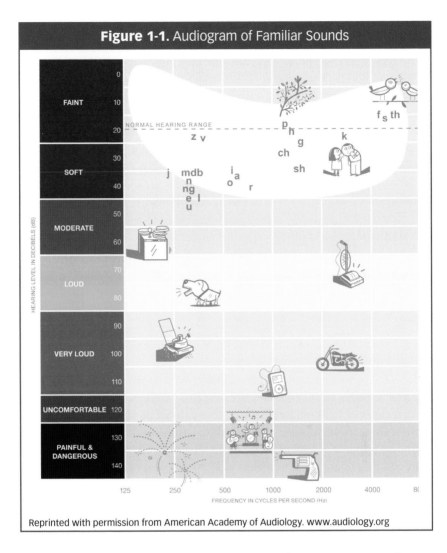

Figure 1-1. Audiogram of Familiar Sounds

Reprinted with permission from American Academy of Audiology. www.audiology.org

about half of all hereditary SNHL in the United States. *GJB2* encodes the protein connexin 26, which is involved in the gap-junction system of the inner ear. Hearing loss from mutations in the *GJB2* gene is autosomal recessive and can vary from mild to profound and be stable or progressive.

Pendred syndrome is the most common form of syndromic hearing loss. Children with Pendred syndrome have SNHL, EVA with or without cochlear aplasia, and goiter. Most cases are caused by mutation in the *SLC26A4* gene. Hearing loss is usually congenital and severe to profound, but milder losses and progressive loss are possible. Goiter does not present until late childhood. Enlarged vestibular aqueduct syndrome (EVAS), which is SNHL and EVA without goiter, is even more common than Pendred syndrome and may account for 5% to 15% of all SNHL. The etiology is multifactorial with environmental and genetic causes. Children with EVAS may be born with normal hearing or have congenital hearing loss. They are at risk for progressive hearing loss, especially from trauma. Thus, all children with progressive or late-onset hearing loss should be evaluated with a CT scan to identify this abnormality. They should also be counseled to avoid head trauma, wear protective helmets when engaged in cycling or skiing, and avoid activities such as contact sports and scuba diving.

ACQUIRED

Most acquired causes of childhood hearing loss are infectious or related to birth complications (Table 1-2). Vaccinations against common causes of congenital hearing loss have nearly eliminated etiologies such as rubella. Congenital CMV is currently the most common infectious etiology of congenital hearing loss and is estimated to cause from 12% to 25% of pediatric hearing loss. Congenital CMV is also a major contributor to delayed and progressive hearing loss in childhood. However, confirmatory diagnosis requires blood samples obtained in the first 4 weeks after birth and because this rarely occurs, most suspected cases of CMV-related hearing loss cannot be verified or treated. Antivirals given in this critical period may prevent the development or limit progression of hearing loss. More recently, polymerase chain reaction analysis of archived newborn heel stick blood spots has allowed the detection of congenital CMV. Some are now advocating adding CMV testing to the battery of newborn screening measures.

In the perinatal period, the most common causes of acquired hearing loss are related to other postnatal morbidities. Admission to the NICU, while not a direct risk, is a measure of serious perinatal morbidity and is associated with a 10-fold increase in SNHL. Many of the risk factors, such as low Apgar scores and prematurity, are most likely due to hypoxemic injury to the inner ear and cochlear nerve. These children are at particular risk for auditory neuropathy/dyssynchrony and require continued surveillance for progressive loss.

Conductive hearing loss caused by acute otitis media or OME is the most common cause of hearing loss in infants and young children. Bacterial meningitis, though rare with the advent of vaccination for *Streptococcus pneumoniae* and *Haemophilus influenzae* type b, is the most frequent cause of acquired SNHL in this age group. The most common etiologies of new hearing loss in older school-aged children are likely silent congenital CMV infection and noise trauma, although many older children, especially those with unilateral hearing loss, may have had unrecognized hearing loss since birth or early childhood.

> **Pearl:** Identifying the cause of hearing loss can help families process the diagnosis and make treatment decisions. However, some families will opt to not obtain this information.

■ Treatment for Sensorineural Hearing Loss

AMPLIFICATION

No medical treatment exists for SNHL. The first step for these children is amplification. All children with bilateral SNHL and many with unilateral SNHL are candidates for amplification. Even those with profound loss on ABR may still experience some benefit and, at the very least, need to undergo a trial with hearing aids prior to being considered for cochlear implantation. Often considerable time delay occurs between identification of a hearing loss and fitting of hearing aids. This can be because of issues with cost, access to audiologic services, or parental concern about the use of hearing aids. Clinicians should emphasize to parents the extreme importance of children with hearing impairment to wear hearing aids and that this is essential for excellent speech and language development and good school performance. Social recognition by peers of "differentness" does not usually occur until 5 or 6 years of age; this may reassure some parents about the appearance of wearing hearing aids. As children get older, they may decide not to wear their aids for various reasons, including lack of perceived benefit and social issues. Clinicians and caregivers should respect the concerns of these children, while at the same time continuing to assess whether they are having difficulties in school or communication by not wearing the aids. Some families may request smaller aids, but because the ear canal is constantly growing, children can only wear behind-the-ear (BTE) hearing aids and not the smaller aids available to adults.

Hearing aids are fitted by creating a properly sized mold for the external ear and canal. The hearing aid rests over and BTE. The amplification is adjusted to optimize hearing while avoiding pain from sound pressure on the tympanic membrane.

Types of Hearing Amplification

Behind the Ear

Most children wear BTE hearing aids. Some who cannot tolerate wearing a device on the ear will use a body aid. The advantages of BTE aids are that they are the most durable; as the child grows only the ear mold must be replaced; they are less likely to produce feedback; and they can be coupled to assistive technology. Adolescents whose ears are fully grown may use smaller aids that are partly or completely in the ear canal, but these cost more, cannot be coupled to other devices, and are more easily damaged.

Contralateral Routing of Signal

Children with severe to profound unilateral loss are unlikely to gain significant benefit from BTE aids. Contralateral routing of signal (CROS) systems have a microphone on the impaired ear that transmits the sound signal to a device worn on the normal-hearing ear. Some children do not tolerate this because they do not wish to wear an aid in the normal-hearing ear. Children with severe to profound hearing loss in one ear and hearing that can be aided in the other can use a similar system called the BiCROS.

Bone-Anchored Hearing Aids

Several types of hearing loss are not suitable for wearing BTE aids. Children with microtia or external auditory canal atresia with CHL or MHL cannot wear traditional aids. In addition, some children who have chronic ear drainage that cannot be treated by surgery cannot wear aids in the ear. Children with single-sided severe to profound SNHL also will not benefit from BTE aids. For these children a hearing aid can be inserted in the cranial bone. This involves the surgical implantation of a titanium strut in the temporal bone BTE. This implant protrudes through the skin and connects to a sound processor. Sound is transmitted through the bone directly to the cochlea, bypassing the external and middle ear. Children cannot obtain this implant until they are 5 years of age. Until then, they can wear a headband (soft band) that holds the sound processor firmly against the skull. Some children prefer the soft band to surgery and opt to continue to use it instead of undergoing surgery, though most find the hearing quality better with the bone-anchored hearing aid. New, surgically implantable bone conducting hearing aids avoid the visible and sometimes troublesome titanium screw abutment on the skull. However, because they are not osseointegrated into the skull bone, hearing improvement is slightly less than BAHA by 10 to 15 dB.

SPEECH THERAPY

Many children, especially those who have experienced a delay in diagnosis of their hearing impairment, have significant issues with speech and language development. Speech therapy can be a helpful resource for these children. Many schools offer brief sessions 1 or 2 times per week, but children with significant delays may require more intensive therapy outside of school.

SCHOOL ACCOMMODATIONS

Children with hearing impairment should be preferentially seated nearest to the teacher. Because many teachers move about the classroom and background noise can interfere with optimal hearing aid performance, an FM system is often helpful. With an FM system, the teacher wears a microphone that communicates to a speaker on the child's desk or directly to the child's hearing aid or cochlear implant. Closed captioning for films and videos can also be beneficial. Children with hearing impairment should always be supplied with an individual education plan to ensure they are receiving the services they require.

> **Pearl:** Early intervention and multidisciplinary collaboration are necessary for the best outcomes for children with hearing impairment.

COCHLEAR IMPLANTS

Cochlear implantation has revolutionized the care of children with severe to profound hearing loss. Numerous studies have shown a clear benefit of implantation over amplification or other modes of communication. It cannot be underestimated that time is of the essence when evaluating infants with congenital SNHL for implantation. Children who experience delays in receiving an implant beyond their first birthday are at increasing risk for poor speech and language development, whereas children who receive implants at or near 12 months of age have the potential to function at the level of their normal-hearing peers. Children who have developed late-onset hearing loss after the development of language (postlingually deaf) are also excellent candidates.

While implants were initially performed in only one ear, growing research supports bilateral implantation in children. Children who are prelingually deaf are assessed for candidacy based on their ABR results as well as failure to develop auditory skills. Older children will be evaluated by audiometry as well as several more specific tests that assess the development of speech and language. All children must undergo a 3-month hearing aid trial. This serves to determine if they may have suitable benefit from hearing aids and also to assess if they and their parents will be compliant with wearing an aid device regularly. All children evaluated for cochlear implantation require imaging studies, usually CT and/or MRI, to evaluate the inner ear anatomy and confirm the presence of a cochlear nerve. Children with abnormalities of the inner ear are still candidates for implantation, but modifications in surgical technique and expectations of outcome by parents may be necessary.

Counseling families about expectations for implantation is paramount. While many children have excellent outcomes, it is not possible beforehand to predict how someone will perform with an implant. Children with developmental delay, autism spectrum disorders, or other cognitive issues may not perform as well. This does not preclude them from being implanted, but it is important for parents to tailor their expectations. In addition, families must understand that the aural rehabilitation following implantation is intensive and requires a long-term commitment. The cochlear implant team should determine that adequate resources will be available to have the maximal benefit of the implant. Educational programs for the hearing impaired are varied in their emphasis and quality, and children undergoing implantation should be in programs that promote listening and speaking instead of signed communication, as their ultimate outcome is considerably dependent on the quality of these programs. Continuing assessment and dialogue should occur among audiologists, otolaryngologists, speech pathologists, school, and family to ensure a maximal benefit from the implant.

Children with SNHL have an increased risk of meningitis; undergoing cochlear implantation increases this risk. The 13-valent pneumococcal conjugate vaccine (PCV13, Prevnar13) and the 23-valent pneumococcal polysaccharide vaccine (PPV23, Pneumovax 23) should be administered. Children cannot undergo PPV23 vaccination until they are 24 months old; thus, children implanted prior to that age must receive the immunization after implantation.

> **Pearl:** Children with congenital hearing loss who are candidates for cochlear implantation should ideally receive an implant by their first birthday.

Treatments for Conductive Hearing Loss

Children with OME that has not resolved after 3 months are candidates for bilateral myringotomies and pressure-equalization tubes. Depending on the degree of hearing loss and presence of speech delay, developmental delay, mental retardation, or MHL, the length of time that OME with hearing loss should be observed varies. In general, children who have or are at risk for speech or cognitive delay should have tubes placed earlier, while those who do not can be observed longer.

Children who use cotton-tipped applicators to clean their ear are at risk for cerumen impaction, as well as retaining part of the applicator in their ear. These should be removed promptly to restore hearing.

External auditory canal atresia, tympanic membrane perforation, and ossicular pathologies can lead to CHL that may benefit from surgery or hearing amplification.

Natural History and Prognosis

Immunizations and antibiotics have contributed substantially in decreasing many causes of pediatric hearing loss. Prior to vaccines, mumps and rubella were leading causes of pediatric hearing loss. In the developing world, congenital rubella syndrome contributes heavily to the burden of SNHL, especially in countries without vaccination programs. The proportion of hearing loss due to other causes has shifted to genetic mutations and complications in the neonatal period.

Even children with mild hearing loss are at risk for delays in speech and language development. In particular they may have difficulty acquiring new words and may require visual and auditory input to develop language at the rate of their peers. The more severe the hearing loss, the greater the risk for deficient speech acquisition and poor academic performance. Infants with severe to profound loss will develop no spoken language at all without amplification or cochlear implantation. These children may use sign language, but because 90% of children with hearing loss are born to hearing parents, tremendous effort will be involved for parents and child to learn this new language.

Historically, sign language was an essential form of communication for people with severe to profound hearing loss. Children who were prevented from learning sign language and relied on lipreading and acquiring oral speech were often exhausted by the intensity of the therapy required. Children born into deaf families easily learn sign language in the same way that hearing children learn oral language. However, for a host of factors, deaf children who sign lag behind their hearing peers and children who have received cochlear implants. The median reading level of deaf adults is fourth grade. In addition, sign language isolates individuals from the world community and limits vocational opportunities. Children with developmental delay or autism spectrum disorders and those with severe to profound loss who are not candidates for cochlear implantation may never develop spoken language, even with the use of amplification or cochlear implantation. For those children, sign language is an essential communication modality.

Unilateral hearing loss gives additional insight into the natural history of pediatric hearing impairment, as these children are less likely to be helped. Thirty-five percent of children with unilateral loss failed at least one grade; 50% showed some difficulty in educational progress; and 20% were believed by teachers to have a behavioral problem.

Children who are identified with hearing loss early and receive appropriate intervention in a timely manner are still at risk for academic and social problems. Ongoing assessment and collaboration among schools, parents, speech therapists, and physicians are essential to improving developmental and academic achievement.

■ Selected References

American Speech-Language-Hearing Association. How does your child hear and talk? http://asha.org/public/speech/development/chart.htm. Accessed July 6, 2011

Bess FH, Tharpe AM, Gibler AM. Auditory performance of children with unilateral sensorineural hearing loss. *Ear Hear.* 1986;7(1):20–26

Early identification of hearing impairment in infants and young children. NIH Consensus Development Conference. *Int J Pediatr Otorhinolaryngol.* 1993;27(2):201–202

Fowler KB, Boppana SB. Congenital cytomegalovirus (CMV) infection and hearing deficit. *J Clin Virol.* 2006;35(2):226–231

Jerry J, Oghalai JS. Towards an etiologic diagnosis: assessing the patient with hearing loss. *Adv Otorhinolaryngol.* 2011;70:28–36

Joint Committee on Infant Hearing. Year 2007 position statement: principles and guidelines for early hearing detection and intervention programs. *Pediatrics.* 2007;120(4):898–921

Katbamna B, Crumpton T, Patel DR. Hearing impairment in children. *Pediatr Clin North Am*. 2008;55(5):1175–1188

Korver AM, Admiraal RJ, Kant SG, et al. Causes of permanent childhood hearing impairment. *Laryngoscope*. 2011;121(2):409–416

Mehra S, Eavey RD, Keamy DG Jr. The epidemiology of hearing impairment in the United States: newborns, children, and adolescents. *Otolaryngol Head Neck Surg*. 2009;140(4):461–472

Misono S, Sie KC, Weiss NS, et al. Congenital cytomegalovirus infection in pediatric hearing loss. *Arch Otolaryngol Head Neck Surg*. 2011;137(1):47–53

National Institute on Deafness and Other Communication Disorders. Enlarged vestibular aqueducts and childhood hearing loss. http://www.nidcd.nih.gov/health/hearing/eva.htm. Published October 2006. Accessed July 6, 2011

Palo Alto Medical Foundation. Hearing loss in children. http://www.pamf.org/hearinghealth/facts/children.html. Accessed July 6, 2011

Shah RK, Lotke M. Hearing impairment. Medscape References. http://emedicine.medscape.com/article/994159-clinical. Updated April 8, 2011. Accessed July 6, 2011

Smith RJ, Bale JF Jr, White KR. Sensorineural hearing loss in children. *Lancet*. 2005;365(9462):879–890

Toriello HV, Reardon W, Gorlin RJ. *Hereditary Hearing Loss and Its Syndromes*. 2nd ed. New York, NY: Oxford University Press; 2004

Traxler CB. The Stanford Achievement Test, 9th Edition: National Norming and Performance Standards for Deaf and Hard-of-Hearing Students. *J Deaf Stud Deaf Educ*. 2000;5(4):337–348

Wang RY, Earl DL, Ruder RO, Graham JM Jr. Syndromic ear anomalies and renal ultrasounds. *Pediatrics*. 2001;108(2):E32

CHAPTER 2

Management and Treatment of Patients With Acute and Chronic Otitis Media

Yamilet Tirado, MD, and Blake Papsin, MD

■ Introduction

Otitis media (OM) is a broad term given to any inflammatory process within the middle ear. There are multiple diagnoses that can be included under this general term, but typically they are classified as acute or chronic, based on the period from onset of the disease. A disease that persists more than 3 months usually is considered chronic. Otitis media can be subclassified as suppurative, nonsuppurative, or recurrent (Box 2-1). The main focus of this chapter is the management and treatment of patients with acute OM (AOM) and chronic OM (COM), including chronic suppurative OM (CSOM) and OM with effusion (OME). Current guidelines are reviewed and advances in epidemiology and pathogenesis are included, as well as the facts necessary to make a certain diagnosis, provide adequate management, and prevent complications.

Acute OM and COM are probably the most common ear diseases that general pediatricians, as well as pediatric otolaryngologists, encounter in their daily clinical practice. Sometimes, distinguishing each condition can be a challenging process for the clinician. This can lead to overdiagnosis, inappropriate use of antibiotics, and overtreatment, which in turn can have a significant effect on children's health and direct cost of health care. Therefore, it is important to recognize and classify each condition accordingly and understand the pathophysiology and treatment options available.

Acute OM is defined by the American Academy of Pediatrics and American Academy of Family Physicians as an infection of the middle ear with acute onset, along with presence of effusion and signs of middle-ear inflammation, such as otalgia, and distinct erythema of the tympanic membrane (TM). The presence of middle-ear inflammation can be indicated by any of the following: bulging of the TM, limited or absent mobility of the TM with pneumatic otoscopy, air-fluid

---

Box 2-1. Classification of Otitis Media

Acute Otitis Media
  Suppurative
  Nonsuppurative
  Recurrent (≥3 episodes)

Chronic Otitis Media
  Suppurative
  Nonsuppurative
  Otitis media with effusion

---

level behind the TM, or otorrhea. Acute OM is the most common diagnosis given to a febrile child, and it is commonly overdiagnosed (often because the TM cannot be visualized due to the presence of cerumen, so the diagnosis becomes speculative). The high incidence and high rate of spontaneous recovery from uncomplicated AOM suggest that it is a natural event and part of the gradual maturation of the child's immune system. On the other hand, an untreated complicated AOM can lead to complications, such as acute mastoiditis, subperiosteal abscess, meningitis, and brain abscess, among others.

Chronic suppurative OM is defined as a TM perforation with chronic ear drainage. Signs of middle-ear inflammation are usually present. If not treated successfully with medical or surgical intervention, CSOM can lead to complications similar to AOM.

Otitis media with effusion is more common than AOM and is defined as middle-ear effusion (MEE) without signs or symptoms of an acute infection. Otitis media with effusion can occur spontaneously because of eustachian tube (ET) dysfunction or may be the result of or sequel to AOM. Even though both disorders require MEE for diagnosis, the main difference is the absence of acute signs and symptoms of middle-ear inflammation in OME. Otitis media with effusion differs from CSOM because there is no TM perforation. Otitis media with effusion commonly resolves spontaneously within 3 months (if there is no reinfection) but if persistent and untreated, conductive hearing loss can occur and may affect behavior and delay communicative development.

> **Pearl:** *Acute otitis media* refers to an acute infection or inflammation in the middle ear with local or systemic signs and symptoms and the presence of an effusion in the middle ear.

■ Epidemiology of Otitis Media

Despite advances in public health and medical care, OM is still prevalent globally and the incidence in North America has actually increased over the past 2 decades. The overall use of antibiotics has also remained high over this interval. In 2006, 9 million children aged 0 to 17 years were reported having an ear infection; of those, 8 million visited a physician or obtained a prescription drug for treatment.

Otitis media occurs in all age groups but is considerably more common in children between the ages of 6 months and 3 years. This is presumably because of immunologic and anatomic factors. Children with significant predisposing factors (eg, cleft palate, Down syndrome) acquire infections more frequently. Generally, by age 3 years, nearly all children have experienced an episode of OM. Males are more susceptible to OM (no specific causative factors identified) and there is a very high incidence of middle-ear infections in Native Americans and Eskimos. Overall, mortality is rare and it is nearly uncommon in countries where treatment of complications is available. However, morbidity is high and may be significant for infants who develop complications and in those in whom persistent effusion results in communicative deficits (perceptive and productive).

Otitis media is most commonly associated with exposure to large numbers of other children (often with upper respiratory infections [URIs]) via child care or crowded households, decreased breastfeeding, and exposure to secondhand smoke. Seasonal increase in the incidence of OM also has been reported, most commonly in winter, fall, and spring. An increased incidence in AOM and COM has been found in children who live in low socioeconomic conditions, who have poor medical care, or both. These factors are not well established; they may represent an increased exposure to other children with URIs. Farjo et al, among others, have shown a well-established relationship between attending child care and an increased incidence of OM in children younger than 3 years. Casselbrant et al showed a strong genetic predisposition to OM, with a higher incidence in children who have older siblings or parents with a significant history of OM.

> **Pearl:** Acute otitis media is the second most frequent diagnosis made by pediatricians and is the most common indication for antibiotic use in children in North America.

■ Pathogenesis of Otitis Media

The pathogenesis of OM is multifactorial. Immunologic and environmental factors have an important role, and any imbalance between them can predispose the host to OM. Age, genetic predisposition, and atopy are host factors that can impair immune response, whereas older siblings, child care, and season of the year are environmental factors related to microbial load (Figure 2-1). For the inflammatory process to develop in the middle ear, the pathogens must adhere to the nasopharyngeal epithelium, enter the middle-ear cavity through the ET, and be able to overcome the defensive mechanisms of the middle ear.

The ET provides clearance of secretions and pressure regulation to the middle ear. It is also the port of entry for middle-ear pathogens from the nasopharynx. Abnormal function of the ET is the cornerstone of the pathogenesis of OM. Dysfunction of the ET can be caused by a URI with decreased mucous clearance and increased obstruction, which predisposes bacteria growth and subsequent middle-ear inflammation. Infants and children are predisposed to MEE and OM secondary to a more horizontal and functionally less mature ET.

Other conditions associated with ET dysfunction and MEE are presented in Box 2-2. Children with craniofacial anomalies affecting ET function, such as cleft palate or craniofacial disorders, have a statistically higher incidence of OM at all ages, especially during the first 2 years of life. These patients will need to be followed until adolescence because the incidence of middle-ear disease does not decrease after surgical repair. Children with congenital or acquired immunodeficiency are at a higher risk secondary to decreased middle ear clearance, including conditions such as hypogammaglobulinemia, IgA deficiency, DiGeorge syndrome, HIV, and drug-induced immunodeficiency (eg, chemotherapy, steroids).

Allergy, nasal obstruction (eg, sinusitis, adenoid hypertrophy, nasal or rare pediatric nasopharyngeal tumors), ciliary dysfunction,

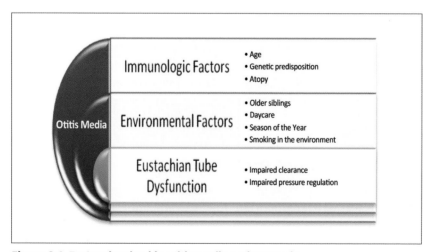

Figure 2-1. Factors involved in otitis media pathogenesis

Box 2-2. Risk Factors Associated With Middle-Ear Effusion

♦ **Middle-ear effusion**
— Craniofacial disorders
  ▪ Cleft palate
  ▪ Midface deformity
  ▪ Down syndrome
  ▪ Apert syndrome
— Immunodeficiencies
  ▪ Hypogammaglobulinemia
  ▪ IgA deficiency
  ▪ DiGeorge syndrome
  ▪ HIV
  ▪ Drug-induced immunodeficiency
— Allergy
— Nasal obstruction
  ▪ Sinusitis
  ▪ Adenoid hypertrophy
  ▪ Nasopharyngeal tumor
  ▪ Ciliary dysfunction

---

prolonged nasal intubation or nasogastric tube placement, and possibly gastroesophageal reflux are other conditions associated with an increased incidence of MEE. Gastroesophageal reflux is common in children and therefore has been implicated in the pathophysiology of OM. Pepsin has been found in the middle ear of patients with OM in 20% of cases and is considered an independent risk factor for OM. A role for allergy in the etiology of OM has long been postulated. However, there is no data supporting antihistamine–decongestant combinations in treating OME. Also, there is an increased incidence in those patients exposed to secondhand smoking and those who use a pacifier.

Children attending child care centers are predisposed to antibacterial-resistant organisms in their nasopharynx, leading to AOM that may be refractory to antibacterial treatment. The environment at child care centers facilitates the development and spread of resistant organisms because of the large number of children, frequent close person-to-person contact, and the wide use of antibiotics. Crowded living conditions, poor sanitation, and inadequate medical care have been all associated with OM.

There is increasing evidence that biofilm formation may play a role in the inflammatory changes observed in the middle ear of patients with OME. There is also accumulating evidence that gastric acid may act as a cofactor in the inflammatory process by facilitating biofilm formation. In fact, the common factor of inflammation suggests that diverse types of insult can influence different stages of the immune cascade that results in persistent MEE.

> **Pearl:** The pathogenesis of acute otitis media is multifactorial. Immunologic and environmental factors have an important role, and any imbalance between them can predispose the host to otitis media.

■ Acute Otitis Media (AOM)

Acute otitis media is the second most frequent diagnosis made by pediatricians and is the most common indication for antibiotic use in children in North America. In general, most children will have at least one episode of AOM by age 1 year, with peak incidence between ages 6 and 11 months. Approximately 10% to 20% of children by age 1 year will have recurrent episodes of AOM, and 80% have had at least one episode by 3 years of age. After an episode of AOM, as many as 45% of children have persistent effusion at 1 month, but this number decreases to 10% after 3 months.

MICROBIOLOGY OF AOM

The pathogens most frequently associated with AOM are *Streptococcus pneumoniae* (30%–50%), *Haemophilus influenzae* (20%–30%), *Moraxella catarrhalis* (10%–20%), and group A streptococci (1%–5%) (Table 2-1). Block et al found that children aged 7 to 24 months with recurrent episodes of AOM who were vaccinated with heptavalent pneumococcal vaccine had twofold more gram-negative bacteria than *S pneumoniae*. Anaerobic bacteria play a minor role in the pathogenesis of AOM.

The exact percentage of bacterial resistance for any particular organism varies with the geographic area and the population studied. Incidence of penicillin-resistant pneumococcus in the United States ranges from 10% to 40%, and more than 80% in Korea and the Middle East. Beta-lactamase is produced by 20% to 50% of *H influenzae* and nearly all *M catarrhalis*. Possible clinical factors in the development of bacterial resistance to antibiotics include multiple and prolonged courses and incomplete or inappropriate administration.

Table 2-1. Microbiology of Acute Otitis Media	
Population	**Most Common Pathogens**
Neonates	*Streptococcus pneumoniae* *Haemophilus influenzae* *Staphylococcus aureus* *Escherichia coli* Group B *Streptococcus*
Infants	*S pneumoniae* *H influenzae* *S aureus* *E coli* Group B *Streptococcus*
Children	*S pneumoniae* *H influenzae* *Moraxella catarrhalis*
Immunocompromised	*Mycobacterium tuberculosis* *Mycoplasma pneumonia* *Chlamydia trachomatis*

Viruses have been suspected increasingly of causing AOM, possibly by acting alone or as bacterial co-pathogens. Viral AOM is most frequently caused by respiratory syncytial virus or rhinovirus, but influenza virus, adenovirus, enterovirus, and parainfluenza viruses have also been isolated from middle-ear fluid. Viral infection can substantially worsen clinical and bacteriological outcomes of AOM.

> **Pearl:** The pathogens most frequently associated with acute otitis media are *Streptococcus pneumoniae, Haemophilus influenza,* and *Moraxella catarrhalis.*

■ Assessment and Diagnosis of AOM

PRESENTING SYMPTOMS

Clinical history alone is poorly predictive of the presence of AOM, especially in younger children. Children with AOM usually present with a history of rapid onset of signs and symptoms such as otalgia or pulling of the ear in an infant, irritability, otorrhea, or fever. These findings, except for otorrhea, are nonspecific and frequently present during an uncomplicated viral URI. However, these symptoms in combination with the presence of MEE and inflammation in the physical examination increases the likelihood of AOM diagnosis.

Less common signs and symptoms in children are hearing loss, dizziness, and tinnitus. Fever is present in up to two-thirds of children with AOM, but fever (temperature above 40°C) is uncommon and may represent bacteremia or other complications. A protruding ear with swelling behind the ear may represent mastoiditis with developing subperiosteal abscess.

The diagnosis of AOM, particularly in infants and young children, is often made with a degree of doubt, most frequently by inability to confirm the presence of MEE. Common factors that increase uncertainty include the inability to clear the external auditory canal of cerumen, a narrow ear canal, or inability to maintain an adequate seal for successful pneumatic otoscopy or tympanometry. Despite all efforts made by the clinician to differentiate AOM from OME or a normal ear, uncertainty is almost always unavoidable.

A certain diagnosis of AOM meets all 3 of the criteria: rapid onset, presence of MEE, and signs and symptoms of middle-ear inflammation. The clinician should maximize diagnostic strategies, particularly to establish the presence of MEE, and should consider the certainty of diagnosis in determining management.

> **Pearl:** A certain diagnosis of acute otitis media meets all 3 of the criteria: rapid onset, presence of middle-ear effusion, and signs and symptoms of middle-ear inflammation.

PHYSICAL EXAMINATION

A complete head and neck examination is essential for diagnosis. To establish a definite diagnosis of AOM, it is important to identify MEE and inflammatory changes of the TM. Therefore, the physical examination of a child with AOM should include otoscopy and pneumatic otoscopy. For an adequate visualization of the TM, the ear canal should be cleared of any cerumen obscuring the TM and the otoscope lighting must be adequate. Depleted batteries and dim lights will make the clinician's job even more difficult and will sometimes alter perception of the image. For an accurate pneumatic otoscopy, a speculum of proper shape and diameter must be selected to obtain a good seal in the external auditory canal. At the same time, if necessary, it is important to appropriately restrain the child to permit adequate examination.

A normal eardrum, such as the one shown in Figure 2-2, will provide the opportunity to identify landmarks such as the annulus, pars flaccida, pars tensa, malleus handle and lateral process, umbo, light reflex, and long process of the incus. The color is quite translucent and does not really appear to be any color except perhaps grey. Also, it is important to distinguish normal variants from pathology. A crying child can have increased TM vascularity, which can be easily mistaken with an erythematous and bulging TM and lead to an incorrect diagnosis and treatment. As the child quiets down, the TM erythema becomes less intense and fades away, while the TM erythema in a patient with AOM persists.

The findings on otoscopy indicating the presence of MEE and inflammation associated with AOM include erythema, opacification, fullness or bulging of the TM, along with loss of TM landmarks, such as the malleus handle and pars flaccida (Figure 2-3). Bulging of the TM is often present and has the highest predictive value for the presence of MEE. Reduced or absent mobility of the TM during performance of pneumatic otoscopy is additional evidence of fluid in the middle ear.

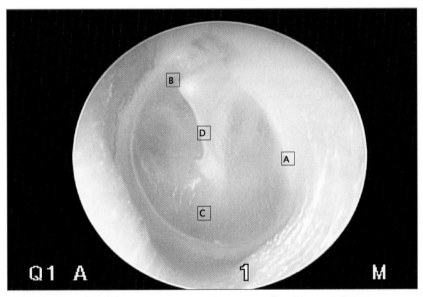

Figure 2-2. Normal left eardrum. A, annulus; B, pars flaccida; C, pars tensa; D, malleus.

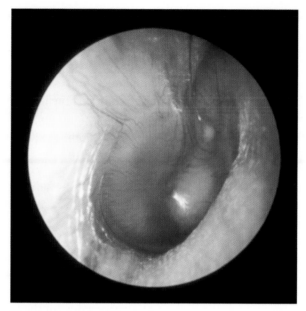

Figure 2-3. Acute otitis media.

> **Pearl:** The findings on otoscopy associated with acute otitis media include erythema, opacification, fullness or bulging of the tympanic membrane, along with loss of tympanic membrane landmarks.

DIAGNOSTIC TESTS

Hearing Evaluation

Pure tone audiometry or visual reinforcement audiometry can be used to diagnose the conductive hearing loss associated with AOM in young children. Tympanometry is a simple, objective, quantitative method of assessing TM mobility and middle-ear function, with similar sensitivity but lower specificity to pneumatic otoscopy. It must be remembered that impedance tympanometry does not provide a diagnosis but merely confirms what the clinician suspects based on the physical examination. It should never be used independently. Tympanometry results can be classified with quantitative measures or by pattern curves (A, B, C1, C2) (Figure 2-4). The presence of type B or C2 curves has 94% sensitivity for MEE but only 62% specificity. Acoustic reflectometry can also

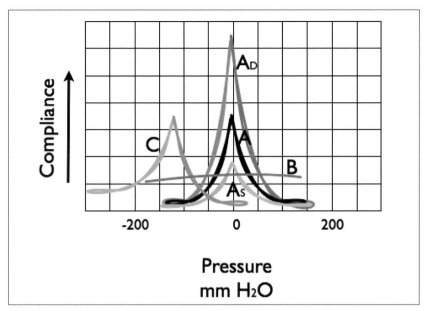

Figure 2-4. One system of tympanogram classification. As, stiffened tympano-ossicular system; AD, disarticulation; B, middle ear effusion, tympanic membrane perforation or impacted cerumen; C, negative middle ear pressure. From Core Curriculum Syllabus: Audiology. The Bobby R. Alford Department of Otolaryngology—Head and Neck Surgery, Baylor College of Medicine. http://www.bcm.edu/oto/index.cfm?pmid=15475

diagnose MEE, but studies are heterogeneous and performance is poorer than pneumatic otoscopy or tympanometry.

Pearl: Tympanometry is useful to identify presence of middle-ear effusion when diagnosis is unclear. Further imaging studies are not necessary unless the patient has developed a complication.

OTHER DIAGNOSTIC PROCEDURES

Other diagnostic procedures, such as lateral neck radiographs, immu-nologic evaluation, and fiber-optic nasopharyngeal examination, are useful in identifying predisposing factors, such as adenoid hypertrophy and associated allergies. Routine imaging of the temporal bone is not warranted unless patients have developed complications. Computed tomography (CT) scanning with intravenous (IV) contrast is the imaging modality of choice in screening for complications of AOM. Magnetic resonance imaging with gadolinium is useful when intracranial involvement is suspected.

■ Treatment Options for AOM

Management of AOM can be somewhat challenging. Evidence-based clinical practice guidelines were published in 2004 for AOM. These guidelines are mostly recommendations and options supported by published evidence on the management of this condition. Current recommendations are available to pediatricians, family physicians, otolaryngologists, physician assistants, nurse practitioners, and emergency department physicians, who treat these conditions on a routine basis.

■ 2004 Guidelines for AOM

RECOMMENDATION 1

To diagnose AOM the clinician should confirm a history of acute onset, identify signs of middle-ear effusion (MEE), and evaluate for the presence of signs and symptoms of middle-ear inflammation. (This recommendation is based on observational studies and a preponderance of benefit over risk....)

RECOMMENDATION 2

If pain is present, the clinician should recommend treatment to reduce pain. (This is a strong recommendation based on randomized, clinical trials with limitations and a preponderance of benefit over risk.)

RECOMMENDATION 3A

Observation without use of antibacterial agents in a child with uncomplicated AOM is an option for selected children based on diagnostic certainty, age, illness severity, and assurance of follow-up. (This option is based on randomized, controlled trials with limitations and a relative balance of benefit and risk.)

RECOMMENDATION 3B

If a decision is made to treat with an antibacterial agent, the clinician should prescribe amoxicillin for most children. (This recommendation is based on randomized, clinical trials with limitations and a preponderance of benefit over risk.)

When amoxicillin is used, the dose should be 80 to 90 mg/kg per day. (This option is based on extrapolation from microbiologic studies and expert opinion, with a preponderance of benefit over risk.)

RECOMMENDATION 4

If the patient fails to respond to the initial management option within 48 to 72 hours, the clinician must reassess the patient to confirm AOM and exclude other causes of illness. If AOM is confirmed in the patient initially managed with observation, the clinician should begin antibacterial therapy. If the patient was initially managed with an antibacterial agent, the clinician should change the antibacterial agent. (This recommendation is based on observational studies and a preponderance of benefit over risk.)

RECOMMENDATION 5

Clinicians should encourage the prevention of AOM through reduction of risk factors. (This recommendation is based on strong observational studies and a preponderance of benefits over risks.)

RECOMMENDATION 6

No recommendations for complementary and alternative medicine (CAM) for treatment of AOM are made based on limited and controversial data.

Medical treatment for AOM includes observation versus immediate antibiotic treatment. The approach for watchful waiting in selected cases is based on the evidence that most children recover uneventfully from AOM without the use of antibiotics (Rosenfeld and Kay, 2003). The decision to observe or treat with antibiotics is based on the child's age, the diagnosis of certainty, and the severity of the disease. In cases in which the child may or may not be able to return for care, observation is not recommended. A certain diagnosis of AOM meets all 3 following criteria: (1) rapid onset, (2) signs of MEE, and (3) signs and symptoms of middle-ear inflammation. An AOM episode is considered severe if the child presents with moderate to severe otalgia or temperature at or above 39°C orally (39.5°C rectally). A child with a non-severe AOM episode presents with mild otalgia and temperature below 39°C orally (39.5°C rectally), or no fever.

A more aggressive approach is recommended for younger children as well as children with underlying medical conditions (eg, Down syndrome, presence of cochlear implant, craniofacial abnormalities).

Children younger than 6 months with an AOM episode should be treated with antibiotics regardless of whether the diagnosis of AOM is certain or uncertain (Table 2-2). Children between the ages of 6 months and 2 years can be observed if they have an uncertain diagnosis with a non-severe illness; otherwise, they should be treated with antibiotics. Children older than 2 years can usually be observed unless they have a certain diagnosis with severe illness. If observation is considered, the clinician should always explain to parents or caregivers the degree of diagnostic certainty and consider their preference. Observation should only be considered when there is ready access to adequate follow-up care. Also, if observation results in clinical failure after 48 to 72 hours, antibacterial therapy should be considered as the next step.

Medical management of AOM should also include pain management. Nonsteroidal anti-inflammatory drugs are effective analgesics and therefore the mainstay of pain management for AOM. Otic analgesic is not reliable (often because of cerumen and TM thickening). Ototopical antibiotics are of no value in cases in which the TM is intact. Suppurative OM (ie, OM of the external canal or as a result of TM perforation) can be treated with ototopical agents, such as ofloxacin and ciprofloxacin with or without steroids. Although often prescribed, there is no proven benefit from oral decongestants and antihistamines in the management of AOM (Flynn et al, 2004). These agents may relieve accompanying nasal symptoms only.

Table 2-2. Criteria for Initial Antibacterial-Agent Treatment or Observation in Children With Acute Otitis Media

Age	Certain Diagnosis	Uncertain Diagnosis
>6 mo	Antibacterial therapy	Antibacterial therapy
6 mo to 2 y	Antibacterial therapy	Antibacterial therapy if severe illness; observation option[a] if nonsevere illness
≥2 y	Antibacterial therapy if severe illness; observation option[a] if nonsevere illness	Observation option[a]

[a]Observation is an appropriate option only when follow-up can be ensured and antibacterial agents started if symptoms persist or worsen. Nonsevere illness is mild otalgia and fever <39°C in the past 24 hours. Severe illness is moderate to severe otalgia or fever ≥39°C. A certain diagnosis of AOM meets all 3 criteria: 1) rapid onset, 2) signs of MEE, and 3) signs and symptoms of middle-ear inflammation.

Rosenfeld RM. Observation option toolkit for acute otitis media. *Int J Pediatr Otorhinolaryngol.* 2001;58:1–8, with permission from Elsevier.

Amoxicillin remains the drug of choice in the treatment of uncomplicated AOM (Table 2-3). This drug remains efficient against *S pneumoniae,* has a favorable pharmacodynamic profile, as well as safety, low cost, acceptable taste, and narrow microbiological spectrum. High amoxicillin doses (80–90 mg/kg/day) can be effectively used in the case scenario where resistant *S pneumoniae* strains or highly resistant *S pneumoniae* strains are the main pathogens.

High-dose amoxicillin-clavulanate (90 mg/kg/day amoxicillin component) is recommended as second-line empirical treatment for non-responding patients treated initially with amoxicillin or other antibacterial agents, or in patients for whom additional coverage for ß-lactamase–producing *H influenzae* and *M catarrhalis* is desired (Table 2-3). Child care attendance and previous antibiotic treatment are risk factors for the presence of bacterial species likely to be resistant to amoxicillin.

Table 2-3. Choice of Antibiotic in the Management of Acute Otitis Media

First-line Therapy

(1) Amoxicillin (80–90 mg/kg/day for 7–10 days)

Empirical treatment of AOM in children having received antibiotics during previous months; in otitis-prone children; in child care attendants
Empirical treatment of AOM in areas with high prevalence of pneumococcal penicillin resistance

(2) Amoxicillin-clavulanate (90 mg/kg/day amoxicillin component, with 6.4 mg/kg/day clavulanate for 7–10 days)

Empirical treatment of AOM in neonates

Empirical treatment of AOM in immunocompromised patients

Empirical treatment of AOM in areas with high prevalence of β-lactamase–producing organisms

Empirical treatment of AOM in patients who received antibiotics for AOM during preceding month

Second-line Therapy[a]

(1) Amoxicillin/clavulanate (90 mg/kg/day amoxicillin component, with 6.4 mg/kg/day clavulanate for 7–10 days)

(2) Intramuscular ceftriaxone (50 mg/kg/day) for 3 days

Abbreviation: AOM, acute otitis media.

[a]Therapeutic failure is considered if no improvement after 72 hours of starting first-line therapy.

Adapted from Segal N, Leibovitz E, Dagan R, Leiberman A. Acute otitis media—diagnosis and treatment in the era of antibiotic resistant organisms: updated clinical practice guidelines. *Int J Pediatr Otorhinolaryngol.* 2005;69(10):1311–1319, with permission from Elsevier.

In cases of non–IgE-mediated penicillin allergy, cefuroxime 50 mg/kg/day in 2 divided doses may be used.

In situations in which the patient cannot tolerate the oral route, a single intramuscular dose of parenteral ceftriaxone (50 mg/kg) has been shown to be effective for the initial treatment of AOM (Table 2-3). In selected cases, macrolides (azithromycin 10 mg/kg/day on day 1 followed by 5 mg/kg/day for 4 days as a single daily dose) or clarithromycin (15 mg/kg/day in 2 divided doses) can be an option. However, resistance to macrolide antibiotics from the 2 main common pathogens involved in AOM, *S pneumoniae* and *H influenzae*, is common.

The optimal duration of antibiotic treatment for AOM remains uncertain. The usual course of treatment remains 7 to 10 days in most cases. Despite the uncertainty of the antibiotic duration, the time course of clinical response should be 48 to 72 hours. Parents should expect improvement of symptoms within this period; if not, reassessment is necessary. Failure to improve clinically to a second-line treatment will lead to need to consider a different antibiotic, such as parenteral ceftriaxone (50mg/kg/day once daily) (Table 2-3). If no improvement despite outpatient treatment, admission to hospital and surgical intervention with myringotomy for cultures and antibacterial-agent sensitivity studies of the fluid are warranted to guide effective treatment and decrease risk of complications. In practice this is rarely required.

Surgical intervention of an uncomplicated AOM episode refractory to treatment consists of tympanocentesis and myringotomy with possible placement of tympanostomy tube. Multiple randomized studies comparing antibiotics versus a combination of antibiotics and myringotomy failed to show any benefit from surgical intervention over medical therapy on symptom resolution. Indications for myringotomy include severe otalgia or high fever, impending complications, AOM in newborns, AOM in patients with immunodeficiency, or unsatisfactory response to antibiotic treatment. Tympanocentesis provides adequate drainage as well as fluid for microbiological analysis.

Tympanostomy tube insertion has been advocated in children with recurrent episodes of AOM. Rosenfeld and Bluestone in 2003 showed that children with recurrent AOM who receive tympanostomy tubes have 67% fewer episodes than controls. Otorrhea is common after tympanostomy tube insertion and may require ototopical antibiotic drops for treatment. Adenoidectomy may be also considered in patients who have recurrent AOM because it reduces the incidence by 0 to 3 episodes per child-year. This procedure also reduces the need for future tympanostomy tube insertion for children aged 2 years or older who have recurrent AOM. In practice, adding adenoidectomy to the treatment of AOM usually occurs at surgery for repeated tympanostomy tube insertion and in the presence of nasal symptoms.

> **Pearl:** Most children recover well from acute otitis media, even without antibacterial therapy. In most patients, the choice of treatment is empirical and should be based on the available local epidemiologic information on the most common pathogens and their susceptibility patterns.

■ Natural History and Complications of AOM

The natural history of most children who experience AOM is clinical resolution within 4 to 7 days of diagnosis. Once the patient has shown clinical improvement, follow-up is based on the usual clinical course of AOM. No therapy is needed for persistent middle ear fluid after resolution of acute symptoms. Middle-ear effusion is a common sequelae of AOM, and approximately 60% to 70% of children will have fluid after 2 weeks from resolution of symptoms, decreasing to 10% after 3 months (Rosenfeld and Kay, 2003). The presence of MEE is not an indication for ototopical or systemic antibiotics because neither will hasten the resolution of the effusion.

Complications of AOM are rare, and the diagnosis depends on a high index of suspicion because antibiotic therapy can mask signs and symptoms. If complications are left untreated, they may rapidly progress with life-threatening consequences. Complications are classified as intratemporal or extratemporal (intracranial and extracranial). Intratemporal complications are more common and include acute TM perforation, mastoiditis, subperiosteal abscess, facial nerve paralysis, and labyrinthitis.

Increased pressure within the middle ear space can lead to TM rupture during an AOM episode. Most of these TM perforations heal spontaneously within 1 to 2 weeks. Patients who develop mastoiditis present with a protruding ear associated with erythema, tenderness, and swelling of the mastoid bone. Fluctuance in this area can suggest coalescent mastoiditis, which involves demineralization of the bone by osteoclastic activity, and the diagnosis can be confirmed with a CT scan of the temporal bone with contrast. Medical treatment with IV antibiotics is preferable in the presence of mastoiditis. In the absence of coalescent mastoiditis, 75% to 90% of the cases can be treated with IV antibiotics along with myringotomy or tympanostomy tube insertion. However, a cortical mastoidectomy and tympanostomy tube placement is advocated in those patients in which a coalescence develops.

Subperiosteal abscess is the most common extracranial complication of AOM. Patients present with a purulent collection lateral to the mastoid cortex. Intravenous antibiotics, tympanostomy tube placement, incision and drainage, and possibly cortical mastoidectomy is the preferred treatment of choice. Acute OM is the most common cause of facial nerve paralysis in children; however, this is an uncommon complication of AOM with an incidence of 0.005%. Treatment consists of IV antibiotics and myringotomy with placement of tympanostomy tube. Complete recovery of facial nerve paralysis occurs in more than 95% of cases. The earlier the tube is placed after the onset of paralysis, the faster the return of function has been our anecdotal experience. Protection of the eye during the paralysis is key to overall management.

When, very rarely, patients with AOM present with acute sensorineural hearing loss and vertigo, labyrinthitis is suspected. This occurs when the infection progresses from the middle ear and mastoid to the inner ear. Labyrinthitis can also be a sequela of meningitis, the most common intracranial complication of AOM. Meningitis presents with lethargy, altered mental status, and fever. A lumbar puncture is necessary for diagnosis and to guide treatment. Other intracranial complications of AOM include sigmoid sinus thrombosis, otitic hydrocephalus, and brain abscess, such as epidural, subdural, and intracranial abscesses.

> **Pearl:** The natural course of acute otitis media is spontaneous resolution. However, the clinician must be aware of the potential complications of acute otitis media and bear in mind that if left untreated, it may rapidly progress with potentially life-threatening consequences.

■ Prevention of AOM

Several environmental control measures based on non-randomized controlled trials have been taken to prevent the onset of AOM episodes. Prolonging breastfeeding, limiting pacifier use, and eliminating exposure to tobacco smoke and child care have been postulated as reducing the incidence of AOM. The benefits of antibiotic prophylaxis on the prevention of recurrent AOM by decreasing the number of episodes per month must be balanced against the risk of drug-induced side effects and the disadvantage of promoting antibiotic resistance. This practice has widely fallen out of favor. Reduction of upper airway infections by changing child care attendance patterns, limiting crowded environments, avoiding full-time child care attendance, or postponing child care until the age of 6 months is often recommended. Intranasal fluticasone administered during viral URIs has no effect and might even increase AOM incidence.

Influenza vaccines given to children older than 2 years have demonstrated more than 30% efficacy in the prevention of AOM during the influenza season, but no efficacy has been seen in younger children. The introduction of the 7-valent pneumococcal conjugate vaccine (PCV7) had a major role in decreasing the number of episodes of S pneumoniae AOM secondary to the serotypes included in the vaccine. It also had a major role in reducing the nasopharyngeal carriage of vaccine-type S pneumoniae, particularly antibacterial-resistant organisms, preventing its spread to contacts in the community. Although the vaccine decreased the proportion of AOM episodes caused by S pneumoniae serotypes by 56% to 67%, it was associated with a shift in serotype distribution from PCV7 types to non-PCV7 types, as well as bacterial pathogens such as H influenzae and Moraxella. Future studies will determine if PCV13 has a greater protective role than PCV7 administration.

> **Pearl:** Recurrent episodes of otitis media can be prevented by applying environmental control measures such as decreased exposure to child care centers and secondhand smoking, and the use of prophylaxis antibiotics. Vaccines are known to be effective in preventing acute otitis media.

■ Chronic Otitis Media

SUPPURATIVE

Chronic Suppurative Otitis Media (CSOM)

Chronic suppurative OM is defined as a perforated TM with persistent drainage from the middle ear lasting more than 12 weeks. Chronic suppurative OM most commonly follows an episode of acute infection but can also occur after trauma or iatrogenic injury (tympanostomy tubes). During an acute infection, a TM perforation can develop secondary to irritation, subsequent inflammation of the middle ear mucosa, and the resulting increased pressure behind an intact drum. Chronic suppurative OM is also associated with granulation tissue, which can develop into polyps within the middle ear space. The cycle of inflammation, ulceration, infection, and granulation tissue formation may continue, destroying surrounding bony margins and ultimately leading to subsequent complications, such as a chronic draining ear or cholesteatoma.

> **Pearl:** *Chronic suppurative otitis media* is defined as a perforated tympanic membrane with persistent drainage from the middle ear and is most commonly initiated after an episode of acute otitis media but can also occur after trauma or tympanostomy tubes.

MICROBIOLOGY OF CSOM

Understanding the unique microbiology of CSOM allows creation of a treatment plan with the greatest efficacy and least morbidity. *Pseudomonas aeruginosa, Staphylococcus aureus, Proteus* species, *Klebsiella pneumoniae,* and diphtheroids are the predominant bacteria cultured from chronically draining ears. Anaerobes and fungi can also be found within the MEE.

P aeruginosa is the most commonly recovered organism from the chronically draining ear (48%–98%). *P aeruginosa* can be found in areas of necrotic or diseased epithelium of the middle ear and can produce proteases, lipopolysaccharide, and other enzymes that inhibit normal immunologic defense mechanisms. Pseudomonal infections commonly resist macrolides, extended-spectrum penicillin, and first- and second-generation cephalosporins. This can complicate treatment plans, especially in children.

S aureus is the second most common organism isolated from chronically draining ears (15%–30%). The remainder of infections are caused by a large variety of gram-negative organisms. *Klebsiella* (10%–21%) and *Proteus* (10%–15%) species are slightly more common than other gram-negative organisms. Approximately 5% to 10% of infections are polymicrobial in etiology, often demonstrating a combination of gram-negative organisms and *S aureus*. Anaerobes *(Bacteroides, Peptostreptococcus,* and *Peptococcus)* and fungi *(Aspergillus, Candida)* complete the spectrum of colonizing organisms in CSOM.

> **Pearl:** *Pseudomonas aeruginosa, Staphylococcus aureus, Proteus* species, *Klebsiella pneumoniae,* and diphtheroids are the most common bacteria cultured from chronically draining ears.

■ Assessment and Diagnosis of CSOM

PRESENTING SYMPTOMS

Patients with CSOM present with otic drainage lasting longer than 3 months and premorbid history of recurrent AOM with perforation, traumatic perforation, or placement of ventilation tubes. Additionally, they commonly present with hearing loss in the affected ear and occasionally can report fever, vertigo, and pain. A history of persistent CSOM after appropriate medical treatment or unilateral CSOM should alert the physician to the possibility of an underlying cholesteatoma.

PHYSICAL EXAMINATION

Patients with CSOM generally have a TM perforation associated with otorrhea that can range from clear or serous to purulent or foul smelling. Physical examination findings can also reveal signs of external auditory canal and middle-ear inflammation. Granulation tissue can be found in the ear canal or middle ear space. The middle ear mucosa that can be visualized through the TM perforation is commonly polypoid, pale, or edematous. It will easily bleed if touched.

An acutely perforated TM is often erythematous and thickened, with otorrhea discharging through the perforation. Other findings of the TM can include tympanosclerosis, retraction pockets, or areas of atelectasis (collapse of the TM). Tympanosclerosis appears as white and thickened areas of the TM (Figure 2-5) but uncommonly affects hearing independently. Retraction pockets can be located anywhere in the TM and may represent areas of atelectasis or the result of persistent negative middle-ear pressure (Figure 2-6). Retraction pockets in the superior quadrant, especially if filled with debris, can be associated with a pars flaccida cholesteatoma (Figure 2-7).

DIAGNOSTIC TESTS

Hearing Evaluation

An audiogram with impedance should be obtained in patients with CSOM to evaluate for any associated hearing loss and corroborate the presence of a perforation. Most patients present with conductive hearing loss secondary to middle-ear inflammation (eg, fluid, polyps, adhesions) or ossicular chain erosion. Although rarely, some patients present with mixed hearing loss, indicating more extensive damage to the inner ear.

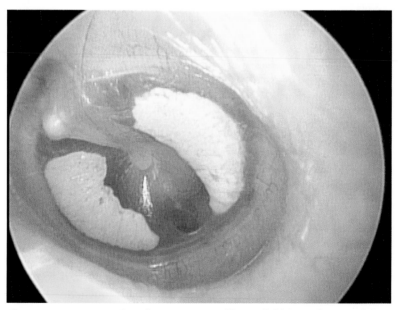

Figure 2-5. Tympanosclerosis appears as white and thickened areas of the tympanic membrane.

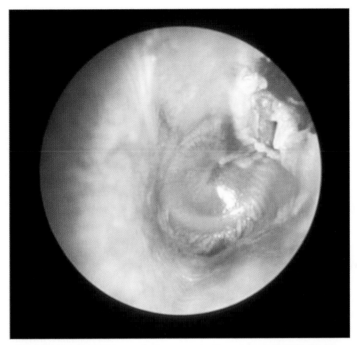

Figure 2-6. Retraction pockets representing areas of atelectasis.

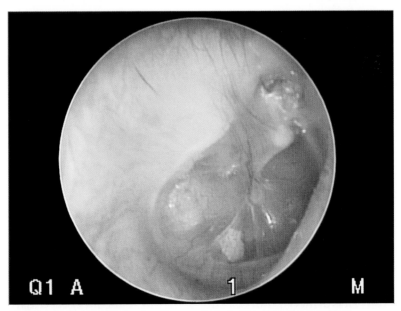

Figure 2-7. Debris-filled retraction pockets in the superior quadrant associated with a pars flaccida cholesteatoma.

OTHER DIAGNOSTIC PROCEDURES

The otorrhea in CSOM can be treated successfully in most cases with ototopical antibiotic drops. The most common cause of treatment failure when using ototopical antibiotic drops is improper administration. The drops will only affect material with which they are in contact, so gentle retraction of the pinna posteriorly and light tragal pressure ensures admixture of the drops with the infected otorrhea and significantly increases effectiveness of the drops. However, in the unusual case in which the patient fails medical therapy with properly administered antibiotic drops, a culture of ear drainage should be obtained for sensitivity. The results from the culture sensitivities can modify systemic therapy and guide treatment successfully.

A CT scan of the temporal bone can also be considered when CSOM is unresponsive, quickly recurrent, or unilateral. This can provide information about any occult cholesteatoma, foreign body, intratemporal and intracranial complications, or other diseases to be considered, such as Langerhans cell histiocytosis or rare neoplasia. A fine-cut CT scan can provide more details about the temporal bone anatomy and reveal any complications of the disease, such as ossicular erosion, bone erosion, petrous apex involvement, coalescent mastoiditis, and subperiosteal abscess. Magnetic resonance imaging can be obtained when intracranial complications are suspected.

> **Pearl:** Chronic suppurative otitis media can present with a serous or purulent ear drainage, signs of middle-ear inflammation, and granulation tissue. An audiogram can reveal hearing loss secondary to drainage occluding the ear canal or from ossicular erosion.

■ Treatment Options for CSOM

Treatment of CSOM is aimed at controlling otorrhea, restoring the integrity of the TM, and improving any associated hearing loss. Control of the ear discharge can be temporary only and patients may opt to undergo surgical intervention to treat the structural changes involved and for better long-term results. However, if proper control of otorrhea is achieved, early closure of the TM is not always necessary and can be postponed.

Topical antibiotic therapy, regular and aggressive aural toilet, and control of granulation tissue are frequently the first treatment options for treating CSOM. Unfortunately, there are no available guidelines for the management of CSOM. However, 2 studies offer a guide to evidence-based treatment of otorrhea in children with CSOM. Smith et al demonstrated that topical and systemic antibiotics after aural toilet resulted in better resolution of otorrhea than aural toilet alone. Macfadyen et al demonstrated that topical antiseptics, such as boric acid and alcohol, are less effective at drying discharging ears than topical quinolones. Based on their conclusions, following are some guidelines for the medical treatment of CSOM in children:

1. *It seems probable that topical treatment with antibiotics after aural toilet is more effective than systemic treatment with antibiotics. The importance of adequately cleaning the ear prior to properly instilling drops cannot be overemphasized.*

2. *It is not clear whether topical quinolones are more effective than other topical antibiotics for the control of CSOM. However, topical quinolones do not carry the potential for ototoxicity associated with aminoglycosides. When possible, topical antibiotic preparations free of potential ototoxicity should be used in preference to ototopical preparations that have the potential for otologic injury if the middle ear and mastoid are open.*

3. *The use of aminoglycoside ear drops should be for short periods, never more than 2 weeks at a time, and only used in the presence of active CSOM, where the risk of ototoxicity from pus in the middle ear cleft probably outweighs that from aminoglycoside drops. The child's parents should be counseled about the risks of using aminoglycosides when the middle ear is exposed.*

4. *Microbiology guidance should be required, especially if there is failure to respond after an initial course of treatment.*

The most common antibiotic drops used are aminoglycosides and fluoroquinolones. These antibiotics have an appropriate spectrum of activity against the most common organisms involved in CSOM, *Pseudomonas* and *S aureus*. Gentamicin- and tobramycin-containing ophthalmic drops have been widely used off-label for the treatment of otologic infections. All aminoglycosides have significant potential ototoxicity, causing vestibular dysfunction or hearing loss. Studies designed to detect hearing loss from use of ototopical aminoglycosides demonstrate that such incidence is very low and dose related and occur following prolonged courses. See Table 2-4 for more information about topical antibiotics used for CSOM.

Antibiotic	Dosing	Contraindications	Precautions
Ciprofloxacin otic suspension	5–10 drops instilled in affected ear twice a day	Hypersensitivity	Headache and pruritus
Tobramycin	5–10 drops instilled in affected ear twice a day	Hypersensitivity	Monitor for auditory or vestibular toxicity.
Ciprofloxacin	10–20 mg/kg orally every 12 h	Hypersensitivity	Increased risk of tendinitis and tendon rupture in all ages
Piperacillin	200–300 mg/kg/d IV divided every 4–6 h; not to exceed 24 g/d	Hypersensitivity	Caution in renal impairment and history of seizures
Ceftazidime	1–2 g IV every 8–12 h	Hypersensitivity	Adjust dose in severe renal insufficiency.

Table 2-4. Antimicrobials Used for Chronic Suppurative Otitis Media

Abbreviation: IV, intravenous.

The anti-inflammatory effect of steroids is an important advantage when a significant amount of granulation tissue is present on physical examination. Granulation tissue can exacerbate otorrhea and prevent topical antibiotic agents from adequately penetrating the middle ear. Topical steroids are effective in treating granulation tissue and hasten resolution. A fixed-ratio combination of tobramycin and dexamethasone (TobraDex) has been especially popular in the United States, while gentamicin-containing drops have been more popular in Canada and Europe. When topical steroids are not effective, silver nitrate can be used, along with cautery or excision technique under the microscope.

Aural toilet is an essential part of the medical treatment of CSOM. Ear drainage must be removed from the ear canal to permit better topical antibiotic penetration. Traditionally, this is performed using the microscope and micro-instruments available at an otolaryngologist's office. Aural irrigation with a solution of 50% peroxide and 50% sterile water is another alternative that is generally painless and effective. This should be performed prior to instilling ototopical antibiotics.

Treatment failures are almost always secondary to incomplete penetration of the topical antimicrobials to the middle ear (often because of inadequate instructions given by the prescribing physician) and almost never because of an antimicrobial resistance to the organisms causing CSOM. In true cases of failure, an underlying cholesteatoma, foreign body, and other diseases in the differential must be ruled out. If the patient has failed to respond to topical antimicrobial therapy, cultures for sensitivities should be performed and a CT scan of the temporal bone should be considered. A trial of systemic antibiotics that exceed the minimal inhibitory concentration of most relevant organisms can be given for a period of 3 to 4 weeks. Most patients experience cessation of otorrhea soon after proper administration of systemic antibiotics. Currently, the most effective and most commonly used oral antibiotics in patients with CSOM are fluoroquinolones. These antibiotics are not approved for use in children because of potential joint injury in juvenile experimental animals. However, this side effect has not been reported in the large database available from children with cystic fibrosis treated with high doses of systemic quinolones. Most parents are agreeable to the off-label use of oral fluoroquinolones if they understand the relative risks and potential benefits that this class of drugs offers.

Surgical intervention should be considered in the rare instance in which CSOM does not respond to medical therapy. A tympanomastoidectomy can eliminate the infection and stop otorrhea in approximately 80% of the cases. Surgical intervention with tympanoplasty is the treatment of choice to close the TM perforation. There is controversy about the best time to perform tympanoplasty in children. Vrabec et al found a significant association of greater success of tympanoplasty with advancing age, from 6 to 13 years. In the pediatric population, choosing the perfect timing to perform a tympanoplasty is a balance between the morbidity of leaving the perforation open and the decreasing risk of surgical failure as the child grows older.

> **Pearl:** The initial treatment of chronic suppurative otitis media should include topical antimicrobial therapy, aural toilet, and topical steroids for any associated granulation tissue. Treatment failures to topical antimicrobials should be evaluated with culture sensitivities and treated with a trial of systemic therapy. Surgical intervention with tympanoplasty or tympanomastoidectomy can be considered in medical therapy failures.

■ Natural History and Complications of CSOM

If not treated successfully, CSOM can cause conductive hearing loss from ossicular erosion and occasionally social stigma secondary to the foul-smelling fluid draining from the affected ear. Other sequelae include acquired cholesteatoma and tympanosclerosis. Complications of CSOM are very similar to AOM complications previously discussed. Chronic suppurative OM without prompt proper treatment can progress into a variety of mild to life-threatening complications that can be separated into 2 subgroups: intratemporal and intracranial. Intratemporal complications include petrositis, facial paralysis, and labyrinthitis. Intracranial complications include lateral sinus thrombophlebitis, meningitis, and intracranial abscess.

■ Prevention of CSOM

In patients with a known TM perforation, CSOM can be prevented by practicing dry ear precautions when washing and swimming with diligent use of earplugs. Tympanoplasty, a surgical intervention that recreates the TM by sealing the perforation with a graft, is another option available to prevent any further drainage and improve hearing with good long-term results. It is important to refer a patient with CSOM with symptoms of aural fullness, otalgia, fever, or headaches to an otolaryngologist for further evaluation and management.

■ Nonsuppurative Otitis Media

OTITIS MEDIA WITH EFFUSION (OME)

The lack of acute symptoms with OME makes prevalence difficult to estimate. However, the point prevalence of MEE on screening test is approximately 20%. Approximately 50% of children will experience OME in the first year of life, increasing to 60% by 2 years. About 90% of children have OME at some time before school age. The incidence seems to peak during the second year of life, is most prevalent during the winter months, and is associated with URIs. The majority of OME episodes will resolve spontaneously within 3 months; however, 30% to 40% of children have persistent episodes. The recurrence rate within 24 months is 50%.

> **Pearl:** Otitis media with effusion is defined as middle-ear effusion without signs or symptoms of an acute infection. It can be secondary to eustachian tube dysfunction or a sequel to acute otitis media.

MICROBIOLOGY OF OME

In the past, chronic MEE was often thought to be sterile. However, several studies have isolated *S pneumoniae, H influenzae, M catarrhalis,* and group A streptococci in 30% to 50% of children with chronic MEE. Although bacterial isolation from middle ear fluid is not proof of an active bacterial infectious process, Post et al reported that bacteria may be present in a higher percentage of OME specimens than was previously thought. In chronic OME, anaerobic organisms such as *Peptostreptococcus* species, *Prevotella* species, and *Propionibacterium acnes* have been isolated. *Helicobacter pylori* has recently been studied and found in middle ear, tonsillar, and adenoid tissues in patients with OME, indicating a possible role in pathogenesis of OME.

> **Pearl:** Otitis media with effusion appears to peak during the second year of life, is most prevalent during the winter months, and is associated with upper respiratory infections.

■ Assessment and Diagnosis of OME

PRESENTING SYMPTOMS

The presence of fluid in the middle ear without acute signs of MEE inflammation is characteristic of OME. As patients do not present with acute onset signs, such as fever, otalgia, or irritability, the diagnosis of OME is usually made by screening or as an incidental finding on routine physical examination. However, some children manifest noninfectious discomfort (commonly, tugging or itching of the ears), hearing loss, clumsiness, or sleep disruption, but most children are usually referred from school as they failed screening hearing programs. Physical examination along with a formal audiogram can confirm the presence of MEE and mild hearing impairment.

> **Pearl:** Because of the lack of acute symptoms, diagnosis of otitis media with effusion is usually made by screening or as an incidental finding on routine physical examination.

PHYSICAL EXAMINATION

To establish a definite diagnosis of OME, it is important to identify MEE without inflammatory changes of the TM. Therefore, physical examination should include otoscopy and pneumatic otoscopy if possible. Adequate visualization of the TM should be obtained.

Air-fluid levels or bubbles without signs of middle-ear inflammation are the usual physical examination findings in OME. Air-fluid levels will indicate intermittent aeration of the middle ear through the ET (Figure 2-8). Pneumatic otoscopy has a sensitivity of 94% and specificity of 88% for diagnosis of MEE when compared with myringotomy, which is the gold standard. In difficult cases, the presence of MEE can be supplemented by tympanometry or impedance (acoustic reflex measurements).

> **Pearl:** The usual findings on physical examination in otitis media with effusion include air-fluid levels or bubbles without signs of middle-ear inflammation.

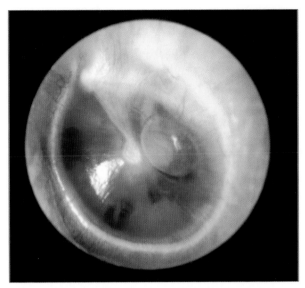

Figure 2-8. Air-fluid levels or bubbles without signs of middle-ear inflammation are usually found in otitis media with effusion. Note the bubble on the right side of the tympanic membrane.

DIAGNOSTIC TESTS

Hearing Evaluation

Pure tone audiometry or visual reinforcement audiometry can be used to diagnose the conductive hearing loss associated with OME in young children. Tympanometry can assess TM mobility and middle-ear function, and the results can be classified with quantitative measures or by pattern curves, as previously mentioned.

OTHER DIAGNOSTIC PROCEDURES

Other diagnostic procedures, such as lateral neck radiographs, immunologic evaluation, and fiber-optic nasopharyngeal examination, may be useful in identifying predisposing factors, such as adenoid hypertrophy and associated allergies, but are not routinely performed. Routine imaging of the temporal bone is not warranted for OME.

■ Treatment Options for OME

Evidence-based clinical practice guidelines were published in 2004 for OME. These guidelines are mostly recommendations and options supported by published evidence on the management of this condition.

Current recommendations are available to pediatricians, family physicians, otolaryngologists, physician assistants, nurse practitioners, and emergency department physicians, who treat OME on a routine basis. They offer evidence-based recommendations to make the appropriate diagnosis and provide options available for management.

■ 2004 Guidelines for OME

RECOMMENDATION 1A

Pneumatic otoscopy: Clinicians should use pneumatic otoscopy as the primary diagnostic method for OME, and OME should be distinguished from AOM. This is a strong recommendation based on systematic review of cohort studies and the preponderance of benefit over harm.

RECOMMENDATION 1B

Tympanometry: Tympanometry can be used to confirm the diagnosis of OME. This option is based on cohort studies and a balance of benefit and harm.

RECOMMENDATION 1C

Screening: Population-based screening programs for OME are not recommended in healthy asymptomatic children. This recommendation is based on randomized, controlled trials and cohort studies, with a preponderance of harm over benefit.

RECOMMENDATION 2

Documentation: Clinicians should document the laterality, duration of effusion, and presence and severity of associated symptoms at each assessment of the child with OME. This recommendation is based on observational studies and strong preponderance of benefit over harm.

RECOMMENDATION 3

Child at risk: Clinicians should distinguish the child with OME who is at risk for speech, language, or learning problems from other children with OME and should evaluate hearing, speech, language, and need for intervention more promptly. This recommendation is based on case series, the preponderance of benefit over harm, and ethical limitations in studying children with OME who are at risk.

RECOMMENDATION 4

Watchful waiting: Clinicians should manage the child with OME who is not at risk with watchful waiting for 3 months from the date of effusion onset (if known) or diagnosis (if onset is unknown). This recommendation is based on systematic review of cohort studies and the preponderance of benefit over harm.

RECOMMENDATION 5

Medication: Antihistamines and decongestants are ineffective for OME and are not recommended for treatment; antimicrobials and corticosteroids do not have long-term efficacy and are not recommended for routine management. This recommendation is based on systematic review of randomized, controlled trials and the preponderance of harm over benefit.

RECOMMENDATION 6

Hearing and language: Hearing testing is recommended when OME persists for 3 months or longer or at any time that language delay, learning problems, or a significant hearing loss is suspected in a child with OME; language testing should be conducted for children with hearing loss. This recommendation is based on cohort studies and the preponderance of benefit over risk.

RECOMMENDATION 7

Surveillance: Children with persistent OME who are not at risk should be reexamined at 3- to 6-month intervals until the effusion is no longer present, significant hearing loss is identified, or structural abnormalities of the eardrum or middle ear are suspected. This recommendation is based on randomized, controlled trials and observational studies with a preponderance of benefit over harm.

RECOMMENDATION 8

Referral: When children with OME are referred by the primary care clinician for evaluation by an otolaryngologist, audiologist, or speech-language patholo-gist, the referring clinician should document the effusion duration and specific reason for referral (evaluation, surgery) and provide additional relevant infor-mation such as history of AOM and developmental status of the child. This option is based on panel consensus and a preponderance of benefit over harm.

RECOMMENDATION 9

Surgery: When a child becomes a surgical candidate, tympanostomy tube insertion is the preferred initial procedure; adenoidectomy should not be performed unless a distinct indication exists (nasal obstruction, chronic adenoiditis). Repeat surgery consists of adenoidectomy plus myringotomy, with or without tube insertion. Tonsillectomy alone or myringotomy alone should not be used to treat OME. This recommendation is based on randomized, controlled trials with a preponderance of benefit over harm.

RECOMMENDATION 10

CAM: No recommendation is made regarding CAM as a treatment for OME. There is no recommendation based on lack of scientific evidence documenting efficacy and an uncertain balance of harm and benefit.

RECOMMENDATION 11

Allergy management: No recommendation is made regarding allergy management as a treatment for OME. There is no recommendation based on insufficient evidence of therapeutic efficacy or a causal relationship between allergy and OME.

The initial management of patients with OME is to provide reassurance to parents of the self-limiting nature of OME and the likelihood that surgical treatment will not be required. The child needs monitoring over a 3- to 6-month period to identify if the effusion is persistent and to determine if surgical intervention is needed.

Medical treatment for OME does not provide lasting resolution of symptoms. Multiple studies have reviewed and compared antibiotics versus a combination of antibiotics and oral corticosteroids, but none have found a lasting benefit from these treatments. The role of intranasal corticosteroids has been evaluated and some studies have shown that they are unlikely to be a cost-effective treatment or clinically effective in the long term. Fluticasone and mometasone are minimally systemically absorbed, free of major side effects, and helpful in treating any associated rhinitis in children older than 4 years.

Nasal auto-insufflation of the ETs has proven to be a benefit if used regularly; however, almost 12% of children between 3 and 10 years are unable to use it on a regular basis. There is no recommendation addressing complementary and alternative medicine, as well as allergy management, as treatment for OME.

A child with OME becomes a surgical candidate when the effusion persists longer than 4 months with persistent hearing loss; if the effusion is recurrent or persistent in children at risk for speech, language, or learning problems regardless of hearing status; and if there is evidence of structural damage to the TM or middle ear. Ultimately, the decision for surgery must be made on a case-by-case basis with consensus among the primary care physician, otolaryngologist, and parent or caregiver.

Tympanostomy tube is the preferred treatment for initial surgery in patients with OME. Myringotomy alone is ineffective for chronic OME. There is a 62% relative decrease in effusion prevalence and an absolute decrease of effusion days per child. Standard ventilation tube will normally extrude between 6 to 9 months after insertion. Unfortunately, approximately 20% to 50% of children who have had tympanostomy tubes have OME relapse after tube extrusion. These patients might benefit from adenoidectomy at the time of repeat placement of tympanostomy tubes, especially if there are symptoms of nasal obstruction present. Adenoidectomy provides a 50% reduction in the need for future surgeries and it has comparable efficacy in children aged 4 years or older. The benefit of adenoidectomy is apparent at age 2 years, greatest at age 3, and independent of adenoid size. There is a clear preponderance of benefit over harm when considering the effect of surgery for OME. Surgical and anesthesia costs are offset by reduced OME after tube placement and reduced need of reoperation after adenoidectomy.

Surgical intervention comes with potential risks, which include anesthesia, adenoidectomy, and sequelae of tympanostomy tubes. Anesthesia risks include laryngospasm, bronchospasm, and anesthesia mortality, which has been reported to be about 1 in 50,000. Tympanostomy tube sequelae are more common and include otorrhea (which is common and therefore hard to classify as a complication), tympanosclerosis, or retraction pockets, among others. Tympanic membrane perforation has a prevalence of 2% with short-term tubes and 17% after placement of long-term tubes. Adenoidectomy has a 0.2% to 0.5% incidence of hemorrhage and 2% incidence of velopharyngeal insufficiency. There is a predominance of benefit over harm among the surgical treatments of OME; however, all these potential risks should be explained in detail to parents and caregivers after the decision for surgical intervention is made.

> **Pearl:** Medical treatments have not been proven to be effective in the management of otitis media with effusion. Insertion of ventilation tubes for children with bilateral hearing impairment associated with otitis media with effusion, who have failed watchful waiting, is effective in restoring hearing thresholds. Adenoidectomy, when performed in conjunction with repeat placement of tympanostomy tubes, reduces the incidence of recurrent otitis media with effusion.

■ Natural History and Complications of OME

As previously stated, OME will usually resolve spontaneously without need of any intervention. Children with persistent OME are at risk of developing hearing loss and early language acquisition impairment. Conductive hearing loss may adversely affect binaural processing, sound localization, and speech perception in noise. Clinicians should ask parents about specific concerns regarding their child's language development. There is evidence that untreated OME may produce lasting effects on behavior and development, particularly attention and hyperactivity.

Damage to the TM and middle ear are common in patients with persistent OME. There is no evidence that treating OME surgically reduces the risk of cholesteatoma formation or permanent damage to the TM.

> **Pearl:** Otitis media with effusion resolves spontaneously in the majority of cases; however, persistent effusion can cause hearing loss and early language acquisition impairment.

■ Prevention of OME

Modifications that may help decrease the frequency of OME include breastfeeding whenever possible, limiting pacifier use, avoiding feeding in a supine position, as well as eliminating exposure to tobacco smoke and child care.

■ Conclusion

The various types of AOM and COM comprise a significant percentage of the patients seen in emergency departments, urgent care, and walk-in practices, and in patients visiting primary care physician and pediatrician offices. A working understanding of the disease, its pathophysiology, diagnosis, and treatment are essential to the physician looking after children. This chapter summarizes the information required to manage these patients but has been forced to divide and subdivide what is a physiologic continuum into non-physiologic entities. Otitis media represents a contiguous spectrum of disease within which several distinct clinical entities have been identified. The truth is that there is no fine line at which point AOM and OME transform in to one or the other, appear or disappear, and many patients will present with components of both (the same goes for temporal delineations, especially when the concept of acute on chronic disease is introduced).

The diagnostic principles and algorithms of treatment for OM, however, are well developed, and higher and higher levels of evidence are emerging with which clinicians can manage this spectrum of disease. The key points and pearls included in this chapter are derived from our experience and will helpfully allow the reader to fine-tune his or her own management practice. The known standard treatment protocols have been reprinted to allow the practitioner to refer to this chapter as a bedside handbook. In addition, we hope this chapter provides a solid foundation and reference to add to the reader's understanding of OM in children.

■ Selected References

American Academy of Family Physicians, American Academy of Otolaryngology–Head and Neck Surgery, American Academy of Pediatrics Subcommittee on Otitis Media With Effusion. Otitis media with effusion. *Pediatrics.* 2004;113(5):1412–1429

American Academy of Family Physicians, American Academy of Pediatrics Subcommittee on Management of Acute Otitis Media. Diagnosis and management of acute otitis media. *Pediatrics.* 2004;113(5):1451–1465

Belshe RB, Gruber WC. Prevention of otitis media in children with live attenuated influenza vaccine given intranasally. *Pediatr Infect Dis J.* 2000;19(5 Suppl):S66–S71

Block SL, Hedrick J, Harrison CJ, et al. Community-wide vaccination with the heptavalent pneumococcal conjugate significantly alters the microbiology of acute otitis media. *Pediatr Infect Dis J.* 2004;23(9):829–833

Casselbrant ML, Mandel EM, Fall PA, et al. The heritability of otitis media: a twin and triplet study. *JAMA.* 1999;282(22):2125–2130

Farjo RS, Foxman B, Patel MJ, et al. Diversity and sharing of *Haemophilus influenzae* strains colonizing healthy children attending day-care centers. *Pediatr Infect Dis J.* 2004;23(1):41–46

Flynn CA, Griffin GH, Schultz JK. Decongestants and antihistamines for acute otitis media in children. *Cochrane Database Syst Rev.* 2004;3:CD001727

Friedmann I. The pathology of otitis media. *J Clin Pathol.* 1956;9(3):229–236

Gates GA, Klein JO, Lim DJ, et al. Recent advances in otitis media, 1: definitions, terminology, and classification of otitis media. *Ann Otol Rhinol Laryngol.* 2002;188:8–18

Graham JM, Scadding GK, Bull PD, eds. *Pediatric ENT.* Heidelberg, Germany: Springer-Verlag Berlin Heidelburg; 2007

Greenberg D, Hoffman S, Leibovitz E, Dagan R. Acute otitis media in children: association with day care centers—antibacterial resistance, treatment, and prevention. *Paediatr Drugs.* 2008;10(2):75–83

Kay DJ, Nelson M, Rosenfeld RM. Meta-analysis of tympanostomy tube sequelae. *Otolaryngol Head Neck Surg.* 2001;124(4):374–380

Leibovitz E, Piglansky L, Raiz S, Press J, Leiberman A, Dagan R. Bacteriologic and clinical efficacy of one day vs. three day intramuscular ceftriaxone for treatment of nonresponsive acute otitis media in children. *Pediatr Infect Dis J.* 2000;19(11):1040–1045

Macfadyen C, Gamble C, Garner P, et al. Topical quinolone vs. antiseptic for treating chronic suppurative otitis media: a randomized controlled trial. *Trop Med Int Health.* 2005;10(2):190–197

O'Reilly RC, He Z, Bloedon E, et al. The role of extraesophageal reflux in otitis media in infants and children. *Laryngoscope.* 2008;118(7 Part 2 Suppl 116):1–9

Park SY, Moore MR, Bruden DL, et al. Impact of conjugate vaccine on transmission of antimicrobial-resistant *Streptococcus pneumoniae* among Alaskan children. *Pediatr Infect Dis J.* 2008;27(4):335–340

Post JC, Hiller NL, Nistico L, Stoodley P, Ehrlich GD. The role of biofilms in otolaryngologic infections: update 2007. *Curr Opin Otolaryngol Head Neck Surg.* 2007;15(5):347–351

Roberts JE, Rosenfeld RM, Zeisel SA. Otitis media and speech and language: a meta-analysis of prospective studies. *Pediatrics.* 2004;113(3 Pt 1):e238–e248

Roland PS, Stewart MG, Hannley M, et al. Consensus panel on role of potentially ototoxic antibiotics for topical middle ear use: introduction, methodology, and recommendations. *Otolaryngol Head Neck Surg.* 2004;130(3 Suppl):S51–S56

Rosenfeld RM. Diagnostic certainty for acute otitis media. *Int J Pediatr Otorhinolaryngol.* 2002;64(2):89–95

Rosenfeld RM, Bluestone CD. Clinical efficacy of surgical therapy. In: Rosenfeld RM, Bluestone CD, eds. *Evidence-Based Otitis Media.* 2nd ed. Hamilton, Ontario, Canada: BC Decker; 2003:227–240

Rosenfeld RM, Kay D. Natural history of untreated otitis media. *Laryngoscope.* 2003;113(10):1645–1657

Segal N, Leibovitz E, Dagan R, Leiberman A. Acute otitis media—diagnosis and treatment in the era of antibiotic resistant organisms: updated clinical practice guidelines. *Int J Pediatr Otorhinolaryngol.* 2005;69(10):1311–1319

Smith AW, Hatcher J, Mackenzie IJ, et al. Randomised controlled trial of chronic suppurative otitis media in Kenyan schoolchildren. *Lancet.* 1996;348(9035):1128–1133

Teele DW, Klein JO, Rosner B. Epidemiology of otitis media during first seven years of life in children in greater Boston: a prospective, cohort study. *J Infect Dis.* 1989;160(1):83–94

Vrabec JT, Deskin RW, Grady JJ. Meta-analysis of pediatric tympanoplasty. *Arch Otolaryngol Head Neck Surg.* 1999;125(5):530–534

Williams RL, Chalmers TC, Stange KC, Chalmers FT, Bowlin SJ. Use of antibiotics in preventing recurrent otitis media and in treating otitis media with effusion. A meta-analytic attempt to resolve the brouhaha. *JAMA.* 1993;270(11):1344–1351

Zielhuis GA, Heuvelmans-Heinen EW, Rach GH, van den Broek P. Environmental risk factors for otitis media with effusion in preschool children. *Scand J Prim Health Care.* 1989;7(1):33–38

CHAPTER 3

Facial Paralysis

David H. Chi, MD

■ Introduction

Facial paralysis is a significant condition because of its cosmetic and functional effects. The physical inability to move a side of the face is very apparent and difficult to disguise. Moreover, facial motion is essential for ocular protection. Secondary corneal injury from drying may occur because of inability to close the eye. Speech and emotional expression may also be affected. The challenge for physicians is to determine the extent of injury, identify the cause of the disorder, and decide whether medical or surgical intervention is required.

■ Anatomy

Basic knowledge of the anatomy and function of the facial nerve is essential in understanding facial paralysis. The nerve carries fibers for many different functions. The main function is from the special visceral efferent fibers that supply motor innervation to the facial musculature as well as to the stapedius, posterior belly of the digastric, and stylohyoid muscles. Special visceral afferent fibers provide the sensation of taste to the anterior two-thirds of the tongue and hard palate. General visceral efferent fibers function to provide parasympathetic innervation to the lacrimal, submandibular, and sublingual glands. General somatic afferent fibers provide cutaneous sensory innervation to the skin of the concha and small area behind the ear.

■ History

A thorough history is essential in evaluating children with facial paralysis. Important information includes the duration and onset of paralysis (eg, sudden, gradual). Other factors include the severity of the paralysis (ie, partial or complete). Partial paresis is usually associated with a good prognosis for recovery as long as the underlying cause is addressed. The physician should also inquire about associated symptoms. Those with severe otalgia and recent vesicular ear lesions suggest herpes zoster oticus. Ipsilateral facial numbness, altered taste, and decreased tearing occur frequently with Bell palsy. Hearing loss and vertigo may indicate tumors of the internal auditory canal or brain stem.

Recurrent episodes of facial palsy may be present with a tumor but also can occur with Bell palsy. Approximately 7% of Bell palsy patients may have recurrent facial paralysis. Other aspects of history include recent head trauma, otologic surgeries, and autoimmune disorders.

■ Physical Examination

A complete head and neck examination with emphasis on the ear is essential. External ear should be assessed for vesicular lesions. External ear canal and tympanic membrane may demonstrate evidence of otitis, cholesteatoma, or tumor. Children with history of trauma may show hemotympanum, perforation, or otorrhea. Clear fluid may be indicative of cerebrospinal fluid. Battle sign (mastoid ecchymosis) or raccoon eyes may occur with skull base fracture. A cheek or neck mass suggests a tumor, especially if facial paresis has been gradual in onset and segmental paresis is present.

A thorough neurologic examination should be performed. All branches of the facial nerve should be assessed and the 2 sides compared. The patient should be asked to maximally raise the brows, close the eyes tightly, wrinkle the nose, pucker, and smile widely. A unique challenge in the physical examination of newborns and very young children is that cooperation is limited and the clinician may need to observe for facial motion while the baby is crying or playing when spontaneous facial expressions occur. In addition, the young child has good facial muscular tone and may make the clinician underestimate the degree of paresis. Multiple cranial neuropathies suggest extensive trauma, infection, extensive neoplasm, or systemic neurologic disease. The most common scale used and accepted to determine severity of facial paresis is the House-Brackmann classification (Table 3-1).

An important early distinction is to identify facial nerve deficit as a central or peripheral lesion. Central problems usually can be differentiated by a thorough neurologic examination because most brain lesions are not specific to be isolated only to the facial nerve. Because the upper face is innervated bilaterally from facial nerve tracts from the brain cortex, a cortical lesion results in facial paralysis of the lower face only.

■ Pathophysiology

Understanding the degree of injury is important in predicting facial nerve recovery. The Sunderland classification scheme is based on the histologic changes and physiologic implications (Table 3-2).

First-degree injury, or neurapraxia, occurs with increased intraneural pressure such as a compression injury. Continuity of the axon is preserved, and the injury prevents conduction of an action potential. No wallerian degeneration occurs. With relief of compression, complete recovery is expected.

Table 3-1. Facial Nerve Grading System

Grade	Description	Characteristics
I	Normal	Normal facial function in all areas

II	Mild dysfunction	Gross: slight weakness noticeable on close inspection; may have very slight synkinesis
		
		At rest: normal symmetry and tone
		
		Motion
		
		    Forehead: moderate to good function
		
		    Eye: complete closure with minimum effort
		
		    Mouth: slight asymmetry

III	Moderate dysfunction	Gross: obvious but not disfiguring difference between two sides; noticeable but not severe synkinesis, contracture, and/or hemifacial spasm
		
		At rest: normal symmetry and tone
		
		Motion
		
		    Forehead: slight to moderate movement
		
		    Eye: complete closure with effort
		
		    Mouth: slightly weak with maximum effort

IV	Moderately severe dysfunction	Gross: obvious weakness and/or disfiguring asymmetry
		At rest: normal symmetry and tone
		Motion
		    Forehead: none
		
		    Eye: incomplete closure
		
		    Mouth: asymmetry with maximum effort

V	Severe dysfunction	Gross: only barely perceptible motion
		At rest: asymmetry
		Motion
		    Forehead: none
		
		    Eye: incomplete closure
		
		    Mouth: slight movement

VI	Total paralysis	No movement

House JW, Brackmann DE. Facial nerve grading system. *Otolaryngol Head Neck Surg.* 1985;93(2):146–147. Reprinted by permission of SAGE Publications.

Second-degree injury, or axonotmesis, occurs when trauma leads to obstruction of vascular flow and subsequent ischemia and breakdown of axons. If trauma is relieved, recovery requires axons to regenerate. Duration of recovery, thus, is longer and may take weeks to months. Endoneural tubes are intact and no crossover to other axons is expected.

Table 3-2. Sunderland Classification of Peripheral Nerve Injuries			
Injury	**Histologic Findings**	**Physiologic Injury**	**Potential for Recovery**
First degree	Neurapraxia	Increased intraneural pressure	Complete recovery
Second degree	Axonotmesis	Increased intraneural pressure and nerve ischemia	Good to complete recovery
Third degree	Neurotmesis	Loss of endoneural tubes	Incomplete recovery, synkinesis
Fourth degree	Partial transection	Disruption of endoneural tubes and perineurium	Poor recovery, synkinesis
Fifth degree	Complete transection	Disruption of entire nerve	None

Adapted from Sunderland S. A classification of peripheral nerve injuries producing loss of function. *Brain.* 1951;74:491–516

Usually the typical pathologic processes that occur with Bell palsy or herpes zoster oticus are limited to first- or second-order injuries, and satisfactory recovery occurs in these individuals.

With third-degree injury, or neurotmesis, pressure is of enough severity or duration that endoneural sheaths are disrupted. Spontaneous recovery often is incomplete, and synkinesis is expected as regenerating axons may cross.

Fourth- or fifth-degree injury occurs when partial or complete transaction occurs, most often from external trauma. Fourth-degree injury occurs when partial disruption of the nerve occurs. In addition to disruption of the endoneurium, perineural disruption also occurs. The only structure holding the nerve together is epineurium. Recovery potential is poor. Fifth-degree injury occurs when the nerve is completely disrupted. No spontaneous recovery will occur.

DIAGNOSTIC TESTING

Because of the proximity of the seventh and eighth cranial nerves in the posterior fossa, pure tone and speech audiometry is recommended in all cases of facial paralysis. Radiographic imaging assists in delineating the site of lesion along the facial nerve. Computed tomography (CT) is best to assess temporal bone trauma, cholesteatoma, and otitis media. Magnetic resonance imaging helps to assess when tumors or infections are suspected.

When other, less common causes of facial paralysis are suspected, laboratory studies to evaluate for Lyme disease and autoimmune disorders should be considered.

Electrophysiologic tests are useful in establishing the prognosis of facial nerve recovery. Tests are complementary and are indicated when complete paralysis is present. They do not have a role in clinically evident partial paresis because recovery is expectant. Electromyography (EMG) records spontaneous, evoked, and voluntary electrical responses of motor end plates. In the acute setting, presence of voluntary active motor units indicates intact nerve with incomplete injury. In a denervated muscle, spontaneous involuntary contractions appear as fibrillation potentials. These require 14 to 21 days to develop after facial nerve injury, thus limiting the role of EMG until this period when voluntary active potentials are absent. With recovery or regeneration, return of neural activity may be predicted by presence of polyphasic potentials, which may be present even though clinically evident facial motion is absent.

Other current clinically relevant tests to assess prognosis for return of function are nerve excitability test (NET), maximal stimulation test (MST), and electroneuronography (ENoG). These 3 tests may be performed 3 days after the onset of paralysis after wallerian degeneration has occurred. Even a completely transected nerve will conduct distally stimulated impulses for 48 to 72 hours. Thus, these tests have limited applicability during the first 3 days. Nerve excitability test is used to measure the current threshold for a barely perceivable facial motor response. The paralyzed side is compared with the unaffected side. Differences of greater than 3.5 mA are considered significant and indicative of nerve fiber degeneration and potential incomplete recovery. In MST, facial muscle contraction is elicited with the highest electrical current that the patient can tolerate. The response is expressed as the difference between the normal and paralyzed side and graded as minimal, moderate, severe, or no response.

Electroneuronography or evoked EMG is the recording of compound action potentials from the facial musculature in response to transcutaneous electrical stimulation of the facial nerve at the level of the stylomastoid foramen. Responses are compared from the 2 sides. The percentage response compared with the unaffected side is proportional to the degree of degeneration. Surgical decompression is recommended in patients who have greater than 90% degeneration because of the high likelihood that recovery will be incomplete with medical management alone in these cases. The advantage of ENoG over NET or

MST is that the response is quantitated and less dependent on the subjective observation of the tester in visualizing responses.

■ Differential Diagnoses

Presentation and etiology of facial paralysis is variable (Table 3-3). Clinical management of paralyses is determined based on etiology and predicted clinical recovery. Regardless of the cause, one important aspect of facial paralysis is eye care because the most common and significant complication of facial paralysis is corneal desiccation. Parent education of the importance of eye moisturization is essential. Treatment measures include ophthalmic lubricants, eyelid taping at night, and use of moisture chambers. Long-term surgical options are gold weights, canthoplasties, and eyelid springs.

BELL PALSY

Bell palsy is the most common etiology and is defined as spontaneous facial paralysis without other disease or injury that may account for the paralysis. The physician must be careful not to quickly diagnose Bell palsy. Bell palsy is a diagnosis of exclusion once other possible etiologies have been considered and ruled out.

This condition may affect all ages, with peak incidence between the ages of 20 and 40 years. The annual incidence is between 30 to 45 per 100,000. Family history of Bell palsy exists in 8% of patients.

Typical presentation is sudden onset or gradually progressive over a 24- to 48-hour period. Approximately 20% of individuals report ipsilateral ear pain or numbness preceding paralysis. Approximately 30% present with only a paresis and of these, full recovery is expected. The remaining 70% develop complete paralysis. In one of the largest series, including those who did not receive specific therapy, 85% of patients began to recover within 3 weeks of onset. The remaining 15% demonstrated partial recovery within 3 to 6 months. Approximately 71% had normal facial function, 13% had minor sequelae, and 16% had diminished function.

Although the cause of Bell palsy is considered unknown, edema of the facial nerve is thought to be the underlying factor. The swelling leads to progressive neural ischemia and subsequent further edema. Some evidence exists that an underlying factor is viral in origin as 30% to 50% of patients report a viral prodrome. In addition, samples of endoneural fluid showed evidence of herpes simplex virus in patients who had decompression surgery for Bell palsy.

Table 3-3. Differential Diagnoses of Facial Paralysis

Infectious
- Bell palsy
- Acute/chronic otitis media or mastoiditis
- Herpes zoster oticus
- Lyme disease
- AIDS

Trauma
- Birth trauma
- Temporal bone fractures
- Penetrating trauma
- Surgical injury

Congenital
- Möbius syndrome
- CULLP
- Oculoauriculovertebral syndrome

Tumors
- Cholesteatoma
- Facial neuroma
- Schwannoma
- Parotid tumors
- Malignancy: carcinoma, sarcoma

Autoimmune
- Guillain-Barré syndrome
- Sarcoidosis

Idiopathic
- Melkersson-Rosenthal syndrome

Abbreviation: CULLP, congenital unilateral lower lip palsy.

Medical management of Bell palsy includes the use of corticosteroids. The rationale is reduction of inflammation on the facial nerve. Meta-analysis, primarily based on adult literature, has demonstrated the benefit of steroid therapy. Recent *Cochrane Reviews* also support the use of steroids to increase frequency of complete recovery. Acyclovir use may also benefit in reduction of less satisfactory outcomes if treatment is initiated within 3 days of onset.

A recent randomized, double-blind, placebo-controlled study has supported the use of prednisolone compared with a placebo group as well as one that received acyclovir. Surgical management for Bell palsy is indicated in individuals who present with complete paralysis and ENoG testing that shows greater than 90% degeneration. Decompression involves a middle fossa approach to decompress the labyrinthine segment. Evidence to support decompression is based on patients who presented within 14 days of onset. Those who had surgical decompression achieved House-Brackman grade I or II in 91% of cases, while those who opted for medical treatment were 41%. There was no difference if decompression was performed after 14 days.

OTITIS MEDIA

Facial palsy can occur secondary to acute otitis media and mastoiditis. Palsy is secondary to inflammation and neural edema along the course of the nerve. Incidence with acute otitis media is approximately 1 in 20,000 cases.

Treatment involves myringotomy with or without a tympanostomy tube, culture of middle ear fluid, and antibiotics. Prognosis is excellent and recovery of facial function is rapid as underlying inflammation is resolved.

Facial paralysis with chronic otitis media and cholesteatoma has a more guarded outcome and requires more extensive surgery than myringotomy alone. Temporal bone CT is recommended to evaluate the extent of involvement and assess for other intratemporal complications. Surgery consists of tympanomastoidectomy to remove granulation or cholesteatoma that may be contributing to inflammation or erosion of the facial nerve. Prognosis is good as long as the onset of paralysis is rapid and diagnosis and treatment are prompt.

HERPES ZOSTER OTICUS (RAMSAY HUNT SYNDROME)

Incidence is approximately 5 cases per 100,000 annually. This is one-tenth of Bell palsy, with increase in age. The condition is secondary to a latent varicella zoster infection involving the seventh nerve ganglia. Reactivation of the infection results in facial paralysis, severe otalgia, and vesicular lesions in the skin of the external auditory canal and concha. Some patients also experience sensorineural hearing loss and vertigo.

Prognosis of Ramsay Hunt syndrome is worse than Bell palsy, with patients more likely having complete clinical paralysis, complete electrical denervation, and incomplete recovery with synkinesis occurring as a late complication. Treatment consists of antivirals (acyclovir or valacyclovir) and steroid therapy.

LYME DISEASE

This multisystem inflammatory illness is caused by tick-borne spirochete *Borrelia burgdorferi*. The infection is categorized as early localized, early disseminated, or late. Erythema migrans, the early localized presentation, is a painless, reddish lesion with concentric circles with a white center zone. Early disseminated disease occurs when the spirochete spreads hematogenously; neurologic symptoms include cranial neuropathy such as facial paralysis. Late Lyme disease manifests as polyarthralgia, arthritis, or polyneuritis.

Diagnosis is made based on enzyme-linked immunosorbent assay and Western blot techniques. Careful interpretation is necessary as a negative result can occur with disease when immunoglobulin M has not had a chance to develop. Positive test results may also reflect prior exposure but be unrelated to the patient's current complaints. Treatment is based on appropriate antibiotic therapy. Prognosis of facial palsy is excellent with permanent dysfunction in 11% of children.

MELKERSSON-ROSENTHAL SYNDROME

Facial paralysis is recurrent and associated with recurrent facial edema and fissured tongue. This condition typically begins during the second decade of life. Facial swelling may vary in degree from ipsilateral isolated lip swelling to bilateral complete edema. Biopsy of the lip reveals noncaseating epithelioid cell granuloma with surrounding histiocytes, plasma cells, and lymphocytes. Etiology of the syndrome is unknown.

KAWASAKI DISEASE

This multisystem condition may involve mucous membranes, skin, coronary arteries, and skin and lymph nodes. One of the neurologic sequelae is facial paralysis. Median age is 13 months. Prognosis of the palsy is good, as it usually resolved in fewer than 3 months.

TRAUMA

The facial nerve is vulnerable from various mechanisms of trauma, including blunt trauma to the facial nerve from temporal bone fractures. The most common mechanisms of pediatric fractures are motor vehicle crashes and falls.

Initial physical examination is important in establishing prognosis, although this may be limited if the child has other injuries and critical care issues prevent evaluation of function. If only a paresis is present, prognosis is excellent without any surgical intervention. In addition, delayed onset facial paralysis also has good recovery of function.

If initial complete paralysis is present, high-resolution temporal bone CT (Figure 3-1) along with electrophysiologic testing is essential to determine prognosis and need for surgical intervention.

Classically, temporal bone fractures are classified as longitudinal or transverse, relative to the axis of the petrous bone. Longitudinal fractures have been associated with facial nerve injury in 20% of

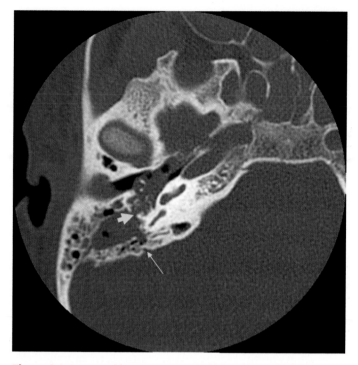

Figure 3-1. Temporal bone computed tomography of fracture through the facial nerve resulting in transection of the nerve. Large arrow depicts fracture through the nerve. Small arrow depicts fracture line.

cases, while transverse fractures may result in damage in 50% of cases. Newer classification schemes have been proposed to help predict the likelihood of facial nerve and inner ear injury with temporal bone fractures. This scheme, otic capsule sparing and violating, may be more predictive of facial nerve injury.

Penetrating trauma with complete facial paralysis should be repaired as soon as the child is medically stable and other potential vascular injuries have been evaluated. This injury typically necessitates end-to-end anastomosis or cable grafting. Early repair within 3 days of injury also allows for distal stimulation of the nerve, which assists in nerve identification because the anatomy is often distorted from penetrating trauma. If facial nerve injury is medial to the lateral canthus, it should be observed, as multiple cross innervation from other nerve fibers are present.

Trauma may also occur iatrogenically during ear or parotid gland surgery. The frequency of facial nerve injury during otologic surgery has been reported to range from 0.6% to 3.6%. The most common site of injury is near the second genu at the tympanic segment. When facial nerve injury is suspected during surgery, site of the injury should be explored and electrically stimulated to verify nerve integrity. Decompression proximal and distal to the injury should be performed. If more than 50% of the circumference of the nerve has been disrupted, the nerve should be repaired.

If facial paralysis is noted after surgery, ear packing should be removed and facial function reassessed after a short period of observation. Incomplete and delayed paralysis indicate that facial nerve integrity is maintained and has a good prognosis. Systemic steroids should be started. If complete facial paralysis is present immediately after surgery, prognosis is worse; surgical exploration is warranted.

Repair of facial nerve trauma depends on the extent of injury; when less than 50% of the diameter of the nerve is involved, the nerve should be decompressed proximal and distal to the site. In more extensive injury, the nerve may be anastomosed without tension. When the extent of injury involves a section of nerve and the nerves cannot be anastomosed without tension, nerve grafting is used. Donor nerves include greater auricular, sural, or median antebrachial cutaneous nerves.

TUMORS

Neoplastic lesions may present as facial paralysis. Factors that suggest a mass lesion and warranting further radiographic imaging are slowly progressive facial paralysis, unilateral middle ear effusion, multiple cranial neuropathies, recurrent paralysis, parotid tumor, cutaneous malignancy, or ipsilateral hearing loss.

Tumors causing facial paralysis in children are rare. Tumors may be benign or malignant, but the most common cause is facial schwannoma. The tumor may occur anywhere along the course of the facial nerve. Malignant tumors that may cause facial paralysis include leukemia, rhabdomyosarcoma, and neuroblastoma.

NEONATAL FACIAL PARALYSIS

The incidence ranges from 0.05% to 0.23%. A key differentiating category is to identify the paralysis as congenital or trauma. Traumatic palsy occurs secondary to intrauterine positioning or injury during delivery.

The distinction of traumatic or congenital palsy can usually be made with history and physical examination. Trauma is usually associated with prolonged or difficult delivery with potential forceps use.

Physical examination may also demonstrate hemotympanum or facial or periauricular ecchymoses. No cases of nerve transection have ever been reported from birth trauma. Congenital facial paralysis is often associated with other facial anomalies such as maxillary defects or auricular anomalies. Other cranial nerve deficits or dysmorphic features of the chest, limbs, and cardiovascular or genitourinary systems may also be presenting findings. Möbius syndrome is a rare condition that is associated with unilateral or bilateral palsy, often sparing the lower half of the face. Abducens palsy often is also present. The cause of the syndrome is unknown, with potential explanations as agenesis of facial musculature or the facial nucleus. Hemifacial microsomia or oculoauriculovertebral syndrome is estimated to occur in 1 in 5,600 live births and has a variable presentation of ocular, auricular, mandibular, and facial nerve anomalies. Facial weakness can occur in approximately 20% to 25% of these children. Congenital unilateral lower lip palsy is apparent on physical examination as the baby is unable to depress the lower lip with crying. The incidence is not uncommon, occurring in 1 in 120 to 160 newborns. The condition may be associated with ear anomalies and congenital cardiac defects in 10% of children.

While the history and physical examination may help differentiate between traumatic and congenital causes, in ambiguous cases, CT of the temporal bone is warranted. Electrophysiologic studies also may help to clarify etiologies. Electroneuronography testing is abnormal at birth in those with congenital paralysis; however, they are typically normal within the first 3 days in those secondary to trauma.

Prognosis for recovery with traumatic facial paralysis is excellent, with greater than 90% of cases with spontaneous return of function. Because of this expectant outcome with traumatic paralysis, surgery is reserved for those who have evidence of electrophysiologic dysfunction, temporal bone fracture on CT, and no evidence of recovery for at least 5 weeks.

Unlike traumatic neonatal paralysis, those associated with developmental causes are unlikely to spontaneously resolve. Surgical exploration is not indicated because the nerve generally tapers to thin fibers that preclude decompression or grafting.

CHRONIC FACIAL PARALYSIS

For children with long-standing paralysis (greater than 1 year) despite medical treatment and no physical or electrophysiologic evidence of recovery may be candidates for reparative reanimation surgery. Types of surgery depend on status of the facial musculature and age of the child and his or her development. Repair includes nerve transposition, muscular slings, and microneurovascular free muscle grafts. These repairs are usually deferred until the child's facial growth is complete.

■ Conclusion

- Pediatric facial paralysis is a challenge to physicians to assess etiology and determine those cases that may require surgical intervention.
- All cases require thorough history and physical examination to determine prognosis.
- Bell palsy is the most common cause of facial paralysis, but other etiologies must be ruled out prior to this diagnosis.
- Appropriate and early referral to an otolaryngologist is warranted for the evaluation of pediatric facial paralysis.

■ Selected References

Adour KK. The true nature of Bell's palsy: analysis of 1,000 consecutive patients. *Laryngoscope.* 1978;88(5):787–801

Adour KK. Otological complication of herpes zoster. *Ann Neurol.* 1994;35(Suppl): S62–S64

Adour KK, Ruboyianes JM, Von Doersten PG, et al. Bell's palsy treatment with acyclovir and prednisone compared with prednisone alone: a double-blind, randomized, controlled trial. *Ann Otol Rhinol Laryngol.* 1996;105(5):371–378

Barrs DM. Facial nerve trauma: optimal timing for repair. *Laryngoscope.* 1991;101(8): 835–848

Bergman I, May M, Wessel HB, Stool SE. Management of facial palsy caused by birth trauma. *Laryngoscope.* 1986;94(4):381–384

Brodie HA, Thompson TC. Management of complications from 820 temporal bone fractures. *Am J Otol.* 1997;18(2):188–197

Ellefsen B, Bonding P. Facial palsy in acute otitis media. *Clin Otolaryngol Allied Sci.* 1996;21(5):393–395

Fisch U. Surgery for Bell's palsy. *Arch Otolaryngol.* 1981;107(1):1–11

Gallagher PG. Facial nerve paralysis and Kawasaki disease. *Rev Infect Dis.* 1990;12(3): 403–405

Gantz BJ, Rubinstein JT, Gidley P, Woodworth GG. Surgical management of Bell's palsy. *Laryngoscope.* 1999;109(8):1177–1188

Gorlin RJ, Cohen MM, Levin LS. *Syndromes of the Head and Neck.* 3rd ed. New York, NY: Oxford University Press Inc; 1990:641–652

Green JD Jr, Shelton C, Brackmann DE. Iatrogenic facial nerve injury during otologic surgery. *Laryngoscope.* 1994;104(8 Pt 1):922–926

Greene RM, Rogers RS. Melkersson-Rosenthal syndrome: a review of 36 patients. *J Am Acad Dermatol.* 1989;21:1263–1270

House JW, Brackmann DE. Facial nerve grading system. *Otolaryngol Head Neck Surg.* 1985;93(2):146–147

Ishman SL, Friedland DR. Temporal bone fractures: traditional classification and clinical relevance. *Laryngoscope.* 2004;114(10):1734–1741

Lee D, Honrado C, Har-El G, Goldsmith A. Pediatric temporal bone fractures. *Laryngoscope.* 1998;108(6):816–821

Little SC, Kesser BW. Radiographic classification of temporal bone fractures: clinical predictability using a new system. *Arch Otolaryngol Head Neck Surg.* 2006;132(12): 1300–1304

May M, Fria TJ, Blumenthal F, Curtin H. Facial paralysis in children: differential diagnosis. *Otolaryngol Head Neck Surg.* 1981;89(5):841–848

McHugh HE, Sowden KA, Levitt MN. Facial paralysis and muscle agenesis in the newborn. *Arch Otolaryngol.* 1969;89(1):131–143

Murakami S, Mizobuchi M, Nakashiro Y, Doi T, Hato N, Yanagihara N. Bell palsy and herpes simplex virus: identification of viral DNA in endoneurial fluid and muscle. *Ann Intern Med.* 1996;124(1 Pt 1):27–30

Peitersen E. Bell's palsy: the spontaneous course of 2,500 peripheral facial nerve palsies of different etiologies. *Acta Otolaryngol Suppl.* 2002;549:4–30

Pitts DB, Adour KK, Hilsinger RL Jr. Recurrent Bell's palsy: analysis of 140 patients. *Laryngoscope.* 1988;98(5):535–540

Ramsey MJ, DerSimonian R, Holtel MR, Burgess LP. Corticosteroid treatment for idiopathic facial nerve paralysis: a meta-analysis. *Laryngoscope.* 2000;110(3 Pt 1):335–341

Robillard RB, Hilsinger RL Jr, Adour KK. Ramsay Hunt facial paralysis: clinical analyses of 185 patients. *Otolaryngol Head Neck Surg.* 1986;95(3 Pt 1):292–297

Salinas RA, Alvarez G, Daly F, Ferreira J. Corticosteroids for Bell's palsy (idiopathic facial paralysis). *Cochrane Database Syst Rev.* 2010;3:CD001942

Skogman BH, Croner S, Nordwall M, Eknefelt M, Ernerudh J, Forsberg P. Lyme neuroborreliosis in children: a prospective study of clinical features, prognosis and outcome. *Pediatr Infect Dis J.* 2008;27(12):1089–1094

Sullivan FM, Swan IR, Donnan PT, et al. Early treatment with prednisolone or acyclovir in Bell's palsy. *N Eng J Med.* 2007;357(16):1598–1607

Sunderland S. *Nerve and Nerve Injuries.* 2nd ed. London, England: Churchill Livingstone; 1978:88–89, 96–97, 133

Wiet RJ. Iatrogenic facial paralysis. *Otlaryngol Clin North Am.* 1982;15(4):773–780

CHAPTER 4

Diseases and Anomalies of the Auricle and External Auditory Canal

Robert F. Yellon, MD, and Raymond Maguire, DO

Auricle	External Auditory Canal
Congenital	Congenital
Traumatic Lesions	Traumatic
Infectious	Infectious
Inflammatory	Acute Otitis Externa
	Inflammatory
	Neoplastic
	Other

■ Auricle

CONGENITAL

Prominent Ears

Having prominent ears may negatively affect a child's self-image because the child looks different and may be teased by peers. This can lead to poor development of interpersonal relationships, social withdrawal, and even depression. For minor degrees of deformity, no intervention may be needed. For severe degrees of congenital deformity (or birth defect), otoplasty or surgical correction (Figure 4-1) is warranted in children who are not at undue risk of anesthesia and surgery. The auricle is 85% of adult size by the time a child is 4 years old; therefore, otoplasty can be considered then. The procedure is not very painful or risky and generally yields good results, although occasionally, revision surgery is needed. Unfortunately, medical insurance companies frequently consider otoplasty to be a cosmetic procedure and will not provide payment for the operation.

Microtia and Congenital Aural Atresia

Microtia means small ear. The extreme case is anotia, or no ear. Microtia is usually, but not always, associated with congenital aural atresia, which is absence of the ear canal and tympanic membrane (TM). In contrast with otoplasty for prominent ears, with a normal ear canal and TM, surgery for microtia and atresia is usually covered by insurance companies because microtia and atresia are associated with

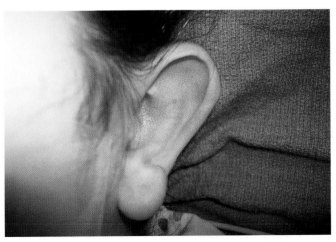

Figure 4-1. Prominent auricle. This congenital anomaly is severe enough to warrant surgical correction.

hearing loss. Grade 1 microtia is a slightly small or malformed ear. Often there is no surgery required since the malformation is mild. Grade 2 microtia (Figure 4-2) is a significant congenital ear deformity usually consisting of absence of most of the superior half of the auricle, often with a small folded-over "lop ear." Grade 3 microtia (Figure 4-3) is a severe auricular deformity with the presence of only a lobule and a small sausage-shaped auricular remnant. Grade 2 and 3 microtia and anotia usually carry significant associated hearing loss due to ear canal stenosis or atresia and cosmetic deficits. The nerve hearing function is usually normal, but in the absence of an ear canal and TM, there is a maximal conductive hearing loss. This maximal conductive hearing loss is 60 dB and is a significant handicapping loss, especially when bilateral. When unilateral, it is often associated with oculoauriculovertebral dysplasia (hemifacial microsomia, Goldenhar syndrome). Ophthalmologic, cervical spine, and cardiac evaluations are required to rule out commonly associated congenital problems. When bilateral, the defect is often associated with Treacher Collins or Nager syndrome. Airway and feeding problems are common in patients with microtia and mandibular hypoplasia.

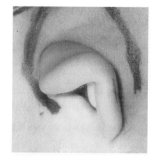

Figure 4-2. Grade 2 microtia. The inferior portion of the auricle is well formed but the superior portion is deficient and folded over. This patient also has a stenotic external auditory canal.

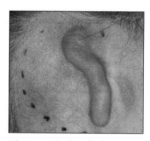

Figure 4-3. Grade 3 microtia with congenital aural atresia. This patient has the cosmetic deformity of absence of the auricle except for a lobule and very small rudimentary auricular remnant. The associated congenital aural atresia results in a handicapping 60-dB conductive hearing loss.

Once airway, feeding, and cardiac problems have been addressed or ruled out, the patient should be referred to an otolaryngologist skilled in the evaluation and treatment of microtia and aural atresia. Early evaluation of patients with severe microtia focuses on determining hearing levels with otoacoustic emission testing and auditory brain stem response testing. Early hearing rehabilitation is accomplished with a strap-on hearing aid known as the bone-anchored hearing aid (BAHA) Soft Band. Patients who have bilateral microtia are referred for speech and language therapy.

A temporal bone computed tomography (CT) scan is obtained to determine whether the patient has sufficient anatomic structures to be a future candidate for surgical opening of the ear canal (aural atresiaplasty). If there are insufficient anatomic structures for atresiaplasty, a BAHA may be implanted into the skull when the child reaches 5 years of age, which will significantly improve hearing. If the CT scan of the temporal bones indicates favorable anatomy, the child is a candidate for surgical aural atresiaplasty, which is opening the ear canal for hearing (Figure 4-4). This is an advanced surgical procedure performed only by a few surgeons. Another option is surgical implantation of the BAHA, which is a transcutaneous titanium osseointegrated implant that allows a clip-on hearing aid to be placed for hearing restoration (Figure 4-5). The decision of BAHA versus atresiaplasty is made on a case-by-case basis, depending on anatomy, medical comorbidities, and family wishes. Conventional hearing aids and special bone conduction hearing aids with a metal headband are also options for some patients. Of course, a child with unilateral atresia and hearing loss has much less urgency for surgical rehabilitation than a child with bilateral aural atresia.

The second significant issue for a child who has microtia is the cosmetic absence of the auricle. An acceptable auricle may be provided in several ways. The simplest method is use of a glued on prosthetic auricle that has the advantage of no surgery but may be easily dislodged during play, which can be embarrassing. A second method is surgical placement of 2 BAHA osseointegrated implants in the area of the microtia

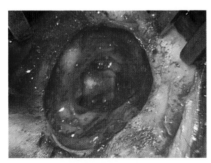

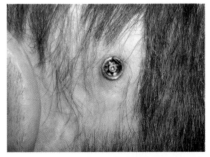

Figure 4-4. Surgery for congenital aural atresia. This patient has had surgical opening of the absent external auditory canal. The malleus-incus complex (center) has been freed for hearing reconstruction.

Figure 4-5. Bone-anchored hearing aid (BAHA). This child with Treacher Collins syndrome has bilateral microtia and congenital aural atresia. The BAHA titanium osseointegrated transcutaneous implant is seen here. The special hearing aid is clipped on to the implant.

to be used as anchors for a clip-on prosthetic auricle that is more secure. A third option is staged surgical reconstruction with rib grafts (Figure 4-6), which provides a permanently attached secure auricle (Figure 4-7). However, there are risks of surgery and the operation is usually performed in several stages. A final option is surgical implantation of a prefabricated synthetic auricle that is covered with a temporal local flap and skin grafts. Again the decision for or against each of these options depends on the individual patient's anatomy, medical comorbidities, family, and surgeon's preference.

External Auditory Canal Stenosis

Another variation of congenital ear anomalies is external auditory canal stenosis or the presence of very narrow ear canal. Mild cases can usually be managed by an otolaryngologist but may require cleaning of the ear with a microscope under general anesthesia to avoid unnecessary and potentially dangerous trauma to the ear canal and TM. Some ear canals are so narrow that surgical reconstruction will be required for improved hearing, for adequate examination, and to prevent constant impaction of cerumen and desquamated epithelium. Referral to an experienced otologic surgeon is required.

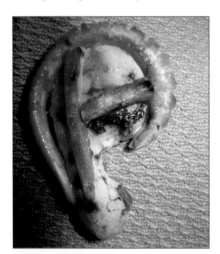

Figure 4-6. Rib cartilage graft for microtia reconstruction. Ribs were harvested and sculpted into this cartilaginous auricle, which was implanted under the scalp in the first stage of the multistage auricular reconstruction.

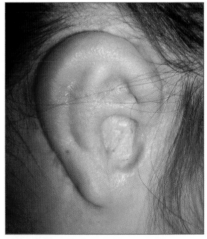

Figure 4-7. Final result of 4-stage auricular reconstruction with rib cartilage for grade 3 microtia. The patient had insufficient anatomic structures to allow congenital aural atresia reconstruction.

TRAUMATIC LESIONS

Lacerations

Minor lacerations of the auricle may be repaired by any competent surgeon. However, more severe injuries should be referred to an experienced auricular surgeon. Whenever cartilage is exposed, prophylactic antimicrobial agents that cover *Staphylococcus aureus* and *Pseudomonas aeruginosa* should be administered. Torn cartilage, missing portions of the auricle, and avulsed auricles should be attended to by experienced surgeons to ensure the best outcomes.

Auricular Hematoma

Trauma to the auricle may avulse the skin from the cartilage, and hematomas may form in the resultant space. If left untreated, several problems may occur. The hematoma may be replaced by scar, and a cosmetic deformity known as cauliflower ear may result. In this condition a raised scar fills the hematoma site and the auricle is permanently deformed; thickened portions may resemble a cauliflower.

An untreated hematoma may also become infected, and cartilage reabsorption of the auricle may result in significant auricular deformity. The treatment of auricular hematoma is initial needle aspiration or incision and drainage of the blood, followed by placement of sterile dental rolls or gauze packing over the area that is fixed with sutures for 3 to 5 days. The dental rolls act as a bolster or packing that holds the avulsed skin in close proximity to the underlying cartilage. This prevents the reaccumulation of blood or serous fluid and recurrence of the lesion. Culture and sensitivity studies are sent and prophylactic antibiotics are administered. Several weeks are required for healing and prevention of recurrence. A problem with auricular hematomas is that they often reoccur in wrestlers and boxers who often resume the sport shortly after the injury.

INFECTIOUS

Perichondritis and Chondritis

Trauma and infection of the auricle may be accidental or caused by piercing with non-sterile equipment. It may also follow piercing with poor hygiene during the healing period. Traumatic auricular hematomas and seromas may become infected and lead to perichondritis and chondritis. Perichondritis implies infection limited to the perichondrium, while chondritis implies deeper infection of the cartilage and is often associated with permanent auricular deformity. *S aureus* and *P aeruginosa* are often involved; antimicrobial treatment should cover these pathogens. Intravenous antimicrobials are required for severe cases. The auricle is erythematous, edematous, indurated, and exquisitely tender. If there is abscess or seroma formation, needle aspiration or incision and drainage may be required, followed by placement of antibiotic-impregnated cotton or gauze, and a gentle mastoid-type pressure dressing is applied to prevent reaccumulation. Culture and sensitivity studies are sent. The ear must be examined regularly and the dressing changed frequently to check for improvement and avoid complications.

INFLAMMATORY

Relapsing Polychondritis

Relapsing polychondritis is a multisystem disease targeting cartilage and connective tissue. Autoantibodies against type 2 collagen are implicated in this disease, which may affect elastic cartilage of the ear, hyaline cartilage of the peripheral joints, and fibrocartilage of the spine. Symptoms of this disease begin with pain, erythema, and swelling of the auricle sparing the lobule, followed by joint pain. Tracheal cartilage involvement is the most serious manifestation of relapsing polychondritis, affecting 20% to 50% of patients resulting in cartilage disintegration and increased morbidity due to airway obstruction. Mild episodes of polychondritis are managed with nonsteroidal anti-inflammatory medications. More serve occurrences are treated with prednisone, 1 mg/kg, with a taper after clinical improvement is observed. Other therapies include administration of immunosuppressive medications such as methotrexate, dapsone, or cyclosporine for more aggressive disease.

Wegener Granulomatosis

Wegener granulomatosis with primary involvement of the auricle is rare and presents with similar clinical findings as relapsing polychondritis, with the exception that the lobule may be involved with inflammation. The diagnosis requires a clinical history with findings of nasal, pulmonary, or renal involvement and serology results positive for centrally accentuated antineutrophil cytoplasmic antibody. Tissue biopsies may be indicated to confirm the diagnosis and are usually obtained from the nasal disease. Otologic involvement may result in otitis media with effusion secondary to eustachian tube obstruction in the nasopharynx. Primary involvement of the middle-ear mucosa with necrotizing granulomas may result in chronic otitis media. Also, sensorineural hearing loss and vertigo may present secondary to involvement of the disease, affecting cochlear and vestibular blood vessels. Early treatment includes trimethoprim-sulfamethoxazole, with more extensive disease requiring immunosuppressive treatments such as corticosteroids, methotrexate, or cyclophosphamide. Side effects of cyclophosphamide include cystitis, myelodysplasia, infections, and infertility; therefore, this medication should be reserved for the most severe cases and should be used with caution.

Allergic Reactions

Allergic reactions of the auricle are common in susceptible patients from nickel-rimmed eyeglasses or earrings. Only the portion of the ear in direct contact with the implicated material is involved in the reaction. Treatment involves removal of the causative material and local treatment in the form of mild steroid creams.

Insect Bites

Insect bites may cause an inflammatory reaction of the auricle that may at first appear to be suspicious for relapsing polychondritis. Careful examination of the skin needs to be performed to search for any signs of cutaneous puncture indicating a possible insect bite. Most insect bites heal well with local treatments, including cold compresses, and do not require any medical intervention. Certain insect bites may be more serious, such as brown recluse spider bites, where the venom may cause tissue necrosis requiring debridement. If the causative insect can be captured it should be placed in a closed, clear container and brought in for proper identification.

■ External Auditory Canal

CONGENITAL

First Branchial Cleft Anomalies

Cystic or firm lesions that occur around the area of the lobule may represent first branchial cleft anomalies. They may remain unchanged, grow slowly, or become acutely or recurrently infected. Treatment of infections includes antimicrobial agents, but needle aspiration or incision and drainage may be required for nonresponsive lesions or large abscesses. Computed tomography or magnetic resonance imaging may show a cystic or infected structure with surrounding inflammatory changes. Deep extension and recurrent infections suggest first branchial cleft anomalies. Surgical excision is warranted for large lesions or recurrent infections. There are 2 types of lesions. A Work type 1 first branchial cleft anomaly contains only ectoderm. It is considered to be a duplication of the external auditory canal and it may have an opening into the external auditory canal. A Work type 2 branchial cleft anomaly contains ectoderm and mesoderm (often cartilage) (Figure 4-8). For both anomalies, there may be a deep extension that requires excision for definitive treatment of the lesion. The interesting and challenging part is that the deep extension or tract of these lesions may be juxtaposed with the bifurcation or trunk of the facial nerve. Thus, proper technique requires facial monitoring, nerve dissection, and preservation before resection of the deep portion of the lesions (Figure 4-9).

Preauricular Sinuses and Cysts

Embryologically, the auricle is derived from the first and second branchial arches. Failure of union of the remnants of the first and second arches results in the formation of preauricular cysts and sinuses. The 6 hillocks of His fuse to form the auricle. Failure of fusion of the first and second hillocks near the root of the helix results in a closed cyst or a sinus with an opening to the skin.

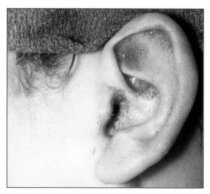 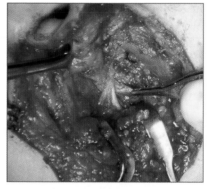

Figure 4-8. First branchial cleft cyst. Note that the cystic structure is just below the lobule, which should alert the clinician to the possibility of a first branchial cleft anomaly.

Figure 4-9. Deep portion of first branchial cleft cyst. The bifurcation of the facial nerve is found to be immediately lateral and juxtaposed to the deep portion of the first branchial cleft anomaly. To avoid nerve injury, facial nerve dissection and preservation are required prior to safe removal of the deep portion of this anomaly.

Preauricular cysts and sinuses may remain asymptomatic and require no treatment. Alternatively, they may drain, be painful, or be a site of recurrent infection (Figure 4-10). Infections may be managed with antimicrobial agents, needle aspiration, or incision and drainage as needed, depending on response to therapy and severity. Recurrent infections, constant drainage, or persistent enlargement of the lesion are indications for referral for surgical excision.

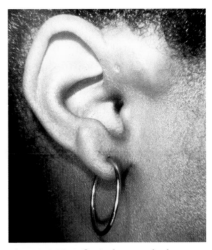

Figure 4-10. Infected preauricular sinus. Note the pit of the preauricular sinus anterior to the root of the helix. The swelling and erythema are caused by infection of the sinus.

Branchio-oto-renal Syndrome

Branchio-oto-renal (Melnick-Fraser) syndrome is an autosomal-dominant genetic syndrome with a phenotype of bilateral preauricular sinuses, bilateral branchial cleft anomalies in the neck, and renal dysplasia. There may be associated microtia, aural atresia, and sensorineural or conductive hearing loss. The kidneys may be normal, dysplastic, or absent. Otologic evaluation, hearing tests, and renal studies are indicated for such patients and for affected family members. Genetic testing and consultation are advised.

TRAUMATIC

Foreign Bodies

Foreign bodies of the external auditory canal may be inert (beads), organic (peas), or biological (insects). Patients with foreign bodies of the external auditory canal must be evaluated for changes in their hearing, vertigo, and facial paralysis. Inert, organic, and biological foreign bodies of the ear canal are often removed in the office with careful restraint of the patient using instruments such as curettes, alligator forceps, right-angle hooks, and suction. Care is taken to avoid traumatizing the surrounding skin to avoid tissue edema, which may complicate foreign body removal. Bracing of hands on the child's head while the child is restrained is required to safely control the instruments (see

"Cerumen Impaction" on page 102). The use of saline irrigation to flush out foreign bodies is discouraged because the status of the TM is often unknown, and if a perforation is present, it may result in further injury or infection. Otologic drops are contraindicated in cases of organic foreign bodies because the solution may cause the object to swell, preventing its removal. In situations in which removal in the office is not possible or when middle ear injury is suspected, it is appropriate to perform an examination of the ear in the operating room under anesthesia. A middle-ear exploration may be necessary to diagnosis and repair ossicular disarticulation, perilymphatic fistulae, or facial nerve injury.

Lacerations

Minor lacerations of the external auditory canal may occur while attempting to remove foreign bodies and often heal spontaneously with aural antibiotic drops. More severe lacerations may result from extensive injuries involving the soft tissues of the head, with circumferential lacerations of the external auditory canal often requiring internal stenting to prevent stenosis. Stenting of the external auditory canal may be accomplished in many ways, including packing with antibiotic-impregnated gauze, ear sponges, or appropriately sized Foley catheters or endotracheal tubes that are cut and sutured in place to the tragus. After stenting for 1 to 3 weeks, removal of the stent is performed in the office to assess for healing. Patients are then reevaluated for stenosis after 1 to 2 weeks and are retreated as needed.

Temporal Bone Fractures

The temporal bone houses many important structures, including the carotid artery and jugular vein, cochlear and vestibular organs, and facial nerve. Therefore, temporal bone fractures have the potential of being quite devastating if any of these structures are injured. The temporal bone is very dense and to fracture it requires great force, often resulting in other serious bodily injury. Temporal bone fractures are categorized as longitudinal (80%) and transverse (20%) injuries as they relate to the position of the petrous pyramid. Longitudinal fractures occur secondary to lateral forces applied to the head. These fractures often result in TM perforation or hemotympanum, ossicular disarticulation with conductive hearing loss, cerebral spinal fluid (CSF) leak from the middle cranial fossae, and facial nerve injury 20% of the time. Transverse fractures of the temporal bone are caused by forces applied in the frontal or occipital directions. Transverse fractures commonly cause intense vertigo from vestibular injury, sensorineural hearing loss due to cochlear damage, and facial nerve injury 50% of the time. Evaluation of patients with temporal bone fractures includes a full neurologic and otologic examination with special attention directed toward signs of CSF otorrhea, through a TM perforation or in the nasopharynx through the Eustachian tube. Computed tomography of the temporal bones with fine cuts is essential in diagnosis of the position and extent of temporal bone fractures. Surgical treatment is rarely required except in cases with persistent CSF fistulae, or in facial nerve paralysis where decompression or repair may be indicated. Disruption of the ossicles with conductive hearing loss may also require surgical repair.

■ Infectious

ACUTE OTITIS EXTERNA

Diffuse acute otitis externa or swimmer's ear is diagnosed by the rapid onset of symptoms including otalgia, pruritus, and aural fullness, with tenderness to manipulation of the auricular cartilage. There may be associated otorrhea, cervical lymphadenitis, or cellulitis of the surrounding skin or pinna. These signs and symptoms must manifest within 48 hours to arrive at this diagnosis. A thorough debridement of the external auditory canal (see "Cerumen Impaction" on page 102), when possible, confirms the diagnosis and begins the treatment. First-line medical therapy for otitis externa not complicated by abscess formation, osteitis, middle-ear disease, or recurrent episodes of infection is topical otic preparations consisting of antibiotics and corticosteroids. When external auditory canal edema is severe it may be necessary to place a wick in the narrowed ear canal to enhance topical drug delivery. Systemic antibiotics and cultures may be required in persistent or severe cases, when there is an associated otitis media, or in immunocompromised patients. Ear drainage following swimming with a tympanostomy tube or perforation is *not* otitis externa or swimmer's ear but rather otorrhea or suppurative otitis media through a tube or perforation. Culture and sensitivity studies are important for refractory cases.

Recurrent Otitis Externa

Recurrent otitis externa may be secondary to predisposing host factors that affect adequate treatment of the condition. Individuals with untreated dermatologic conditions, such as atopic dermatitis and seborrhea, and immunocompromised patients with diabetes, cancer, or HIV may require improved management of their systemic illness to effectively control recurrent otitis externa. Other factors contributing to recurrent infections include repeated local trauma to the external auditory canal with removal of protective cerumen with cotton swabs. The protective properties of cerumen include its hydrophobic nature, acidic pH, and lysozyme content, which inhibit bacterial and fungal growth. Culture and sensitivity studies are important for recurrent and refractory cases.

Otomycosis

Otomycosis is a superficial fungal infection of the external auditory canal. Symptoms include pruritus, otalgia, and otorrhea that tends to be fluffy and white; however, it may also be black, gray, bluish-green, or yellow depending on the causative organism. Cultures are important to identify the pathogens. On otoscopy, black or white conidiophores on white hyphae are associated with *Aspergillus* infections. Ninety percent of otomycosis infections are caused by *Aspergillus* species and typically result from the treatment of prolonged bacterial otitis externa with the overzealous use of topical steroid preparations rendering the external auditory canal vulnerable to opportunistic infections. Uncomplicated presentations are best treated with local debridement and topical antifungal drops such as clotrimazole for *Candida* species or acidifying drops such as acetic acid for *Candida* and *Aspergillus* species. Restoration of external auditory canal pH, adequate and often repeated debridements, and moisture reduction are essential for the resolution of the infection. Cultures are required for refractory or severe cases.

Necrotizing (Malignant) External Otitis

Necrotizing otitis externa is osteomyelitis of the skull base involving the cancellous bone of the skull, periosteum, dura, blood vessels, and cranial nerves. Individuals with compromised immunity, such as diabetics and those undergoing chemotherapy, are at increased risk of this disease. The presence of granulation tissue in the external auditory canal at the bony cartilaginous junction, with disproportionate pain despite adequate topical treatment, are signs of necrotizing otitis externa. Facial paralysis may result from involvement of the bone surrounding the stylomastoid foramen. Thrombosis of the sigmoid dural sinus may also occur with resultant septic emboli and cranial nerve palsies. The major diagnostic criteria for necrotizing otitis externa are

- Pain
- Exudate
- Edema
- Granulation tissue
- Microabscesses
- Positive technetium-99 scan
- Failure after 1 week of topical therapy
- Presence of *P aeruginosa*

Treatment of necrotizing otitis externa includes prolonged systemic antibiotic therapy in the form of intravenous third-generation cephalosporins or oral fluoroquinolones along with appropriate management of any correctable metabolic derangements. Adjunctive treatments include use of hyperbaric oxygen treatments to increase the phagocytic oxidative killing of aerobic organisms and promotion of osteoneogenesis.

Furunculosis

Furunculosis may be differentiated from acute otitis externa in that it involves a focal segment of the external auditory canal. A single infected hair follicle in the lateral auditory canal results in pain and possibly drainage. *S aureus* is the usual etiologic pathogen, and treatment involves warm compresses, incision, and drainage with topical and possible systemic antibiotics.

INFLAMMATORY

Dermatologic conditions such as seborrhea, contact dermatitis, and eczema may result in inflammation of the external auditory canal. These conditions will predispose individuals to secondary infections of the external auditory canal. Neomycin is the most common otic preparation resulting in sensitization reactions in susceptible individuals with chronic otitis externa. Treatment with aural corticosteroid drops is indicated for these dermatologic conditions of the external auditory canal. Dermatologic consultation may be helpful in refractory cases.

NEOPLASTIC

Adenoma of Cerumen Glands

Ceruminous adenomas are rare tumors that present in the lateral third of the external auditory canal where sebaceous and apocrine glands are present. These lesions may be present for years as non-ulcerated masses of the external auditory canal and often manifest with canal obstruction. Extension of this disease may involve the bony external auditory canal or middle ear. Treatment involves complete surgical excision, and the prognosis of the disease is favorable with rare local recurrences.

Exostoses/Osteomas

Exostoses and osteomas are common lesions of the external auditory canal. Exostoses are bony growths of the external auditory canal arising from the bony cartilaginous junction. There is a high association of exostosis formation in individuals with cold-water exposure (from chronic periostitis) in individuals such as surfers and swimmers. These lesions occur bilaterally and may result in conductive hearing loss secondary to auditory canal obstruction. When severe, surgical canaloplasty may be indicated to remove these lesions that may recur if cold-water exposure continues. Osteomas differ from exostoses in that they do not have any association with cold-water exposure. Osteomas are most common in middle-aged men and are generally unilateral, pedunculated growths based on the temporal-squamous suture line in the external auditory canal. As with exostoses, osteomas may require surgical canaloplasty to treat conductive hearing loss associated with their growth.

OTHER

Cerumen Impaction

Special cerumen-producing glands secrete an acidic substance that belongs in the external auditory canal to inhibit the growth of bacteria and yeast, which may cause external otitis if some cerumen were not present. Cerumen in different individuals may be soft or hard, scant or excessive. The cerumen and desquamated epithelium in the external auditory canal are usually self-cleaning due to natural exfoliation and water exposure during swimming and bathing. In some individuals, cerumen is hard or excessive, or the external auditory canal may be stenotic. These factors may lead to accumulation of cerumen and impaction with hearing loss and possible secondary external otitis. Some individuals may cause impactions by pushing the cerumen in with cotton-tipped swabs during attempted cleaning. The old saying, "Nothing smaller than your elbow should ever be put in your ear," should be evoked for such patients.

For routine cerumen removal an otoscope and curettes, alligator forceps, or ear suctions may be used. A variety of sizes of curettes and suctions are required to treat patients with different-sized ear canals. The patient is instructed to "hold still like a statue." Uncooperative patients may be restrained by parents or nurses or with a papoose board, which uses restraining straps. Immobility of the patient is absolutely required because patient motion may lead to significant accidental trauma, such as ear canal laceration with bleeding, TM perforation, facial nerve injury, or dislocation of the malleus, incus, or stapes. A second critical point is that the clinician must rest part of his or her hands that are holding the otoscope and instrument on the head of the child. This is called *bracing*. Bracing is critical to ensure that if the child moves during a cerumenectomy the hand and ear-cleaning instrument move with the child to avoid injury to the ear. Very few clinicians have hands that are steady enough to clean a narrow ear canal gently, and this is especially true when working with a young, frightened child who is constantly trying to move. If the child makes a major sudden movement and the clinician is not bracing properly on the child's head, the uncontrolled instrument my cause serious injury to the ear. If a child cannot be satisfactorily restrained, the ear cleaning procedure must be aborted and referral to an otolaryngologist is required. In some cases, a brief general anesthetic is required for a thorough, safe ear cleaning and microscopic examination.

Bleeding from minor lacerations of the ear canal can be controlled with oxymetazoline nasal drops; ototopical antimicrobial drops should be prescribed to prevent secondary infection and to help clear out any residual blood clot. The injured ear canal should be kept dry for one week and an earplug should be used during bathing and swimming.

If the cerumen is hard and cannot be removed easily with curettes, alligator forceps, or ear suctions, a course of mineral oil or antimicrobial ototopical drops is prescribed and the patient is brought back to the office for ear canal cleaning at a second visit. If a cerumen impaction has caused a secondary external otitis, thorough ear canal cleaning is necessary, followed by a course of ototopical antimicrobial drops.

For individuals with a history of repeated cerumen impactions and a physical examination documenting intact TMs, 3 drops of mineral oil may be applied to each ear canal at bedtime once a week. This may help to soften the cerumen and allow spontaneous egress or at least easier cleaning of the softened cerumen. Peroxide-containing over-the-counter preparations that help to disperse and displace cerumen may also be useful. Irrigations performed in the office using syringes and gentle pressure with warmed saline may be useful. It is critical to note that if the clinician is not certain whether the patient's TM is intact, saline irrigation, peroxide, and mineral oil are contraindicated. If infection is present in the ear canal or middle ear and the TM is not intact, irrigation of the ear canal may drive infection into the inner ear and possibly result in sensorineural hearing loss, labyrinthitis, and otogenic meningitis.

Keratosis Obturans

Keratosis obturans is a disease resulting from abnormal epithelial migration from the TM. The resulting collection of desquamated debris develops into a dense obstructive mass in the external auditory canal. There is widening of the bony external auditory canal without erosion of the osseous structures, thereby differentiating these lesions from external auditory canal cholesteatomas. Many patients with this disorder also have a history of sinusitis and bronchiectasis.

Cysts

Sebaceous cysts may occur in the external auditory secondary to the occlusion of a follicular ostium with the accumulation of sebaceous material. Theses lesions are prone to superinfection with *S aureus* or other normal skin flora. The pinna may be tender to manipulation, and surgical incision and drainage followed by excision is occasionally required to manage these lesions. Other similar lesions include epidermal inclusion cysts and dermoid cysts. Epidermal inclusions cysts result from the introduction of dermal elements into the subcutaneous tissues by trauma or piercings. Dermoid cysts are congenital lesions in which epidermal tissue becomes trapped under embryologic skin flaps. These lesions are similarly treated with complete surgical excision.

■ Selected References

Brent B. Technical advances in ear reconstruction with autogenous rib cartilage grafts: personal experience with 1200 cases. *Plast Reconstr Surg.* 1999;104(2):319–334

Cohen D, Friedman P. The diagnostic criteria of malignant external otitis. *J Laryngol Otol.* 1987;101(3):216–221

Jahrsdoerfer RA. Congenital atresia of the ear. *Laryngoscope.* 1978;88(9 Pt 3 Suppl 13):1–48

Kim HJ, Patronas NJ, Goldstein BS, Oliverio PJ. Imaging studies of the temporal bone. In: *Head and Neck Surgery – Otolaryngology.* 3rd ed. 2001:1694

Melnick M, Bixler D, Nance WE, Silk K, Yune H. Familial branchio-oto-renal dysplasia: a new addition to the branchial arch syndromes. *Clin Genet.* 1976;9(1):25–34

Powell RH, Burrell SP, Cooper HR, Proops DW. The Birmingham bone anchored hearing aid programme: paediatric experience and results. *J Laryngol Otol Suppl.* 1996;21:21–29

Rafeq S, Trentham D, Ernst A. Pulmonary manifestations of relapsing polychondritis. *Clin Chest Med.* 2010;31(3):513–518

Roland PS, Smith TL, Schwartz SR, et al. Clinical practice guideline: cerumen impaction. *Otolaryngol Head Neck Surg.* 2008;139(3 Suppl 2):S1–S21

Takagi D, Nakamaru Y, Maguchi S, Furuta Y, Fukuda S. Otologic manifestations of Wegener's granulomatosis. *Laryngoscope.* 2002;112(9):1684–1690

Triglia JM, Nicollas R, Ducroz V, Koltai PJ, Garabedian EN. First branchial cleft anomalies: a study of 39 cases and a review of the literature. *Arch Otolaryngol Head Neck Surg.* 1998;124(3):291–295

Verhagen CV, Hol MK, Coppens-Schellekens W, Snik AF, Cremers CW. The BAHA Softband. A new treatment for young children with congenital aural atresia. *Int J Pediatr Otorhinolaryngol.* 2008;72(10):1455–1459

Yellon RF. Congenital external auditory canal stenosis with partial atretic plate. *Int J Pediatr Otorhinolaryngol.* 2009;73(11):1545–1549

Nose and Sinus

CHAPTER 5

Neonatal Nasal Obstruction

Tulio A. Valdez, MD, and Tiffiny Ainsworth, MA, MD

■ Introduction

Infants are obligate nasal breathers for at least 6 weeks and up to 6 months. Nasal obstruction can be unilateral or bilateral and intranasal or nasopharyngeal. The spectrum of symptoms and presentation are the result of the degree of obstruction and location. Unilateral or mild symptoms (eg, unilateral rhinorrhea, mild work of breathing) suggest an intranasal or unilateral level of obstruction. Nasopharyngeal or processes affecting both nostrils will present with significant, even life-threatening respiratory distress, cyclical cyanosis, and feeding difficulties. Cyclical cyanosis describes the process by which infants with nasal obstruction develop increasing work of breathing culminating in crying, which allows the infant to breathe through the mouth. Feeding difficulties include fatigue secondary to the inability to breathe while feeding, and poor coordination secondary to potential mass effect on the palate.

> **Pearl:** Cyclical cyanosis is a key feature of bilateral nasal obstruction.

■ Physical Examination and Diagnosis

Physical examination of the infant with respiratory distress must focus first on assessing the need for stabilizing the airway. Children with severe respiratory distress may require intubation or placement of an oral airway before undergoing further examination. Also, patients with congenital nasal obstruction may have other congenital anomalies such as severe cardiac and neurologic anomalies, which may contribute to cyanosis and poor respiratory effort.

Examination of the infant with nasal obstruction includes anterior rhinoscopy and possible flexible fiber-optic nasopharyngoscopy. A non-otolaryngologist practitioner may use a mirror or passage of a 6F suction catheter to evaluate for posterior obstruction. A dental mirror that does not fog when placed under a nostril with the opposite nostril occluded denotes a complete obstruction on the tested side. The failure to pass a 6F suction catheter through the nares into the oropharynx with a normal anterior nasal examination suggests an obstruction at the nasopharynx (eg, choanal atresia), while difficulty passing the catheter in the anterior aspect of the nasal cavity would suggest a narrow pyriform aperture. Identifying the level of obstruction with physical examination imaging may be required to further verify the nature of obstruction. Magnetic resonance imaging (MRI) will provide better soft-tissue detail of an obstructing mass such as encephaloceles or gliomas. Computed tomography (CT) provides the bony detail ideal for diagnosis of choanal atresia and pyriform aperture stenosis (Figure 5-1). The advent of fetal MRI allows clinicians the opportunity to plan for life-threatening respiratory distress in newborns with large obstructing lesions.

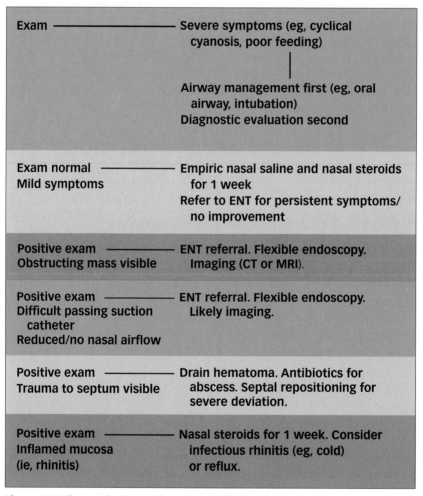

Figure 5-1. Diagnostic approaches to nasal obstruction

■ Nasal Embryology and Anatomy

Around the fifth week of gestation, paired ectodermal nasal placodes develop on the frontonasal process. These placodes are the beginning of the neonatal nose. Grooves form on the medial and lateral sides of the placodes and the nose projects forward. By the seventh week the grooves form blind-ending pits. The medial grooves form the septum and midline nasal structures. The lateral grooves form the lateral nasal sidewall and ala. As the nasal pits deepen, they form the nasal sac. At the posterior portion of the nasal sac, an epithelial membrane separates the nares from the developing oropharynx. By days 42 to 44, the oronasal membrane ruptures to provide a direct communication from the nose to the oropharynx. A cartilaginous capsule encases the developing nasal cavity. This cartilage develops into the turbinates and lateral nasal wall, which will eventually ossify. The lateral nasal wall evaginates to form the paranasal sinuses.

The nasal cavity is divided by the nasal septum. The septum is composed of bony and cartilaginous structures. In the neonate most of the septum is cartilage; ossification begins during childhood. Additionally, the mostly cartilaginous septum is thicker in the neonate to support the nasal dorsum. The nasal septum is composed of the quadrilateral cartilage anteriorly with the premaxilla. Posteriorly the septum is formed by the perpendicular ethmoidal plate and sphenoidal crest. Inferiorly the vomer articulates with maxillary and palatine bones.

The external nose is composed of paired nasal bones, upper lateral cartilages, and lower lateral cartilages. The internal and external nasal valves are the narrowest portions of airway. The internal nasal valve is defined by the septum medially, the upper lateral cartilage laterally, and anterior head of the inferior turbinate posteriorly. The external nasal valve (ie, nasal vestibule) is formed by the lower lateral cartilages and the nasal septum. The internal nasal valve is the narrowest segment of the 2 and is responsible for two-thirds of nasal airway resistance.

> **Pearl:** The internal nasal valve is the narrowest portion of the nasal airway. Borders include the septum, upper lateral cartilages, and inferior turbinate.

■ Differential Diagnosis

There are multiple etiologies of neonatal nasal obstruction, which can be categorized as congenital anatomic deformities, obstructing masses, traumatic obstructions, and inflammatory mucosal changes. Congenital anatomic deformities are aberrations of normal anatomy, present since birth, that alter normal nasal physiology. They can be further subdivided into external and internal nasal malformations. External malformations include unilateral nostril agenesis, arhinia, and nostril hypoplasia. External nasal malformations are exceedingly rare and easily diagnosed by visual inspection. Internal nasal cavity malformations include choanal atresia and pyriform aperture stenosis. Obstructing nasal masses include vascular anomalies (eg, infantile hemangiomas, vascular malformations), dermoid cysts, encephalocele, gliomas, dacryocystoceles, and teratomas. Of the obstructing lesions, encephalocele, glioma, and dermoid are the most common. Malignant neoplasms of the nasal cavity and nasopharynx are most commonly lymphoma and rhabdomyosarcoma. However, these lesions are exceptionally uncommon in neonates. Traumatic neonatal causes of obstruction are septal deviation and septal hematoma.

Inflammatory etiologies, while not a cause of complete obstruction, will often worsen a fixed obstruction. Allergic rhinitis and rhinitis medicamentosa are examples of inflammatory etiologies. Adenoid hypertrophy is a rare cause of neonatal obstruction. It is significantly more common in children. It should be remembered that as a child grows, inflammatory etiologies (eg, allergic rhinitis) become the most common cause of obstruction.

■ Congenital Anatomic Deformities

CHOANAL ATRESIA

Choanal atresia is a congential obstruction of the posterior nasal aperture on one or both sides. The incidence is approximately 1 in 5,000 to 1 in 8,000 live births. Other congenital anomalies are associated with choanal atresia 50% of the time.

These include coloboma, heart defects, choanal atresia, retardation of growth and development, genital, and ear malformations (CHARGE) syndrome; Treacher Collins syndrome; Crouzon syndrome; polydactyly; and nasal, auricular, and palatal deformities, CHARGE being the most commonly associated congenital anomaly. The exact point of disruption in embryologic development that leads to choanal atresia is not known.

Theories include failure of the oronasal membrane to rupture or abnormal migration of neural crest cells.

Signs and symptoms of choanal atresia can be varied depending on the presence of unilateral or bilateral disease. In unilateral choanal atresia, patients can present later in life with unilateral rhinorrhea and obstruction. In bilateral disease, infants present as early as neonates with complete nasal obstruction and cyclic cyanosis. Diagnosis is confirmed with the inability to pass a 6F suction catheter through the nose into the nasopharynx. Endoscopic evaluation further validates a fixed obstruction suggested by the failed passage of a suction catheter (Figure 5-2). Fine-cut craniofacial CT confirms the diagnosis and more importantly provides anatomic information about the thickness of the atresia.

> **Pearl:** Failure to pass a 6F suction catheter can signify anterior or posterior levels of obstruction.

Treatment for choanal atresia is surgical. Two surgical approaches are available for repair. The first is the more classically described transpalatal approach. In this approach, incisions are made to gain access to the hard palate. Portions of the posterior hard palate are removed to allow resection of the membranous or bony atresia plate. While the exposure is superior in this approach, it has a greater risk of dental and facial growth abnormalities. The transnasal approach uses

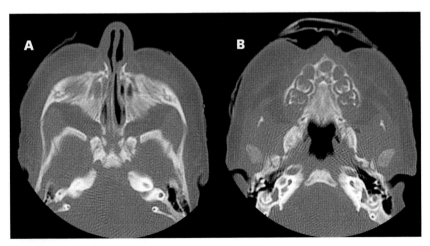

Figure 5-2. Choanal atresia

endoscopes to puncture and resect the membranous or bony atresia plate. Because this technique does not involve the palate, it does not have adverse risk to palatal and dental growth. Recent literature examining surgical approaches in 73 patients noted comparable restenosis rates in the transpalatal and endoscopic transnasal approaches (12.5% and 17%, respectively). Endoscopic transnasal approaches are becoming the standard of care in most urban settings.

Timing of surgical repair and airway management in the interim are areas of controversy. Unilateral atresia treatment is delayed to allow for growth to decrease operative risk and potential restenosis. Most children with unilateral atresia have surgical repair by the time they are 4 or 5 years of age. In patients with bilateral atresia, airway concerns and management necessitate an earlier repair time. Establishing a secure airway may necessitate a tracheotomy in these patients while they await further nasal growth and a definitive repair. Most of these children have definitive surgical repair within 12 months. Classically, nasal stenting of the choana was used to prevent restenosis. However, more recently, no increased risk of restenosis with stentless endoscopic approaches has been noted in various studies. Oral and nasal steroids are also used to help prevent restenosis. Patients with bilateral atresia and those with syndromes (eg, CHARGE) have greater risks of restenosis.

> **Pearl:** Neonates with syndromic disorders (eg, CHARGE) are at greater risk of restenosis after choanal atresia repair.

CONGENITAL PYRIFORM APERTURE STENOSIS

Congenital pyriform aperture stenosis (CPAS) is an anterior nasal obstruction of the nasal valve area. It is caused by excessive bony growth of the nasal process of the maxilla into the nasal cavity (Figure 5-3). Congenital pyriform aperture stenosis has an association with holoprosencephaly (ie, forebrain abnormality) and other congenital midline anomalies (eg, hypertelorism, flat nasal bridge, a central incisor, pituitary disorders).

Congenital pyriform aperture stenosis generally presents in the neonatal period. Like choanal atresia, CPAS presents with cyclical cyanosis. This is more pronounced during feeding as the infant tries to increase nasal airflow against a fixed obstruction. In older infants and children,

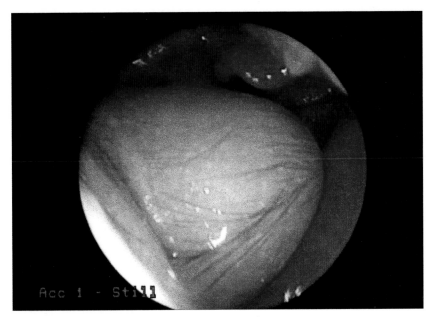

Figure 5-3. Congenital pyriform aperture stenosis

a respiratory infection may trigger exacerbation of milder obstructive symptoms and therefore come to the attention of the clinician.

Diagnosis is made on physical examination and by performing nasal endoscopy or CT. Although a suction catheter may or may not be passable through the nares on a CPAS patient, the site of obstruction in CPAS is directly visible on physical examination, whereas the anterior nares seem patent in choanal atresia. Radiographic diagnosis requires less than 11 mm of space between the medial aspects of the maxilla at the level of the inferior meatus as measured on axial CT cuts. Further imaging (ie, MRI), endocrine and neurologic consultations, and laboratory analysis for pituitary function should be considered given the association with holoprosencephaly and pituitary disorders.

Congenital pyriform aperture stenosis management and treatment are guided by the degree of stenosis and symptoms. Mild cases can be managed with topical vasoconstrictive drops, nasal steroids, and humidification until further growth increases the size of the nasal airway. Surgical indications for correction include sleep apnea, repeated intubation, frequent difficulties feeding, persistent or frequent respiratory distress, and failure of medical management.

> **Pearl:** Congenital pyriform
> aperture stenosis is associated with
> holoprosencephaly and central incisor. There is
> also an association with pituitary disorders.

Surgical management includes a sublabial approach to expose the pyriform aperture. Typically an endoscopic drill or a microdebrider is used to widen the lateral and inferior margin. Care is taken to prevent damage to tooth buds. Nasal stents are commonly placed postoperatively to prevent restenosis.

■ Obstructing Masses

DERMOID CYST OR SINUS

A dermoid cyst or sinus is derived from ectoderm and mesoderm. The sinus tract or cyst cavity is lined by squamous epithelium and contains adnexal structures (eg, hair follicles, sebaceous glands, sweat glands). Nasal dermoids are responsible for 10% to 12% of all head and neck dermoids. Nasal dermoids occur as a midline pit or mass on the nasal dorsum. It may be associated with a widened nasal bridge. When presenting as a dorsal nasal mass they are firm, often lobulated, non-compressible, and non-pulsatile. If associated with a sinus opening, keratin-like discharge is common. A protruding hair from the sinus is pathognomic for nasal dermoid. A dermoid may extend into the nasal septum.

> **Pearl:** The most common obstructing
> lesions in a neonate are encephalocele,
> glioma, and dermoid.

A dermoid cyst or sinus is thought to occur as a persistent connection between the prenasal space and intracranium during fetal development. The prenasal space is located posterior to the nasal bones and anterior to the nasal and septal cartilages. This space has a connection with the intracranium through a defect between the developing frontal bones. During development the dura extends through this defect in the prenasal space and attaches to ectoderm on the dorsal nose. As the defect closes, the dural attachment to the ectoderm releases and the dura retracts into the cranium. A nasal dermoid cyst or sinus represents a failure of separation and obliteration of the connection between the ectoderm and cranium through the prenasal space. As a result, a nasal dermoid may be found anywhere along this connection, including intracranially. Additional intracranial extension occurs in 4% to 45% of these lesions.

> **Pearl:** Brain magnetic resonance imaging is necessary in nasal dermoids to rule out intracranial extension.

Workup of these lesions includes a CT and an MRI. Thin-slice CT with contrast examines for potential skull-base defects. In particular, anomalies of the crista galli and foramen caecum are suggestive of possible intracranial extension. A contrast-enhanced MRI provides information about intracranial extension in addition to delineating normal soft tissue from dermoid. Nasal dermoid is hyperintense on T1-weighted imaging.

Management of nasal dermoids is via surgical excision. If intracranial extension is present, a combined intracranial-extracranial approach is pursued in conjunction between the otolaryngologist and neurosurgeon. If a sinus is present, the skin surrounding the sinus is excised with the tract. The complete excision of the cyst is required to prevent recurrence.

TERATOMA

Teratomas are typically benign lesions that include tissue from all 3 germ layers (ie, ectoderm, mesoderm, and endoderm). Less than 5% of all teratomas occur in the head and neck. Of those that occur in the head and neck, a frequent location includes the nasopharynx. Nasopharyngeal teratomas typically protrude into the oropharynx (Figure 5-4). As a result of the mass effect on surrounding development, nasopharyngeal teratomas are associated with palatal defects.

Presentation in the prenatal period is common. Polyhydramnios secondary to impaired swallowing and elevated alpha-fetoprotein levels can lead to diagnosis of large lesions via ultrasound. If not diagnosed prenatally, presentation in the early neonatal period is common. Acute severe respiratory distress is common. Typically the degree of respiratory distress necessitates endotracheal intubation or tracheotomy. If diagnosed prenatally, an ex utero intrapartum treatment procedure may be

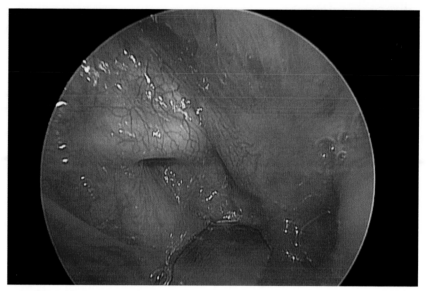

Figure 5-4. Nasopharyngeal teratoma

performed that uses maternal-fetal circulation to provide oxygenation to the neonate while the airway is secured. However, if the teratoma is small, feeding difficulties may be the only presenting symptom.

After adequate airway control, the management of these lesions is surgical excision. The approach to these lesions is dictated by their size. Alpha-fetoprotein can be used to monitor for recurrence.

> **Pearl:** Teratomas include tissue from all 3 germ layers (ie, ectoderm, mesoderm, and endoderm).

ENCEPHALOCELE

Encephaloceles are displaced intracranial contents through a bony defect in the skull. A meningocele is an encephalocele that includes only meninges. A meningoencephalocele contains brain and meninges. Given that a skull-base defect is present, encephaloceles may present with meningitis or cerebrospinal fluid leak. Encephaloceles can present as glabellar or dorsal nasal masses. As masses they appear bluish, soft, pulsatile, and compressible. Encephaloceles that herniate through a defect in the cribriform plate or through the junction of the posterior ethmoid air cells and sphenoid sinus present as an unilateral intranasal mass. Computed tomography and MRI help to make the diagnosis. Thin-cut CT characterizes the bony defect; MRI distinguishes a meningocele from meningoencephalocele. Management is surgical repair of the bony defect with reduction of herniated contents. Typically surgical intervention is performed early to prevent risk of meningitis and cosmetic deformities with large external encephaloceles.

GLIOMA

Gliomas are masses of heterotopic glial tissue that lack a patent cerebrospinal fluid intracranial connection. As a result these masses are firm, noncompressible, non-pulsatile, and lobular. In an external nasal location they have cutaneous telangiectasias. Intranasal gliomas often arise from the lateral nasal wall. Given that 15% to 20% are associated with connection to the intracranial space, a CT to assess for a skull-base defect is recommended. An MRI and nasal endoscopy better delineate the location in relation to surrounding structures. Management is via surgical excision, often with a combined otolaryngologic and neurosurgical approach. Surgical intervention is often early to avoid midface growth distortion.

> **Pearl:** Intranasal gliomas most often arise from the lateral nasal wall.

■ Traumatic Obstructions

SEPTAL DEVIATION

The incidence of septal deviation in neonates is approximately 1%. It has been postulated to be attributable to forceps trauma and passage through the birth canal during delivery. Anterior quadrilateral cartilage deviation is more common in newborns delivered vaginally than via cesarean delivery. However, internal rotation of the head toward the pelvic wall during cesarean delivery can also lead to septal deviation. Management of septal deviation is guided by symptoms. If associated with allergic symptoms, topical nasal steroids can be used. However, if there is significant septal deviation and severe obstruction, the septum can be repositioned. For milder cases of deviation, surgical correction via septoplasty at an older age may be helpful in increasing the size of the nasal airway. Indications for surgical correction have been advocated at any age if deformity causes significant obstruction and nasal stenosis.

> **Pearl:** Neonatal septal deviation has an incidence of 1%.

SEPTAL HEMATOMA AND ABSCESS

Septal hematomas form most often as a result of minor nasal trauma. While septal hematomas are far more common in children, minor birth trauma can lead to septal injury and hematomas. The trauma to the septum leads to rupture of blood vessels. As blood collects between septal cartilage and mucoperichondrium, ischemia and pressure necrosis begins to damage septal cartilage. As the cartilage necroses, bacteria can colonize and the developing infection can form an abscess. Cartilage necrosis can lead to significant nasal deformity (ie, saddle nose deformity). The primary presenting symptom of a septal hematoma is nasal obstruction. The resulting deformity leads to a fixed anatomic obstruction. Management of a septal hematoma and abscess involves urgent drainage and placement of nasal packing to prevent recollection. Antibiotics are prescribed to prevent a sinus infection while the drainage ostia are obstructed with nasal packing. In a recent study of the patients who had recollection, all had recollection within 3 days of packing removal.

■ Inflammatory Etiologies

RHINITIS

Allergic rhinitis is the most common cause of nasal obstruction in children. Prevalence increases with age. The incidence is nearly 1% in infants and 15% in adolescents. The inflammatory reaction of the nasal mucosa to inhaled allergens leads to congestion, increased viscous mucous, and obstruction of sinus drainage pathways. As a result, allergic rhinitis is associated with other conditions, such as sinusitis, otitis media with effusion, and asthma. Symptoms in infants include congestion and rhinorrhea. Symptoms such as postnasal drip, sneezing, and itchy, watery eyes are very uncommon in neonates. Rhinitis of infancy tends to be self-limited and symptoms often resolve within weeks. Treatment with topical steroids is only recommended in cases of severe respiratory distress. Diagnosis is made by clinical history and examination. Findings include but are not limited to pale boggy nasal mucosa and watery rhinorrhea.

■ Selected References

April MM, Ward RF, Garelick JM. Diagnosis, management, and follow-up of congenital head and neck teratomas. *Laryngoscope.* 1998;108(9):1398–1401

Belden CJ, Mancuso AA, Schmalfuss IM. CT features of congenital nasal piriform aperture stenosis: initial experience. *Radiology.* 1999;213(2):495–501

Brown OE, Myer CM 3rd, Manning SC. Congenital nasal pyriform aperture stenosis. *Laryngoscope.* 1989;99(1):86–91

Canty PA, Berkowitz RG. Hematoma and abscess of the nasal septum in children. *Arch Otolaryngol Head Neck Surg.* 1996;122(12):1373–1376

Cedin AC, Peixoto Rocha JF Jr, Deppermann MB, Moraes Manzano PA, Murao M, Shimuta AS. Transnasal endoscopic surgery of choanal atresia without the use of stents. *Laryngoscope.* 2002;112(4):750–752

Dispenza F, Saraniti C, Sciandra D, Kulamarva G, Dispenza C. Management of nasoseptal deformity in childhood: long-term results. *Auris Nasus Larynx.* 2009;36(6): 665–670

Hengerer AS, Strome M. Choanal atresia: a new embryologic theory and its influence on surgical management. *Laryngoscope.* 1982;92(8 Pt 1):913–921

Korantzis A, Cardamakis E, Chelidonis E, Papamihalis T. Nasal septum deformity in the newborn infant during labour. *Eur J Obstet Gynecol Reprod Biol.* 1992;44(1):41–46

Losee JE, Kirschner RE, Whitaker LA, Bartlett SP. Congenital nasal anomalies: a classification scheme. *Plast Reconstr Surg.* 2004;113(2):676–689

Losken A, Burstein FD, Williams JK. Congenital nasal pyriform aperture stenosis: diagnosis and treatment. *Plast Reconstr Surg.* 2002;109(5):1506–1512

Min YG. The pathophysiology, diagnosis and treatment of allergic rhinitis. *Allergy Asthma Immunol Res.* 2010;2(2):65–76

Myer CM 3rd, Cotton RT. Nasal obstruction in the pediatric patient. *Pediatrics.* 1983;72(6):766–777

Neskey D, Eloy JA, Casiano RR. Nasal, septal, and turbinate anatomy and embryology. *Otolaryngol Clin North Am.* 2009;42(2):193–205

Osguthorpe JD, Shirley R. Neonatal respiratory distress from rhinitis medicamentosa. *Laryngoscope.* 1987;97(7 Pt 1):829–831

Otteson TD, Hackam DJ, Mandell DL. The ex utero intrapartum treatment (EXIT) procedure: new challenges. *Arch Otolaryngol Head Neck Surg.* 2006;132(6):686–689

Rahbar R, Shah P, Mulliken JB, et al. The presentation and management of nasal dermoid: a 30-year experience. *Arch Otolaryngol Head Neck Surg.* 2003;129(4):464–471

Schoem SR. Transnasal endoscopic repair of choanal atresia: why stent? *Otolaryngol Head Neck Surg.* 2004;131(4):362–366

Stankiewicz JA. The endoscopic repair of choanal atresia. *Otolaryngol Head Neck Surg.* 1990;103(6):931–937

Tewfik TL, Mazer B. The links between allergy and otitis media with effusion. *Curr Opin Otolaryngol Head Neck Surg.* 2006;14(3):187–190

Van Den Abbeele T, Triglia JM, François M, Narcy P. Congenital nasal pyriform aperture stenosis: diagnosis and management of 20 cases. *Ann Otol Rhinol Laryngol.* 2001;110(1):70–75

CHAPTER 6

Rhinosinusitis

Amy S. Whigham, MD, and Maria T. Peña, MD

Background	Evaluation
Definitions	Microbiology
Anatomy	Medical Management
Pathophysiology	Surgical Management
Contributing Factors	Complications

■ Background

Pediatric rhinosinusitis (RS) is one of the most prevalent diseases that can significantly affect a child's quality of life, especially if it is recurrent or chronic. Persistent RS symptoms, including rhinorrhea, cough, headache, and fatigue, are likely to disrupt a child's sleep and concentration at school, which can affect emotional well-being. Caregivers and families of children with recurrent acute RS, chronic RS (CRS), or both, experience considerable disruption in daily routines. Indeed, sinusitis creates a substantial health care burden, with an estimated cost of $5.78 billion per year. Health care costs for children younger than 12 years make up approximately $1.8 billion per year of this estimate. This figure is likely higher because the indirect costs due to lost caregiver workdays, additional child care expenses for patient and siblings, and other related expenses, are inestimable. Additional economic burdens are created by this disease because the prevalence of pediatric RS is increasing and it is known to exacerbate other airway pathologies such as reactive airway disease.

Children average between 6 and 8 upper respiratory tract infections (URTIs) per year, with 0.5% to 5% progressing to acute sinusitis. Symptoms of viral URTIs and acute bacterial RS are similar, which makes it challenging to differentiate between them. The immaturity of the pediatric immune system, the different clinical presentations of RS, and symptoms from associated medical conditions also add to difficulties in making a correct diagnosis. The management of patients with pediatric RS remains controversial as well. Unlike adult patients, there is a lack of consensus in treatment paradigms.

> **Pearl:** Children average between 6 and 8 upper respiratory tract infections per year, with 0.5% to 5% progressing to acute sinusitis.

■ Definitions

The Sinus and Allergy Health Partnership and the American Academy of Pediatrics Subcommittee on Management of Sinusitis and Committee on Quality Improvement have divided RS into 5 categories based on the duration and frequency of symptoms (Table 6-1). Acute RS is a bacterial infection of the nose and paranasal sinuses that lasts less than 30 days, after which symptoms resolve completely. The key signs and symptoms

Table 6-1. Rhinosinusitis Definitions

Term	Definition
Acute bacterial rhinosinusitis	A bacterial infection of the nose and paranasal sinuses lasting *less than 30 days*. Symptoms completely resolve.
Subacute bacterial rhinosinusitis	A bacterial infection of the nose and paranasal sinuses *lasting between 30 and 90 days*. Symptoms completely resolve.
Recurrent acute bacterial rhinosinusitis	Multiple episodes of bacterial infection of the nose and paranasal sinuses, each lasting for *at least 7 to 10 days but less than 30 days* **and** *separated by asymptomatic intervals of at least 10 days.*
Chronic rhinosinusitis	A group of disorders characterized by inflammation of the mucosa of the nose and paranasal sinuses of *at least 12 consecutive weeks' duration.*
Acute exacerbation of chronic rhinosinusitis	When individuals with chronic rhinosinusitis develop new acute respiratory symptoms

of acute bacterial RS are rhinorrhea and cough. The quality of the nasal discharge is variable (eg, clear, mucoid, purulent, thick, thin). Other manifestations include nasal congestion, low-grade fever, otitis media, halitosis, irritability, and rarely, headache. Acute bacterial RS should be suspected when symptoms persist beyond 10 days. Severe acute RS is classified as purulent rhinorrhea for 3 to 4 consecutive days, temperature above 39.0°C, and periorbital edema. Recurrent acute bacterial RS is defined as episodes each lasting less than 30 days, separated by asymptomatic periods of at least 10 days' duration. Subacute RS is defined as signs and symptoms of RS for more than 30 days but less than 90 days. An indolent infection lasting more than 12 consecutive weeks without improvement is defined as CRS. During this time, the respiratory symptoms of rhinorrhea, nasal obstruction, and cough are persistent. Sore throat may result due to chronic mouth breathing secondary to nasal congestion. Headache and fever are uncommon. Individuals with CRS may have abrupt worsening of their symptoms, defined as acute exacerbation of CRS, which resolves with antimicrobial therapy.

> **Pearl:** Pediatric rhinosinusitis is divided into 5 categories based on the duration and frequency of symptoms.

■ Anatomy

The paranasal sinuses consist of 4 paired cavities or collections of air cells—maxillary, ethmoid, frontal, and sphenoid sinuses (Figure 6-1)—that ultimately drain into the nasal cavity via channels called ostia. The ostiomeatal complex is the space between the middle and inferior turbinates where there is a confluence of sinus drainage from the frontal, anterior ethmoid and maxillary sinuses. The paranasal sinuses are lined with pseudostratified ciliated epithelium which contains goblet cells and submucosal glands that produce seromucinous secretions and innate immune mediators.

The maxillary and ethmoid sinuses are present, albeit small, at birth. In neonatal life, the maxillary sinuses begin as a small slit-like cavity inferior to the orbits. They slowly enlarge laterally and vertically. Between ages 8 and 12 years, the floor of the maxillary sinuses reaches the floor of the nose. By age 15, the maxillary sinuses are adult size and have an inverted pyramidal shape. The natural opening of the maxillary sinus is positioned superiorly on the medial maxillary sinus wall and opens beneath the middle turbinate into the middle meatus.

The ethmoid sinuses consist of a honeycomb of air cells that are divided by thin, bony partitions and lie medial to the orbits. They reach their final form when children are between 12 and 14 years of age. The ethmoid sinuses are divided into anterior and posterior. The anterior ethmoids drain into the middle meatus, and the posterior ethmoids

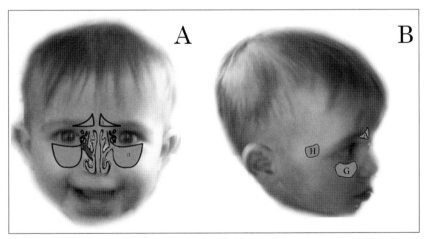

Figure 6-1. Paranasal sinus anatomy. Coronal (A) and sagittal (B) depiction of the nose and paranasal sinuses. A, frontal sinus; B, ethmoid sinus; C, superior turbinate; D, middle turbinate; E, ostiomeatal complex; F, inferior turbinate; G, maxillary sinus.

drain into the superior meatus, which is between the middle and superior turbinates. The orbit is separated from the ethmoid sinuses by a thin bone, the lamina papyracea. Infection of the ethmoids can easily spread to the orbit directly through small congenital bony dehiscences of the lamina, or by traversing neurovascular foramina.

The frontal sinuses arise from an anterior ethmoid air cell and move above the superior orbital rim by age 5 to 6 years. They continue to develop throughout late adolescence and drain into the middle meatus. The walls of the frontal sinuses are shared with the orbit and intracranial cavity. Therefore, frontal sinus infections are capable of spreading directly to these adjacent structures. The diploic veins, a valveless venous system that extends through the posterior wall of the frontal sinus to connect the vasculature of the sinus mucosa with the intracranial sinuses and veins, also provide a potential route of infectious spread. Septic thrombi can easily produce intracranial complications via this venous drainage system.

The sphenoid sinuses begin to develop by 3 to 5 years of age. They are located just posterior to the ethmoids and anterior to the pituitary fossa. The optic nerve and carotid artery are often located on the lateral wall of the sphenoid sinuses. The sphenoid sinuses represent another direct route for infections to spread into the central nervous system. Their strategic position anterior to the pituitary fossa can also be used to access tumors of the pituitary gland intranasally.

> **Pearl:** The paranasal sinuses consist of 4 paired cavities or collections of air cells—maxillary, ethmoid, frontal, and sphenoid sinuses—that ultimately drain into the nasal cavity via channels called ostia. The paranasal sinuses are in close proximity to the orbits and intracranial cavity.

■ Pathophysiology

The normal functioning of the paranasal sinuses depends on 3 factors: patency of the sinus ostia, mucociliary function, and character of sinus secretions. The diameter of the sinus ostia ranges from 1 mm to a few millimeters. Consequently, they are easily occluded by systemic illnesses that cause mucosal inflammation or structural abnormalities of the sinonasal cavities. Allergic rhinitis, immune disorders, extra esophageal reflux disease, and viral infections are commonly encountered pathologies that contribute to mucosal inflammation characteristic of RS with subsequent ostial obstruction. Trauma, intranasal growths such as nasal polyps and tumors, or obstructive sinonasal anatomic abnormalities like a deviated nasal septum are common etiologies causing mechanical obstruction of the sinus ostia. The most common factors causing pediatric RS are viral URTIs and allergic rhinitis.

Prolonged sinus ostial obstruction creates conditions that support unchecked bacterial growth. The secretions produced by the goblet cells and submucosal glands in the sinus mucosa stagnate as sinus outflow tracts are closed off. Over time, sinus oxygenation becomes significantly reduced, which increases the acidity of sinus secretions, creating a nutrient-rich medium for bacteria to thrive. Complete ostial obstruction also creates a negative intrasinus pressure and impairs bacterial export to the nasal cavity. Alterations in intranasal pressure, from sneezing, sniffing, and nose blowing, may allow the heavily colonized intranasal contents to enter the usually sterile sinus cavity.

The mucociliary apparatus of the sinonasal cavities is an essential defense mechanism against bacterial and viral pathogens as well as environmental irritants. It consists of a mucous layer that is moved by cilia located beneath the mucous. The mucous layer itself is subdivided into 2 compartments. The deep compartment is thin and serous, permitting normal cilia motility, while the superficial layer's increased viscosity captures particulate matter and pathogens. The mucous layer and cilia play a pivotal role in normal sinonasal function. Alterations in quality of mucous or cilia morphology and number, as seen with diseases like cystic fibrosis (CF) and primary ciliary dyskinesias (PCD), respectively, interrupt the normal physiology of the paranasal sinuses.

> **Pearl:** The normal functioning of the paranasal sinuses depends on 3 factors: patency of the sinus ostia, mucociliary function, and character of sinus secretions.

CONTRIBUTING FACTORS

Viral URTIs are the most common contributing factor that predisposes children to acute bacterial sinusitis. The average child has between 6 and 8 viral URTIs each year, and this number may increase by a factor of 3 in those children who regularly attend child care. Through the production of various inflammatory and immune mediators, viral infections cause obstructive inflammation of the sinonasal out-flow tracts and inhibition of normal ciliary function, predisposing to increased bacterial overgrowth. Other than supportive measures, there is no standard treatment for viral URTIs. Frequent hand washing is recommended. In severe cases, removing the child from the child care setting for a prolonged period may be necessary.

Second to viral URTIs, allergy is the most common comorbidity associated with bacterial sinusitis. Sixty percent of children with refractory sinusitis were found to have positive allergy testing. These children frequently present with a history of sneezing, copious watery nasal secretions, pruritus of the eyes and throat, and nighttime cough. On physical examination, clear rhinorrhea or pale, boggy inferior turbinates may be identified. These clinical symptoms and signs are thought to be related to the release of major basic protein and histamine by eosinophils and mast cells, respectively. Both substances disrupt mucociliary clearance by causing inflammatory obstruction of the sinus ostia. Major basic protein is thought to be toxic to the sinonasal mucosa. Other environmental pollutants, such as cigarette smoke, may contribute to an increased risk of pediatric RS by directly irritating the sinonasal mucosa. Secondhand smoke exposure has recently been linked with a higher likelihood of sinonasal symptoms and CRS.

> **Pearl:** After viral upper respiratory tract infections, allergy is the most common comorbidity associated with bacterial sinusitis.

Immunodeficiency is present in 0.5% of the general population. Up to a third of refractory RS cases may involve immune deficiencies, especially in patients with a history of frequent bacterial infection or illness soon after discontinuing antibiotics. Children with immune deficiencies will likely have a history of multiple upper and lower respiratory infections, including otitis media, RS, bronchitis, and pneumonia.

Anatomic variations in the nasal and sinus cavities have been postulated to predispose patients to sinus disease by narrowing sinus outflow tracts. However, studies in children have not found a relationship between intranasal anatomic variations and sinus disease. Consequently, contributing factors other than anatomic abnormalities likely play a more integral role in the development of pediatric acute and chronic RS.

Gastroesophageal reflux (GER) has been implicated in many aerodigestive disorders, including RS. Children with a history of chronic cough, hoarseness, and asthma are especially suspect for having GER. Nasopharyngeal reflux has been documented in children with symptoms of CRS and associated with coughing paroxysms. Gastroesophageal reflux may directly injure mucosa, thereby initiating an inflammatory response that leads to sinonasal edema and impaired mucociliary clearance. Evaluation for GER should be considered in patients with a history of reflux as an infant, poor weight gain, and reactive airway disease.

> **Pearl:** Evaluation for gastroesophageal reflux should be considered in patients with a history of reflux as an infant, poor weight gain, recurrent or chronic rhinosinusitis, and reactive airway disease.

Chronic medical diseases that affect the function of sinonasal mucosa, such as CF and PCD, must be considered. In the United States, CF has a prevalence of 1 in 3,200 white newborns. The disease manifests as chronic upper and lower respiratory tract infections, malnutrition, intestinal obstruction, and pancreatic insufficiency. The presentation and manifestations of CF are variable and many children with CF first present with nasal obstruction and CRS with nasal polyps. Primary ciliary dyskinesia, such as Kartagener syndrome, is a rare disorder of ciliary structure or function. Children with PCD will also have recurrent upper and lower respiratory infections.

> **Pearl:** The presentation and manifestations of cystic fibrosis are variable, and many children with cystic fibrosis first present with chronic rhinosinusitis with nasal polyps.

■ Evaluation

The diagnosis of RS is made by a thorough clinical history and supported by findings on physical examination. In infants or young children, irritability and decreased energy may be the only signs. In older children, the diagnosis of acute bacterial RS is strongly suggested by the presence of 2 major symptoms or 1 major and 2 minor symptoms (Table 6-2). The key signs and symptoms of acute bacterial RS are rhinorrhea, nasal obstruction, hyposmia/anosmia, and facial pressure. Minor factors include fever, halitosis, fatigue, ear pressure, dental pain, and headache. Self-limiting viral URTIs may be indistinguishable from acute bacterial RS. Viral etiology is suggested by rhinitis preceded by fever. Lack of improvement or worsening of symptoms at 7 to 10 days is highly suggestive of acute bacterial RS. A careful head and neck examination, while often difficult in children, may corroborate a suspected diagnosis of RS. Turbinate erythema and induration with pooled purulent secretions on the nasal floor may be seen on anterior rhinoscopy. The posterior oropharynx should be examined for erythema and purulent secretions coming from the nasopharynx. Transillumination of the paranasal sinuses poorly correlates with sinus disease. Nasal endoscopy to evaluate for purulence in the middle meatus, intranasal polyps, and adenoid size should be considered. Mucopurulent secretions in the region of the middle meatus is highly suggestive of bacterial RS. Nasal polyps (Figure 6-2) are uncommon in children and should prompt an evaluation for CF.

> **Pearl:** Identification of sinonasal polyps in any child is an indication for cystic fibrosis testing.

Plain radiographs are considered low utility in cases of pediatric RS because of high false-positive rates. Positive signs of acute RS on radiographs are complete opacification of the sinus, thickening (>4 mm) of the sinus mucoperiosteum, and air-fluid levels within the sinus. Correlation of abnormal sinus radiographs with positive culture results (>104 colony-forming units/mL) are reported to range

| Table 6-2. Diagnosis of Rhinosinusitis ||
Major Symptoms	Minor Symptoms
Facial pain/pressure	Headache
Nasal obstruction/congestion	Fever
Nasal discharge	Halitosis
Hyposmia/anosmia	Fatigue
Cough	Dental pain
	Ear fullness/pain

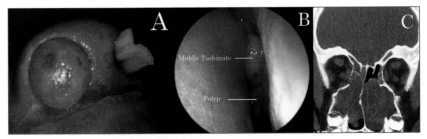

Figure 6-2. Nasal polyposis. Patient with large nasal polyp (A) and nasal endoscopic view of a small nasal polyp (B). Computed tomography scan of a patient with bilateral extensive nasal polyposis (C).

from 70% to 75%. A thorough history identifying symptoms for more than 10 days has been shown to significantly correlate with abnormal radiographs and positive cultures, thereby obviating the need for imaging. While CT is considered the gold standard in imaging, a positive scan alone is not diagnostic of bacterial RS. The CT scans of children with purulent rhinorrhea lasting from 2 to 9 days has demonstrated sinus opacification or air-fluid levels in roughly 70% of the scans. Despite treatment with antibiotics or placebo, 60% were normal and 40% were improved at 3-week follow-up imaging. Computed tomography should be reserved for suspected complications of RS, patients who are unresponsive to medical therapy, and patients under consideration for surgical intervention.

> **Pearl:** Computed tomography scans should be reserved for suspected complications of rhinosinusitis, patients who are unresponsive to medical therapy, and patients who are under consideration for surgical intervention.

The gold standard for the diagnosis of bacterial RS is maxillary sinus puncture with aspiration and culture. However, this procedure is unnecessary in uncomplicated cases of acute RS, as diagnosis is based on a thorough clinical history. Furthermore, maxillary sinus puncture and aspiration is a painful, invasive procedure that typically requires general anesthesia in the pediatric population. In addition, it has potential complications, such as facial numbness and injury to the tooth roots, especially in young children where the floor of the maxillary sinus is above the floor of the nose. Sinus aspiration for culture should therefore be reserved for those patients who fail appropriate medical therapy or in patients with immunodeficiency or toxemia. Nasal cavity bacterial cultures correlate poorly with those from the maxillary sinus. However, an 83% to 94% correlation of endoscopically guided middle meatal cultures with maxillary sinus cultures has been demonstrated. This procedure has few risks and is less painful than maxillary sinus puncture and aspiration.

> **Pearl:** Sinus aspiration for culture should be reserved for those patients who fail appropriate medical therapy or patients with immunodeficiency or toxemia.

Because many factors contribute to RS, testing for associated medical conditions may be indicated. Allergy testing is recommended in all children whose symptoms are unresponsive to medical therapy, especially in children with a strong family history of allergy or those with a history of urticaria. Evaluation for immunodeficiency should be performed in children with recurrent RS, severe symptoms, or an inadequate response to appropriate medical management. Initial immunologic testing includes an assessment of total serum immunoglobulin and IgG subclass levels, and antibody responses to diphtheria, tetanus, and pneumococcal vaccines. In cases of suspected GER, a 24-hour pH probe is considered the gold standard for diagnosis. Alternatively, an empiric trial of antireflux medication may be used as a diagnostic tool. Children with nasal polyps should be evaluated for CF. While an elevated sweat chloride concentration is often found in CF patients, genetic testing is more accurate and reliable. Primary ciliary dyskinesia is diagnosed by biopsy of nasal or tracheal mucosa.

> **Pearl:** Evaluation for associated medical conditions such as allergy, gastroesophageal reflux, cystic fibrosis, primary ciliary dyskinesias, and immune disorders may be indicated in patients with recurrent or chronic rhinosinusitis.

■ Microbiology

The most common pathogens in acute and subacute RS are *Streptococcus pneumoniae,* nontypeable *Haemophilus influenzae,* and *Moraxella catarrhalis. S pneumoniae* is isolated from 30% to 40% of specimens. *H influenzae* and *M catarrhalis* each account for approximately 15% to 20% of cases. Much less frequently identified bacteria include group A streptococci, group C streptococci, *Peptostreptococcus, Moraxella* species, and *Eikenella corrodens.* Chronic RS does not have a well-defined bacterial population but is often polymicrobial. The most frequently cultured bacteria include alpha-hemolytic streptococci, *Staphylococcus aureus,* coagulase-negative staphylococci, nontypeable *H influenzae, M catarrhalis,* anaerobic bacteria (including *Peptostreptococcus, Prevotella, Bacteroides,* and *Fusobacterium),* and *Pseudomonas.* Positive *Pseudomonas* cultures are frequently encountered after multiple courses of antibiotics.

■ Medical Management

Antibiotics should be reserved for those children with respiratory symptoms that persist beyond 10 to 14 days or those with significant purulent rhinorrhea for at least 3 to 4 consecutive days and a temperature of 39°C. In children with mild to moderate symptoms of uncomplicated acute bacterial RS who have not been treated with antibiotics 90 days or more prior to the infection and who do not attend child care, first-line therapy is amoxicillin. The recommended dose is 45 to 90 mg/kg/day divided into 2 doses. For children with penicillin allergy, cefdinir (14 mg/kg/day in 1 or 2 doses), cefuroxime (30 mg/kg/day in 2 divided doses), or cefpodoxime (10 mg/kg/day once daily) is recommended. Clarithromycin (15 mg/kg/day in 2 divided doses) or azithromycin (10 mg/kg/day on 1, then 5 mg/kg/day once daily for 4 days) is suggested in patients with serious allergic reactions to penicillin. If a patient has a culture revealing penicillin-resistant *S pneumoniae,* clindamycin at 30 to 40 mg/kg/day in 3 divided doses is indicated. Duration of antibiotic treatment varies, but treatment of acute bacterial RS for at least 14 days is recommended.

For children whose symptoms do not improve after 48 to 72 hours of treatment with the usual dose of amoxicillin, those who have been treated with antibiotics 90 days or more prior to an infection, children who attend child care, or those with moderately severe symptoms, initial therapy should be high-dose amoxicillin-clavulanate (80–90 mg/kg/day of amoxicillin, 6.4 mg/kg/day of clavulanate, in 2 divided doses). Other therapeutic alternatives include cefdinir, cefuroxime, or cefpodoxime. In patients with vomiting preventing administration of oral antibiotics, a single dose of intravenous (IV) or intramuscular ceftriaxone at 50 mg/kg/day may be used. An oral antibiotic should be initiated 24 hours later to complete therapy. Children who do not improve with a second course of antibiotics or who are acutely ill should be treated with IV cefotaxime or ceftriaxone. Consultation with an otolaryngologist may be necessary to obtain sinus cultures for culture-directed therapy.

> **Pearl:** Children whose symptoms do not improve after 48 to 72 hours of treatment with the usual dose of amoxicillin, who have been treated with antibiotics in the last 90 days, who attend child care, or those with moderately severe symptoms, should receive initial therapy of high-dose amoxicillin-clavulanate.

Children with CRS should be treated with antibiotics and adjunctive medical therapies. A 3- to 4-week course of antibiotics, directed at resistant pneumococci, S aureus, and anaerobic bacteria, has been advocated as part of initial medical treatment in CRS. Since the emergence of community-acquired methicillin-resistant S aureus (MRSA), much attention has been directed toward the management of sinonasal MRSA. While scientific evidence in this area is lacking, no treatment regimen is recommended for cases of sinonasal MRSA colonization. On the contrary, in patients with heavy growth of MRSA in the setting of acute sinonasal inflammation, a 1- to 2-week course of cultured, directed oral antibiotics and topical mupirocin is advocated. First-line oral antibiotics include clindamycin and trimethoprim/sulfamethoxazole.

Studies to evaluate the benefit of nasal saline rinses in children are limited; however, this is a common supplemental therapy, especially in children with CRS. Daily nasal rinses are also particularly helpful in patients with CF and PCD, particularly after functional endoscopic sinus surgery (FESS) because the sinus ostia have been enlarged. Mechanical flushing with nasal saline rinses assists in clearing the nose and paranasal sinuses of stagnant secretions and biofilms reducing bacterial counts, which improves sinus ventilation, drainage, and mucociliary transport. Saline may also aid is reducing nasal edema because of its mild vasoconstrictive properties.

Data on the use of topical nasal steroids in acute bacterial RS reveal marginal benefit. As antibiotics are typically effective within the first 3 to 4 days of treatment, intranasal steroids are not commonly advocated in children with acute bacterial RS. However, in allergic patients, daily use of topical nasal steroids is essential, and they are suggested as initial medical therapy in patients with CRS. Nasal steroids should be applied by aiming the nozzle at the lateral nasal wall, where they are most effective. Complications of nasal irritation and epistaxis are minimized when the spray is directed at the lateral nasal wall, away from the nasal septum. Oral steroids may be considered in patients with acute RS who do not respond to initial therapy, those with nasal polyposis, or those with severe nasal mucosal edema.

Nasal decongestants and mucolytics have limited efficacy. Topical nasal decongestants may improve symptomatic nasal congestion but should be limited to only the first 4 to 5 days of medical treatment to avoid rebound vasodilatation.

Correcting or ameliorating associated comorbidities is essential to the treatment of pediatric RS. In patients with specific environmental allergies, optimizing the home environment to decrease or avoid allergens is vital. Antihistamines are indicated in cases of suspected or documented allergy. Also, secondhand smoke exposure should be avoided. Those patients with diagnosed immunodeficiencies should be referred to an immunologist and may require immunoglobulin therapy. In patients with CRS and suspected GER, an empiric trial of antireflux medications should be considered. Patients with CF or PCD should be managed with the assistance of a pulmonologist.

■ Surgical Management

Surgical therapy is indicated in cases of failure of maximal medical management. Adenoidectomy is usually first-line surgical management. Culture of the middle meatus or maxillary sinus may also be performed at the time of adenoidectomy. The adenoid pad can contribute to recurrent acute bacterial RS and CRS because it acts as a bacterial reservoir that is a nidus for infection. Studies have shown that adenoidectomy alone improves the symptoms of recurrent and chronic RS in 50% to 60% of children. However, those children with asthma or exposed to secondhand smoke did not respond as well to adenoidectomy.

Indications for other surgical interventions remain controversial. Although FESS has been performed safely in children for more than 20 years, pediatric otolaryngologists are performing FESS less often and with a much more conservative dissection than in years prior. Pediatric FESS is currently indicated in patients with persistent sinonasal disease despite maximal medical therapy, adenoidectomy, and culture-directed systemic antibiotics; patients with sinonasal tumors, obstructing nasal polyps, or CF; and patients with intraorbital or intracranial complications of RS. Balloon sinuplasty has recently emerged for the treatment of sinusitis. This procedure uses endoscopic techniques and intraoperative radiographic guidance to dilate the sinus ostia with a balloon instead of a sharp instrument. As it is a novel technique, its experience in children in limited and the indications and long-term outcomes have not yet been studied.

> **Pearl:** The indications for sinus surgery are patients with persistent sinonasal disease despite maximal medical therapy, adenoidectomy, and culture-directed systemic antibiotics; patients with sinonasal tumors or obstructing nasal polyposis; and patients with intraorbital or intracranial complications.

■ Complications

Children are more susceptible to orbital complications of RS due to the thinness of their sinus walls and bony septa, greater bony porosity, open suture lines, and larger vascular foramina. Pediatric patients with orbital infections caused by sinusitis can present with decreased visual acuity, gaze restriction, diminished pupillary reflex, and proptosis. The severity of these infections can range from eyelid edema, to abscess of the orbital soft tissues (Figure 6-3), to cavernous sinus thrombosis. Cavernous sinus thrombosis occurs because of retrograde spread of orbital infection through the valveless orbital veins and is a life-threatening condition. Urgent consultation with an otolaryngologist and an ophthalmologist is indicated in any patient with ophthalmologic findings and sinusitis.

Pearl: Urgent consultation with an otolaryngologist and an ophthalmologist is indicated in any patient with ophthalmologic findings and sinusitis.

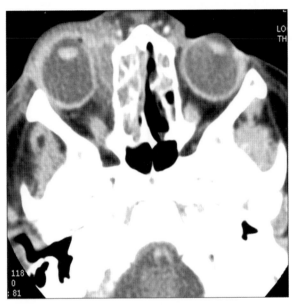

Figure 6-3. Orbital complications of sinusitis. Computed tomography scan of a patient with a right orbital abscess.

Intracranial complications can also be associated with acute sinusitis and include meningitis, epidural and subdural abscesses, cavernous and sagittal sinus thromboses, and intraparenchymal brain abscesses (figures 6-4 and 6-5). The most common presenting symptoms of intracranial complications are fever and headache; lethargy, seizures, and neurologic deficits are ominous signs associated with increased morbidity and mortality. Extension of frontal sinusitis through the valveless diploic veins or direct extension of an infection through osteitic bone are the most common anatomic routes for infections to access the central nervous system. However, the remaining sinuses may be sources of intracranial infection. In cases of potentially life-threatening intracranial complications of RS, prompt neurosurgical and otolaryngologic evaluation is necessary.

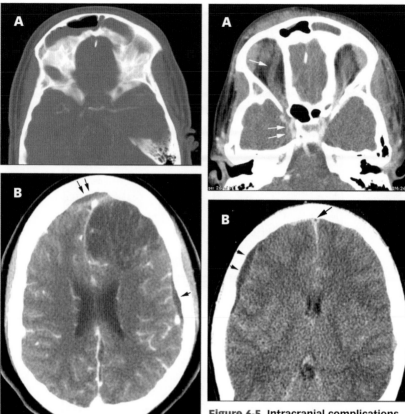

Figure 6-4. Intracranial complications of sinusitis. Contrast computed tomography scan showing (A) frontal sinusitis with an air-fluid level and (B) left frontal cerebritis, left subdural abscess (single arrow), and midline epidural empyema (double arrows) in a 15-year-old with acute mental status changes.

Figure 6-5. Intracranial complications of sinusitis. Axial contrast computed tomography (CT) scan revealing (A) thrombosis of the superior ophthalmic vein (single arrow) and right cavernous sinus (double arrows) in an 11-year-old who presented with right orbital pain and periorbital edema. Contrast CT scan of the brain demonstrates (B) thrombosis of the superior sagittal sinus (single arrow) and a right subdural abscess (double arrows) in the same patient.

Pearl: Patients with fever, mental status changes, and sinusitis need emergent otolaryngologic and neurosurgical intervention.

■ Selected References

American Academy of Pediatrics Subcommittee on Management of Sinusitis and Committee on Quality Improvement. Clinical practice guideline: management of sinusitis. *Pediatrics*. 2001;108(3):798–808

Antimicrobial treatment guidelines for acute bacterial rhinosinusitis. Executive summary. Sinus and Allergy Health Partnership. *Otolaryngol Head Neck Surg*. 2000;123(1 Pt 2):1–4

Becker SS, Russell PT, Duncavage JA, Creech CB. Current issues in the management of sinonasal methicillin-resistant *Staphylococcus aureus*. *Curr Opin Otolaryngol Head Neck Surg*. 2009;17(1):2–5

Brook I. Microbiology and antimicrobial treatment of orbital and intracranial complications of sinusitis in children and their management. *Int J Pediatr Otorhinolaryngol*. 2009;73(9):1183–1186

Chan R, Astor FC, Younis RT. Embryology and anatomy of the nose and paranasal sinuses. In: Younis RT, ed. *Pediatric Sinusitis and Sinus Surgery*. New York, NY: Taylor & Francis Group, LLC; 2006:1–14

Clayman GL, Adams GL, Paugh DR, Koopmann CF Jr. Intracranial complications of paranasal sinusitis: a combined institutional review. *Laryngoscope*. 1991;101(3):234–239

Cunningham JM, Chiu EJ, Landgraf JM, Gliklich RE. The health impact of chronic recurrent rhinosinusitis in children. *Arch Otolaryngol Head Neck Surg*. 2000;126(11):1363–1368

Goldsmith AJ, Rosenfeld RM. Treatment of pediatric sinusitis. *Pediatr Clin North Am*. 2003;50(2):413–426

Herrmann BW, Forsen JW Jr. Simultaneous intracranial and orbital complications of acute rhinosinusitis in children. *Int J Pediatr Otorhinolaryngol*. 2004;68(5):619–625

Leo G, Mori F, Incorvaia C, Barni S, Novembre E. Diagnosis and management of acute rhinosinusitis in children. *Curr Allergy Asthma Rep*. 2009;9(3):232–237

Lippincott LL, Brown KR. Medical management of pediatric chronic sinusitis. *J La State Med Soc*. 2000;152(10):470–474

Lund VJ, Kennedy DW. Quantification for staging sinusitis. The Staging and Therapy Group. *Ann Otol Rhinol Laryngol Suppl*. 1995;167:17–21

Lusk R. Pediatric chronic rhinosinusitis. *Curr Opin Otolaryngol Head Neck Surg*. 2006;14(6):393–396

Lusk RP, Stankiewicz JA. Pediatric rhinosinusitis. *Otolaryngol Head Neck Surg*. 1997;117(3 Pt 2):S53–S57

Passalacqua G, Canonica GW, Baiardini I. Rhinitis, rhinosinusitis and quality of life in children. *Pediatr Allergy Immunol*. 2007;18(Suppl 18):40–45

Phipps CD, Wood WE, Gibson WS, Cochran WJ. Gastroesophageal reflux contributing to chronic sinus disease in children: a prospective analysis. *Arch Otolaryngol Head Neck Surg*. 2000;126(7):831–836

Ramadan HH. Surgical management of chronic sinusitis in children. *Laryngoscope*. 2004;114(12):2103–2109

Ray NF, Baraniuk JN, Thamer M, et al. Healthcare expenditures for sinusitis in 1996: contributions of asthma, rhinitis, and other airway disorders. *J Allergy Clin Immunol.* 1999;103(3 Pt 1):408–414

Reh DD, Lin SY, Clipp SL, Irani L, Alberg AJ, Navas-Acien A. Secondhand tobacco smoke exposure and chronic rhinosinusitis: a population-based case-control study. *Am J Rhinol Allergy.* 2009;23(6):562–567

Rosenfeld RM. Pilot study of outcomes in pediatric rhinosinusitis. *Arch Otolaryngol Head Neck Surg.* 1995;121(7):729–736

Rosenstein BJ, Cutting GR. The diagnosis of cystic fibrosis: a consensus statement. Cystic Fibrosis Foundation Consensus Panel. *J Pediatr.* 1998;132(4):589–595

Schwartz RH, Pitkaranta A, Winther B. Computed tomography imaging of the maxillary and ethmoid sinuses in children with short-duration purulent rhinorrhea. *Otolaryngol Head Neck Surg.* 2001;124(2):160–163

Shapiro GG, Virant FS, Furukawa CT, Pierson WE, Bierman CW. Immunologic defects in patients with refractory sinusitis. *Pediatrics.* 1991;87(3):311–316

Sobol SE, Samadi DS, Kazahaya K, Tom LW. Trends in the management of pediatric chronic sinusitis: survey of the American Society of Pediatric Otolaryngology. *Laryngoscope.* 2005;115(1):78–80

Vogan JC, Bolger WE, Keyes AS. Endoscopically guided sinonasal cultures: a direct comparison with maxillary sinus aspirate cultures. *Otolaryngol Head Neck Surg.* 2000;122(3):370–373

Wald ER. Microbiology of acute and chronic sinusitis in children. *J Allergy Clin Immunol.* 1992;90(3 Pt 2):452–456

Wald ER. Sinusitis. *Pediatr Ann.* 1998;27(12):811–818

Wald ER. Sinusitis in children. *N Engl J Med.* 1992;326(5):319–323

Willner A, Choi SS, Vezina LG, Lazar RH. Intranasal anatomic variations in pediatric sinusitis. *Am J Rhinol.* 1997;11(5):355–360

Younis RT, Anand VK, Davidson B. The role of computed tomography and magnetic resonance imaging in patients with sinusitis with complications. *Laryngoscope.* 2002;112(2):224–229

CHAPTER 7

Epistaxis

Mark S. Volk, MD, DMD

■ Introduction

Epistaxis is a common, usually benign condition of childhood. While simple epistaxis can be a source of inconvenience, chronic or excessive bleeding requires proper diagnosis and management, as nasal bleeding may be a source of morbidity or an indication of serious underlying pathology. Because epistaxis is so common, how extensive the workup and treatment of a child with nasal bleeding should be can be a difficult decision.

■ Epidemiology

Epistaxis is most common in pediatric and geriatric populations. More than 50% of children between 6 and 10 years of age have nosebleeds. The peak age group is between 8 and 9 years. While no doubt common, there have not been a great number of studies that have described the actual incidence of epistaxis. In one study, 30% of children between the ages of 0 and 5 years, 56% of those aged 6 to 10 years, and 64% of those aged 11 to 15 years reported having epistaxis. However, in an Italian study of 1,281 children between 11 and 14 years of age, 8.5% reported having episodes of epistaxis. In addition to the increased incidence of epistaxis during childhood, nosebleeds occur more frequently in cold, dry conditions. In a review of emergency department (ED) visits in a tertiary care general hospital in Boston, MA, it was shown that between the months of December and February nosebleeds accounted for 0.50% of ED visits. This number decreased to 0.34% of ED visits during all other times of the year. Studies show a predisposition to epistaxis after upper respiratory tract infections and in males compared with females.

The site of the bleeding is on the anterior nasal septum in the vast majority (>90%) of patients. This area is prone to bleeding secondary to a network of small blood vessels known as Kiesselbach plexus. These vessels are located in a superficial portion of the septal mucosa, which makes them prone to injury from the slightest mechanical or chemical insult.

■ Presenting Symptoms

The presenting symptom of epistaxis is, of course, bleeding from the nose. Parents bring their children to see the pediatrician for varying degrees of nose bleeding. The bleeding can range in frequency from 1 or 2 episodes every other month to several per day. Quantity of bleeds can also vary from a trace amount that stops spontaneously to copious bleeding that can go on for 30 minutes or more and results in significant blood loss. When bleeding episodes happen, they can occur in one or both nostrils or in alternating nostrils. It is critical to record the location to tailor any needed cauterization in the future. One of the challenges in dealing with this condition is trying to gauge the severity of the bleeding. Katsanis et al developed a grading system that can be a useful guide (Table 7-1). Documentation of frequency and severity of episodes is vital to gauge how aggressive workup and therapy need to be as well as to determine progress during treatment. Any medicines that increase

Table 7-1. Epistaxis Scoring System

Component	Score[a]
Frequency	
5–15/y	0
16–25/y	1
>25/y	2
Duration	
<5 min	0
5–10 min	1
>10 min	2
Amount[b]	
<15 mL	0
15–30 mL	1
>30 mL	2
Epistaxis history/age[c]	
<33%	0
33%–67%	1
>67%	2
Site	
Unilateral	0
Bilateral	2

[a]Mild = 0–6, severe = 7–10.

[b]Estimation of average blood loss per episode: based on fractions or multiples of teaspoons (5 mL), tablespoons (15 mL), or cups (240 mL).

[c]Proportion of the child's life during which nosebleeds have been recurrent (>5 episodes/y).

From Katsanis E, Luke K-H, Hsu E, et al. Prevalence and significance of mild bleeding disorders in children with recurrent epistaxis. *J Paediatr.* 1988;113:73–76, with permission from Elsevier.

the chances of bleeding (eg, ibuprofen, salicylates) should be noted. It is also important to determine if there is a history of any systemic diseases, bleeding, easy bruising, or family history of bleeding problems.

■ Physical Examination Findings

A thorough head and neck examination is important in evaluating any patient with epistaxis. The oral cavity has the largest surface area of mucous membrane that can be examined without an endoscope, so it is important to examine the mouth to look for any petechiae or other generalized mucosal lesions that may be more difficult to see in the nose. Anterior rhinoscopy can be performed using an otoscope. This instrument is well known to children and is usually nonthreatening. On examination of the nose, special attention should be paid to the nasal septum. The anterior septum is the location of a network of vessels known as Kiesselbach plexus. These vessels can be superficial and fragile and are the origin of most episodes of epistaxis. While distended vessels can sometimes be seen in this area, this occurs in only about 40% to 50% of children who present with nasal bleeding. Often there is minimal old blood seen in the area, even shortly after a nosebleed episode.

> **Pearl:** After nasal trauma, a septal hematoma may form. This bulge in the nasal septum can be differentiated from a septal deviation by palpating for fluctuance using a cerumen loop or the wooden end of a cotton swab. A hematoma of the septum requires referral to an otolaryngologist for incision and drainage.

■ Differential Diagnosis

Two-thirds of epistaxis episodes occur spontaneously and without apparent trauma. If there is trauma involved, it is usually secondary to nose blowing, sneezing, nose picking, or application of preparations such as intranasal steroids. Parents often give a history of discovering their child awakening at night or in the morning with blood on the pillowcase or sheets. These have been felt to be secondary to occult trauma such as contact with the pillow or nose picking (intentional or non-intentional). Only about 2% of nosebleeds occur secondary to an obvious blow to the nose such as being struck by a ball or an elbow. Upper respiratory tract infections, dehydration of the nasal mucosa, carriage of *Staphylococcus aureus* in the nasal vestibule, and nose picking all seem to play a part in nasal bleeding. Although some recent data suggest that nose picking may have less of a role than was once thought, the factors mentioned above frequently have a synergistic effect. Thus an upper respiratory infection, dry nasal mucosa, and low-grade *S aureus* infection make it more likely that a child will manipulate or pick his or her nose. Likewise, frequent nose picking makes it more probable that the nose will carry or recolonize with *S aureus*.

Epistaxis can be the first sign of a hematologic disorder. In adult studies, the incidence of hematologic disorders in patients with nosebleeds is somewhere between 0.7% and 3.5%. However, determining which patients would benefit from a hematologic workup has been difficult. In one study a total 36 children with epistaxis were tested and none had any abnormality of their prothrombin time (PT)/partial thromboplastin time (PTT), fibrinogen, or platelet aggregation studies. Two of the 12 patients who were in the severe nose-bleeding group had abnormal von Willebrand factors and were found to have von Willebrand disease (vWd). Another patient who was classified in the severe epistaxis group had a factor VIII:c deficiency. A similar study looking at 20 children with recurrent epistaxis noted that 4 patients had hematologic abnormalities consistent with vWd. Two of the 4 patients had totally normal PT/PTT and the other 2 had only a sight elevation of these values. Given that the prevalence of vWd in the general population is approximately 0.82%, it appears that patients who have recurrent nosebleeds have a significantly increased chance of having this hematologic disorder.

> **Pearl:** Because of the finding of normal prothrombin time/partial thromboplastin time values despite the diagnosis of von Willebrand disease (vWd) in this population, it is recommended that all patients undergoing blood work for coagulation studies have a vWd panel drawn at the same time.

Other causes of nosebleeds include allergies, vascular abnormalities, and nasal or nasopharyngeal tumors (Table 7-2).

Table 7-2. Etiology of Epistaxis

Local Causes of Epistaxis

- ◆ Inflammatory
  - — Allergy
  - — Rhinitis sicca
  - — Vasomotor rhinitis
- ◆ Infectious
  - — Viral (URI)
  - — Bacterial (vestibulitis, sinusitis)
- ◆ Trauma
  - — Nose picking
  - — External trauma (nasal/facial trauma)
  - — Foreign body
  - — Postoperative—sinus surgery, septoplasty, turbinate reduction
- ◆ Anatomic
  - — Acquired
  - — Nasal septal deviation
  - — Congenital
    - ▪ Choanal atresia
    - ▪ Meningocele, encephalocele, glioma

- ◆ Medications (topical)
  - — Decongestants (rhinitis medicamentosa)
  - — Cocaine
- ◆ Inhalants
  - — Tobacco
  - — Toxic fumes
  - — Cannabis
- ◆ Neoplasms
  - — Malignant
    - ▪ Squamous cell carcinoma
  - — Benign
    - ▪ Angiofibroma
    - ▪ Inverting papilloma
    - ▪ Polyp

Systemic Causes of Epistaxis

- ◆ Medications
  - — Aspirin
  - — Anticoagulants
  - — Antibiotics (chloramphenicol)
  - — Antineoplastics (methotrexate)
- ◆ Bleeding disorders
  - — Coagulopathies
    - ▪ Inherited (factor deficiencies)
    - ▪ Acquired (vitamin K deficit)

- ◆ Neoplasms
  - — Leukemia
  - — Lymphoma
- ◆ Inflammatory disorders
  - — Wegener granulomatosis
  - — Lethal midline granuloma
- ◆ Hypertension
- ◆ Other
  - — Sepsis
  - — Liver or bone marrow failure
    - ▪ Biliary atresia
    - ▪ Aplastic anemia
- ◆ Osler-Weber-Rendu disease

Abbreviation: URI, upper respiratory infection.

> **Pearl:** Any significant history of epistaxis in a male between the ages of 10 and 24 years requires consultation by an otolaryngologist for examination of the nasopharynx to rule out the presence of juvenile nasopharyngeal angiofibroma.

■ Treatment

Management of most nosebleeds primarily revolves around educating the parent and patient on treatment at the time of the bleed as well as using ways to prevent bleeding in the future. In general, bleeding will usually stop by applying pressure and occasionally using a vasoconstricting agent. There are a number of common misconceptions as to the best way to stop a nosebleed. In a 1993 study, only 33% of personnel in a Glasgow ED knew the proper anatomic site to apply pressure to the nose. This is consistent with the many ineffective techniques that are suggested by professionals and laypeople to stop an ongoing nosebleed. These include lying down, extending the head, pinching the bridge of the nose, putting a tissue under the upper lip, and applying ice (to the nose or back of the neck). These are not useful because they do not address the common site of bleeding, namely the anterior nasal septum.

> **Pearl:** To control a nosebleed at home, patients should be instructed to place constant pressure on the anterior septum by pinching the caudal (soft) portion of the nose with the fingers for 5 to 10 minutes. Blood clots are a source of fibrinolytic enzymes, so if bleeding persists after 5 to 10 minutes, the nose should be gently blown to evacuate any clots. If available, a vasoconstrictor such as oxymetazoline can be sprayed up the nose and pressure reapplied. These measures are usually effective. However, if bleeding is copious or persists for more than 30 minutes, medical attention at an emergency department is recommended.

Patients who present with persistent nosebleed may benefit from otolaryngologic consultation. However, if an otolaryngologist is not readily available, there are several maneuvers that the pediatrician can do in the office to stop or reduce bleeding. First, the patient or parent should continue to squeeze the caudal portion of the nose. This should be done for 5 minutes by the clock. Leaning back will cause blood to enter and pool in the pharynx, so the patient should sit straight up or lean slightly forward during these maneuvers. In this acute setting, optimum treatment would be localization and cauterization of the bleeding area. This is best accomplished by using a headlight, nasal speculum, and silver nitrate sticks. In lieu of having these equipment and supplies available, the pediatrician can place a rolled-up piece of an absorbable hemostatic agent up against the nasal septum. If bleeding is brisk or unremitting and the patient is showing signs of airway distress or hypovolemia, transfer to an ED. Because most nosebleeds are from small blood vessels in the septal mucosa, this is relatively uncommon in children. It suggests an arterial source of the bleeding or a systemic cause. Patients presenting to the ED in this condition require fluid resuscitation, workup, and definitive management. The first step in this situation is reassessment and if necessary, placement of an anterior or posterior nasal pack. These are usually left in for 24 to 48 hours. If bleeding resumes after pack removal, more definitive therapy is indicated. This can take the form of endoscopic visualization and cautery, angiography with embolization, or surgical clipping of the arteries supplying the bleeding area. All of these treatments require general anesthesia. Depending from where the bleeding is emanating, the latter intervention involves surgical ligation of the anterior or posterior ethmoid arteries or clipping of offending branches of the internal maxillary artery. The first surgical procedure is done through a Lynch incision made just medial and superior to the eye. The second type of surgery involves accessing the internal maxillary artery through the maxillary sinus via an incision under the upper lip (Caldwell-Luc approach).

As previously stated, severe nasal bleeding is rare. The most common presentation of epistaxis is of frequent, easily controlled episodes. In this setting, there are 2 initial management options. One way to control bleeding is to perform a chemical cauterization of the nasal septum. This can be done in the office by an otolaryngologist. It involves spraying lidocaine or placing a lidocaine-soaked pledget against the nasal septum followed by application of silver nitrate to any identifiable ectatic vessels or to the offending vascular plexus.

> **Pearl:** Patients who have continued, severe epistaxis may need placement of an anterior nasal pack. If the bleeding area is located posteriorly, placement of an anterior and posterior pack may be indicated. This type of packing is often quite uncomfortable and frequently requires hospital admission, intravenous hydration, antibiotics, and sedation or pain control.

This technique has the advantage of causing immediate cessation of further bleeding episodes. It unfortunately has some disadvantages— it can be difficult to reliably pinpoint the offending vessels; there can be associated discomfort; the silver nitrate can stain skin and clothing; and it can be difficult to perform with less-than-cooperative pediatric patients. The other technique that can be used is the use of nasal saline followed by antibiotic (ie, Bacitracin or Bactroban) ointment. Saline is instilled in the form of nose drops or spray and ointment is applied with cotton applicators to the anterior nasal septum. This combination should be applied twice a day and serves to hydrate the nasal mucosa as well as reduce the population of S aureus and other bacteria that may be causing inflammation in the nose. This has the advantage of not requiring a specialist and is usually well tolerated by the patient. The disadvantage of the saline/ointment regimen is that it can take as long as 10 to 14 days to start to have an effect and must be done twice daily for at least a month. Several studies have shown that the efficacy of these techniques (silver nitrate cautery alone, cautery and saline/ ointment, and saline/ointment alone) is similar. Interestingly, use of saline with petroleum jelly, a nonantibiotic ointment, showed no reduction in nosebleeds. This supports the theory that nasal vestibulitis may be a cause of epistaxis.

IF REFERRAL TO SPECIALIST IS RECOMMENDED, WHAT IS OPTIMAL TIME FRAME?

Referral to an otolaryngologist should be made in the presence of severe or unremitting bleeding or when conservative measures such as application of saline and antibiotic ointment fail.

NATURAL HISTORY AND PROGNOSIS

It is common for adults to comment that they have had episodes of nose bleeding as children and that these resolved as they grew older. This frequent remark correlates with observations that nose-bleeds show a bimodal peak in incident. Short-term resolution rate is unknown but has been estimated at approximately 30%. Virtually all children who have uncomplicated epistaxis will resolve their nose-bleeds as they mature.

LONG-TERM PROGNOSIS AND POTENTIAL COMPLICATIONS INTO ADULTHOOD

Epistaxis in childhood rarely leads to long-standing complications. Developmentally delayed individuals can obsessively pick their noses as a response to the crusting after epistaxis episodes. The resulting continued trauma to the septum may result in septal perforation. Cocaine users also run the risk of developing a septal perforation. Here the etiology is ischemia of the septal mucoperichondrium that results in ischemia and loss of the underlying cartilage. A septal perforation, no matter what the cause, will often lead to chronic crusting and epistaxis.

PROJECTED TIME TO RETURN TO ACTIVITIES OF DAILY LIVING

Most individuals with epistaxis are able resume their normal activities shortly after treatment. In the case of individuals who are being treated conservatively with saline and antibiotic ointment, they can often continue their normal activities during treatment. Recommendations for children who have been treated for severe epistaxis need to be made on an individual basis.

■ Selected References

Burton MJ, Dorée CJ. Interventions for recurrent idiopathic epistaxis (nosebleeds) in children. *Cochrane Database Syst Rev.* 2004;1:CD004461

Evans J. The aetiology and treatment of epistaxis: based on a review of 200 cases. *J Laryngol Otol.* 1962;76:185–191

Glad H, Vainer B, Buchwald C, et al. Juvenile nasopharyngeal angiofibromas in Denmark 1981-2003: diagnosis, incidence, and treatment. *Acta Otolaryngol.* 2007;127(3):292–299

Joice P, Ross P, Robertson G, White P. The effect of hand dominance on recurrent idiopathic paediatric epistaxis. *Clin Otolaryngol.* 2008;33(6):570–574

Juselius H. Epistaxis. A clinical study of 1,724 patients. *J Laryngol Otol.* 1974;88(4): 317–327

Katsanis E, Luke K-H, Hsu E, Li M, Lillicrap D. Prevalence and significance of mild bleeding disorders in children with recurrent epistaxis. *J Paediatr.* 1988;113:73–76

Kiley V, Stuart JJ, Johnson CA. Coagulation studies in children with isolated recurrent epistaxis. *J Pediatr.* 1982;100(4):579–581

Loughran S, Spinou E, Clement WA, Cathcart R, Kubba H, Geddes NK. A prospective, single-blind, randomized controlled trial of petroleum jelly/Vaseline for recurrent paediatric epistaxis. *Clin Otolaryngol Allied Sci.* 2004;29(3):266–269

McGarry GW, Moulton C. The first aid management of epistaxis by accident and emergency department staff. *Arch Emerg Med.* 1993;10(4):298–300

Pallin DJ, Chng YM, McKay MP, Emond JA, Pelletier AJ, Camargo CA Jr. Epidemiology of epistaxis in US emergency departments, 1992 to 2001. *Ann Emerg Med.* 2005;46(1): 77–81

Petruson B. Epistaxis in childhood. *Rhinology.* 1979;17(2):83–90

Rodeghiero F, Castaman G, Dini E. Epidemiological investigation of the prevalence of von Willebrand's disease. *Blood.* 1987;69(2):454–459

Ruddy J, Proops DW, Pearman K, Ruddy H. Management of epistaxis in children. *Int J Pediatr Otorhinolaryngol.* 1991;21(2):139–142

Wertheim HFL, van Kleef M, Vos MC, Ott A, Verbrugh HA, Fokkens W. Nose picking and nasal carriage of *Staphylococcus aureus. Infect Control Hosp Epidemiol.* 2006;27(8):863–867

CHAPTER 8

Pediatric Nasal and Facial Fractures

T.J. O-Lee, MD

■ Introduction

Despite advances in child protective measures, trauma remains the leading cause of death of children in the United States. Medical care rendered for all traumatic injuries is valued at greater than $15 billion annually. Pediatric ear, nose, and throat (ENT) trauma accounts for only a small share of this total. Most head and neck injuries comprise soft tissue trauma, such as laceration, contusion, or abrasion. Bony injuries occur even less frequently. Pediatric maxillofacial injuries account for approximately 5% of all facial fractures, with reported incidence ranging between 1.5% and 15%. Children younger than 5 years have a significantly lower risk ranging from 1% to 1.5%. With increasing age, the incidence of facial fracture also increases, ultimately reaching the pattern and frequency of adult trauma victims around late adolescence.

■ Diagnosis

In the evaluation of all traumatic patients, airway, breathing, and circulation must first be assessed and restored before initiating treatment. Following this algorithm is especially important in cases of ENT trauma because injuries of the head and neck can produce dramatic bleeding and distract the treatment team from the most important task—securing the airway.

Once the patient is stabilized, a systematic evaluation should be performed. The ears, nose, and throat should be evaluated separately. Organ functions, such as hearing, nasal patency, and voice, can be important predictors of injury site, but they should not be exclusively relied on because it is possible for injuries to have subtle or delayed onset of deficits. Evaluating facial symmetry with the patient at rest and in motion is important to assess facial nerve integrity. Progressive breathing or swallowing difficulty can indicate expanding hematoma of the neck or throat.

When suspicion for bony or deep tissue trauma is high, radiologic imaging often is indicated. Plain film has limited accuracy in evaluating the complex bony structures of the face and therefore has limited applicability. Even in cases of suspected nasal fracture, plain films are infrequently helpful to the treating physician. Even though plain film may be able to visualize fractures of the nasal bone, such visualization does not affect treatment.

Panoramic x-ray (panorex) is a plain film of the mandible that is taken with a rotating x-ray source. The result is a linear picture of an otherwise curved mandible. This is likely the most helpful type of plain film x-ray in traumatic evaluation of the face and neck. It is sensitive for fractures and often demonstrates the relative position of the fracture line to the teeth or teeth buds.

Computed tomography (CT) scans are often the study of choice for pediatric trauma evaluation because of their high resolution and short duration of study. Compared with magnetic resonance imaging (MRI), CT has better bony resolution and can be performed in a few seconds versus a few minutes for MRI, thereby often eliminating the need for general anesthesia. Computed tomography evaluation of trauma is usually performed without contrast unless deep tissue bleeding is suspected.

■ Soft Tissue Injuries

Soft tissue injury to the face is perhaps the most commonly encountered ENT trauma in pediatric patients. Some general treatment guidelines include

1. Judicious cleaning of laceration wounds and careful removal of all foreign bodies that may be embedded in the tissue. This process should take place after the wound is adequately anesthetized to minimize secondary trauma to the child and ensure thorough exploration of the wound.
2. Careful realignment of tissue prior to starting repair. Meticulous preservation of tissue will often make realignment more accurate.
3. Tissue closure in layers when possible. This increases the strength of the repair and also the accuracy of skin approximation. Absorbable sutures should be used whenever possible to avoid the trauma of suture removal for the child.

BITES

Animal and human bites often result in large avulsions of soft tissue. Wounds should be thoroughly irrigated with sterile saline prior to closure to decrease the bacterial load. Prophylactic antibiotic use is indicated and amoxicillin-clavulanate often is used as a first-line drug to cover oral flora. In children with penicillin allergy, clindamycin or azithromycin often are substituted.

TISSUE LOSS

Any significant tissue loss in a wound presents a challenge to the treating physician. In the immediate period after the injury, it may not be possible to distinguish viable and nonviable tissue. After a thorough cleaning of the wound, a moist dressing to preserve tissue viability is a reasonable course of action in wounds in which tissue loss prohibits immediate closure. Once the margins of viable tissue are declared, usually within 24 to 48 hours, the use of advancement or other local tissue rotation methods can be considered. Skin graft also is an option, although the limited tissue thickness, poor color match, and donor site morbidities make grafting less desirable. Vacuum-assisted wound dressing has shown remarkable results in many instances and should be considered for large wounds.

■ Bony Injuries

Great advances have been made in recent decades in treating pediatric facial fractures. Specific techniques used for reconstruction in children must accommodate a child's developing anatomy, rapid healing, psychological development, and potential for deformity as a consequence of altered facial growth. The prevalence of CT scans makes accurately diagnosing facial fractures possible in most instances. Rigid internal fixation has been successfully adapted from adults to pediatric patients with careful modification. Open reduction and rigid internal fixation is indicated for severely displaced fractures. Primary bone grafting is preferred over secondary reconstruction. Alloplastic materials should be avoided when possible.

Associated injuries are a common feature of childhood maxillofacial trauma. Neurologic and orthopedic injuries are seen in 30% of children with facial fractures, which reinforces the importance of a complete initial assessment of a child with facial trauma and highlights the dilemma with regard to the timing of the reconstruction because of the rapid healing of bony injuries in children.

NOSE

Nasal fractures are by far the most common facial bone injuries in children, followed by dentoalveolar injuries. Nose fractures usually are treated in the outpatient setting and do not require surgical intervention. Whether treatment is necessary is not dictated by the presence of fracture but by the presence of functional or cosmetic deficits.

The initial examination of a child with nasal fracture may be very limited due to midfacial swelling. Several days are required for the swelling to subside before the true extent of the deformity can be appreciated. On the other hand, immediate intranasal examination is important to detect the presence of septal hematoma (Figure 8-1). Although

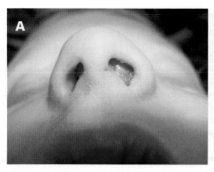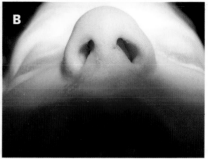

Figure 8-1. A, Nasal septal hematoma visible inside the left nostril. B, Nasal septum after drainage of the hematoma in the same patient.

rarely seen, septal hematoma can be observed on anterior rhinoscopy as an obvious purple bulge on one side of the nose. The bulge is compressible with a cotton tip applicator and does not shrink with topical vasoconstriction. A septal hematoma requires immediate evacuation on detection. An untreated hematoma can become a thick, fibrotic, and obstructive septum. If the hematoma becomes infected, the resulting loss of cartilage can cause a saddle nose deformity.

In cases of nasal fracture without septal hematoma, the patient should return 3 to 4 days after injury, when a more accurate examination is possible. If a cosmetic deformity or a fixed nasal obstruction is detected, definitive surgical treatment is undertaken. Closed reduction of the bony fracture can be performed with intranasal instrumentation and bimanual external manipulation. If significant dislocations are present or if the injury is more than 2 weeks old, open reduction may be necessary.

MANDIBLE

Fractures of the mandible are the most common facial fractures requiring hospitalization. They account for 30% to 50% of all pediatric facial fractures when nasal fractures are excluded. Because pediatric condyles are highly vascularized and thin necks are poorly resistant to impact forces, the most vulnerable part of the pediatric mandible is the condyle. More than 50% of pediatric mandibular fractures involve one of the condyles, whereas only 30% of adult cases show condylar involvement. As patients mature, the frequency of symphyseal, body, and ramus fractures increases.

Clinical signs of mandibular fractures may include displacement of the fragments, mobility, swelling, mucosal tears, limited mouth opening, malocclusion, and pain. Clinical suspicion of a fracture is confirmed by panorex, a complete mandible series, or CT scans. Computed tomography is especially helpful to help determine 3-dimensional displacement of the condyles.

Immobilization is difficult in patients younger than 2 years because of incomplete eruption of the deciduous teeth, although later growth and remodeling frequently compensate for less than ideal post-injury alignment. The primary teeth, which develop firm roots between 2 and 5 years of age, can be used for splints and arch bars. Deciduous roots are resorbed between 6 and 12 years of age; hence arch bars may need extra support from circummandibular wiring and pyriform aperture suspension. Permanent teeth are safe anchors for fixation after 13 years of age.

The central question when treating pediatric condylar fracture is whether the patient needs immobilization. Although minimally invasive endoscopic open reduction with internal fixation (ORIF) is gaining popularity for treating adult condylar fractures, most authors still advocate conservative measures in pediatric patients. If the patient has normal occlusion and normal mandibular movement, only a soft diet and movement exercises are necessary. However, if open bite deformities with retrusion of the mandible and movement limitation are present, a brief period of immobilization lasting 2 to 3 weeks followed by the use of guiding elastics can yield normal function in the end.

Displaced symphysis fractures can be treated by ORIF through an intraoral incision after age 6 years, after the permanent incisors have erupted. Open reduction with internal fixation in parasymphysial fractures is possible once buds of the canines have moved up from the mandibular border after age 9 years. In body fractures, the inferior mandibular border can be plated when buds of the permanent premolar and molar have migrated superiorly toward the alveolus.

Frequent postoperative follow-up visits are necessary to detect and treat early complications such as infection, malocclusion, malunion, and nonunion. Late complications such as damage to permanent teeth, temporomandibular joint dysfunction, or midface deformity with facial asymmetry also need attention and possible treatment.

ORBIT

Fractures of the orbital walls are not infrequent secondary to the very thin bones that are present, accounting for 20% to 25% of pediatric facial fractures. Medial orbital wall and orbital floor fractures are more common for the same reason. The mechanism of injury is often direct trauma to the eye or surrounding structure. Such pressure causes the orbital contents to explode beyond the normal boundary, thus fracturing the bones.

In assessing orbital injuries, it is important to document visual acuity, ocular pressure, and extraocular movements. Diplopia is a sensitive measure of extraocular movement deficit in a cooperative patient. All visual fields need to be inspected before diagnosing diplopia.

The treatment of isolated blowout fractures is symptom dependent. In an asymptomatic patient, no intervention is necessary because fractures will heal spontaneously. If persistent enophthalmos, extraocular muscle restriction, or pain on movement of the eye is present, surgical exploration is indicated. Large fractures also are routinely explored, as are fractures that on CT have obvious muscle entrapment. Absorbable gelatin film usually is sufficient for reconstructing small defects of the floor, although large disruptions are best repaired with calvarial bone grafts.

Orbital roof fractures occur in very young children whose frontal sinuses are still underdeveloped. These are often associated with skull injuries.

Pediatric orbital roof fractures are different than those of adults. They occur more frequently because of the lack of frontal sinus pneumatization. Children have a craniofacial ratio of 8:1 at birth, compared with 2:1 in adults, thus exposing more of their cranium and skull base to potential injuries. Most orbital roof fractures, particularly those that are non-displaced or with fragments displaced superiorly (blowout fractures), can be safely observed in the acute setting. Treatment should be directed by the presence of symptoms, such as extraocular muscle entrapment, enophthalmos, exophthalmos, diplopia, vision changes, or dystopia. Large blow-in fractures have a higher chance for late onset complications; therefore, surgical thresholds should be lower. Depending on the extent and location of the orbital roof fracture, various approaches are available. Cooperation among neurosurgery, ophthalmology, and head and neck surgery are essential to ensure optimal care for these patients.

MIDFACE

Midfacial fractures are rare in children and usually result from high-impact, high-velocity forces such as motor vehicle crashes (MVCs). Zygomaticomalar complex (ZMC) fractures are seen in 10% to 15%, and Le Fort maxillary fractures are seen in 5% to 10%. Free-floating nasal base is a rare injury and indicates a nasoethmoidal fracture.

Zygomaticomalar complex fractures parallel the pneumatization of the maxillary sinus and are uncommon before the age of 5 years. Surgical correction of ZMC fractures is indicated when bony displacement is present. Adequate exposure is essential, and such correction is achieved by a process called triangulation. Three key sites need to be directly visualized: the frontozygomatic suture, infraorbital rim, and anterior zygomaticomaxillary buttress. Access can be achieved via the lateral upper eyelid incision, lower eyelid infraciliary or transconjunctival incision, and transoral buccal sulcus incision. Unlike adults, one-point fixation at the frontozygomatic suture may suffice in children because of shorter lever arm forces from the frontozygomatic suture to the infraorbital rim.

In nasoethmoidal fractures, medial canthal ligament integrity must be assessed. This is done by inserting a hemostat into the nose toward the medial orbital rim. The child should be anesthetized for this examination. Mobility of the underlying fragments suggests that the bone with its canthal attachment has been displaced and that reconstruction of the nasal maxillary buttress and possibly transnasal wiring is necessary. Measurement of soft-tissue intercanthal distance is difficult because ethnic, racial, and gender variations can significantly affect its values. Nevertheless, the average intercanthal distance at 4 years of age is approximately 25 mm; by age 12 years, 28 mm; and by adulthood, 30 mm. One can easily see that near-adult intercanthal distance is achieved at a very early age; hence, an easy mistake is to set the intercanthal distance too wide. Intercanthal distances 5 mm more than the average values tend to be indicative of, and 10 mm confirms the diagnosis of, displaced fractures of the nasoethmoidal complex. Attempts should be made to narrow excessive distance between the eyes and project the nose of a child.

■ Conclusion

Children of all ages can be afflicted by ENT trauma, often resulting in functional and cosmetic deficits. A thorough understanding of pediatric skull and facial growth enables practitioners to focus the search for subtle fractures in the most age-appropriate locations. Soft tissue injuries often can point out possible locations of fracture and should be carefully treated. Anticipation of mandibular growth facilitates repair because most injuries can be treated with intermaxillary fixation. Unerupted dentition requires careful selection of fixation methods and cautious screw placement if rigid fixation is ultimately required. Modern rigid plating systems have greatly enhanced surgeons' ability to reconstruct facial fractures in a 3-dimensional fashion. Depending on the site of injury, a multidisciplinary team approach can ensure that injuries to organs systems around the face are cared for in an optimal manner.

■ Selected References

Caldicott WJ, North JB, Simpson DA. Traumatic cerebrospinal fluid fistulas in children. *J Neurosurg.* 1973;38(1):1–9

Gussack GS, Luterman A, Powell RW, Rodgers K, Ramenofsky M. Pediatric maxillofacial trauma: unique features in diagnosis and treatment. *Laryngoscope.* 1987;97 (8 Pt 1):925–930

Hardt N, Gottsauner A. The treatment of mandibular fractures in children. *J Craniomaxillofac Surg.* 1993;21(5):214–219

Hogg NJ, Horswell BB. Soft tissue pediatric facial trauma: a review. *J Can Dent Assoc.* 2006;72(6):549–552

Holland AJ, Broome C, Steinberg A, Cass DT. Facial fractures in children. *Pediatr Emerg Care.* 2001;17(3):157–160

Kaban LB. Diagnosis and treatment of fractures of the facial bones in children 1943–1993. *J Oral Maxillofac Surg.* 1993;51(7):722–729

Kaban LB, Mulliken JB, Murray JE. Facial fractures in children: an analysis of 122 fractures in 109 patients. *Plast Reconstr Surg.* 1977;59(1):15–20

Koltai PJ. Maxillofacial injuries in children. In: Smith JD, Bumstead RM, eds. *Pediatric Facial Plastic and Reconstructive Surgery.* New York, NY: Raven Press; 1993

Koltai PJ. Pediatric facial fractures. In: *Bailey Head and Neck Surgery-Otolaryngology.* Philadelphia, PA: Lippincott; 2001

Koltai PJ, Rabkin D. Management of facial trauma in children. *Pediatr Clin North Am.* 1996;43(6):1253–1275

Koltai PJ, Rabkin D, Hoehn J. Rigid fixation of facial fractures in children. *J Craniomaxillofac Trauma.* 1995;1(2):32–42

Law RC, Fouque CA, Waddell A, Cusick E. Lesson of the week. Penetrating intra-oral trauma in children. *BMJ.* 1997;314:50–51

Lee D, Honrado C, Har-El G, Goldsmith A. Pediatric temporal bone fractures. *Laryngoscope.* 1998;108(6):816–821

Liu-Shindo M, Hawkins DB. Basilar skull fractures in children. *Int J Pediatr Otorhinolaryngol.* 1989;17(2):109–117

Marom T, Russo E, Ben-Yehuda Y, Roth Y. Oropharyngeal injuries in children. *Pediatr Emerg Care.* 2007;23(12):914–918

McGraw BL, Cole RR. Pediatric maxillofacial trauma. Age-related variations in injury. *Arch Otolaryngol Head Neck Surg.* 1990;116(1):41–45

McGuirt WF Jr, Stool SE. Cerebrospinal fluid fistula: the identification and management in pediatric temporal bone fractures. *Laryngoscope.* 1995;105(4 Pt 1):359–364

McGuirt WF Jr, Stool SE. Temporal bone fractures in children: a review with emphasis on long-term sequelae. *Clin Pediatr (Phila)*. 1992;31(1):12–18

Mitchell DP, Stone P. Temporal bone fractures in children. *Can J Otolaryngol.* 1973;2:156–162

Nicol JW, Johnstone AJ. Temporal bone fractures in children: a review of 34 cases. *J Accid Emerg Med.* 1994;11(4):218–222

Pierrot S, Bernardeschi D, Morrisseau-Durand MP, Manach Y, Couloigner V. Dissection of the internal carotid artery following trauma of the soft palate in children. *Ann Otol Rhinol Laryngol.* 2006;115(5):323–329

Posnick JC, Wells M, Pron GE. Pediatric facial fractures: evolving patterns of treatment. *J Oral Maxillofac Surg.* 1993;51(8):836–845

Rowe IM, Fonkalsrud EW, O'Neil JA, et al. The injured child. In: *Essentials of Pediatric Surgery.* St. Louis, MO: Mosby; 1995

Rowe NL. Fractures of the facial skeleton in children. *J Oral Surg.* 1968;26(8):505–515

Shapiro RS. Temporal bone fractures in children. *Otolaryngol Head Neck Surg.* 1979;87(3):323–329

Stefanopoulos PK, Tarantzopoulou AD. Facial bite wounds: management update. *Int J Oral Maxillofac Surg.* 2005;34(5):464–472

Thorén H, Iizuka T, Hallikainen D, Lindgvist C. Different patterns of mandibular fractures in children. An analysis of 220 fractures in 157 patients. *J Craniomaxillofac Surg.* 1992;20(7):292–296

Troulis MJ, Kaban LB. Endoscopic approach to the ramus/condyle unit: clinical applications. *J Oral Maxillofac Surg.* 2001;59(5):503–509

von Domarus H, Poeschel W. Impalement injuries of the palate. *Plast Reconstr Surg.* 1983;72(5):656–658

Williams WT, Ghorayeb BY, Yeakley JW. Pediatric temporal bone fractures. *Laryngoscope.* 1992;102(6):600–603

SECTION 3

Oropharynx

CHAPTER 9

Disorders of the Tonsils and Adenoid

David H. Darrow, MD, DDS

■ Introduction

Adenotonsillar disorders in children occur as a result of hyperplasia, infection, inflammation, or malignancy. Hyperplasia is a natural consequence of immune activity within these tissues but may become problematic when tissue size becomes excessive for the pharyngeal space they occupy. Infection of the tonsils and adenoid is common in this age group because of their participation in immune processes and continuous exposure to inhaled and ingested antigens. Malignancy of the tonsils and adenoid, in contrast, is exceedingly rare. This chapter will review the functions of the tonsils and adenoid, diagnosis and management of diseases of these tissues, and appropriate indications for their surgical removal.

■ Functions of Tonsils and Adenoid

The palatine tonsils and adenoid are tissues of Waldeyer ring, a group of lymphoepithelial tissues that also includes tubal tonsils in the nasopharynx and the lingual tonsil. Collectively, these tissues participate in the mucosal immune system of the pharynx. Positioned strategically at the entrance of the gastrointestinal and respiratory tracts, the tonsils and adenoid serve as secondary lymphoid organs, initiating immune responses against antigens entering the body through the mouth or nose. The size of the tonsils appears to correlate with their level of immunologic activity, peaking between the ages of 3 and 10 years, and demonstrating age-dependent involution. There is also some evidence that their size increases with bacterial load.

Tonsils are covered by a non-keratinizing stratified squamous epithelium featuring some 10 to 30 deep crypts that effectively increase the surface area exposed to incoming antigens. The crypts occasionally harbor degenerated cells and debris that give rise to so-called tonsilloliths, in which the presence of biofilms has also been implicated. Although tonsils lack afferent lymphatics, the epithelium contains a system of specialized channels lined by M cells that take up antigens into vesicles and transport them to the intraepithelial and subepithelial spaces where they are presented to lymphoid cells. The transport function of M cells serves as a portal for mucosal infections and immunizations; M cells also can initiate immunologic responses within the epithelium, introducing foreign antigens to lymphocytes and antigen-presenting cells (APCs).

After passing through the crypt epithelium, inhaled or ingested antigens reach the extrafollicular region or lymphoid follicles. In the extrafollicular region, APCs process antigens and present them to helper T lymphocytes that stimulate proliferation of follicular B lymphocytes. B lymphocytes ultimately develop into 1 of 2 types of cell—antibody-expressing B memory cells capable of migration to the nasopharynx and other sites, or plasma cells that produce antibodies and release them into crypt lumen. Tonsillar plasma cells can produce all 5 immunoglobulin classes helping to combat and prevent infection. In addition, contact of memory B cells in the lymphoid follicles with antigen is an essential part of the generation of a secondary immune response.

Among immunoglobulin isotypes, IgA may be considered the most important product of the adenotonsillar immune system. In its dimeric form, IgA can attach to the transmembrane secretory component (SC) to form secretory IgA (SIgA), a critical component of the mucosal immune system of the upper airway. This component is necessary for binding of IgA monomers to each other and to the SC and is an important product of B-cell activity in tonsil follicles. While tonsils produce immunocytes bearing the J (joining) chain carbohydrate, SC is produced only in the adenoid and extratonsillar epithelium, and therefore only the adenoid possesses a local secretory immune system.

Pearls

1. Tonsil size peaks between 3 and 10 years of age.
2. The tonsils and adenoid are a secondary source of circulating B lymphocytes.
3. Only the adenoid and extratonsillar lymphoid tissues, not the tonsils, possess a local secretory immune system.

■ Infectious and Inflammatory Diseases of Tonsils and Adenoid

Pharyngotonsillitis is a general term used to describe diffuse inflammation of structures of the oropharynx, including the tonsils. The disorder presents with symptoms of sore throat; however, objective signs of inflammation must be present to make the diagnosis. Pharyngotonsillitis may be classified based on duration of symptoms as acute, subacute, or chronic, with most patients presenting acutely. Alternatively, inflammatory disease of the nasopharynx may be considered *nasopharyngitis,* in which common symptoms include rhinor-rhea, nasal congestion, sneezing, and cough. Inflammation limited to the adenoid pad (adenoiditis) is difficult to diagnose in the primary care setting because of inaccessibility of this tissue to direct visualization.

COMMON VIRAL INFECTION

Nasopharyngitis typically occurs in cold weather months among young children during their early exposures to respiratory viruses. Adenoviruses, influenza viruses, parainfluenza viruses, and entero-viruses are the most common etiologic agents. Rhinovirus and respi-ratory syncytial virus occur almost exclusively in preschool children and are rarely associated with overt signs of pharyngeal inflamma-tion. Adenoviruses are more common among older children and adolescents. Nasopharyngitis of viral etiology may also cause a con-comitant pharyngotonsillitis. The infection is most commonly acute and self-limited, with symptoms resolving within 10 days. Nonviral agents are less frequently associated with nasopharyngitis but may include *Corynebacterium diphtheriae, Neisseria meningitidis, Haemophilus influenzae,* and *Coxiella burnetii.*

Viruses responsible for pharyngotonsillitis are more diverse than those in nasopharyngitis; adenoviruses, influenza viruses, parainflu-enza viruses, enteroviruses, Epstein-Barr virus (EBV), and *Mycoplasma* account for some 70% of these infections. As in nasopharyngitis, most viral pharyngotonsillitis requires no specific therapy.

GROUP A BETA-HEMOLYTIC STREPTOCOCCAL INFECTION

Group A beta-hemolytic streptococcus (GABHS) is the most com-mon bacterium associated with pharyngotonsillitis in children. In the 70 years since the advent of antibiotics, most pharyngeal infections by GABHS are benign, self-limited, and uncomplicated processes. In fact, most patients improve symptomatically without any medical interven-tion whatsoever. However, a small number of affected children continue to develop renal and cardiac complications following GABHS infection, and some authors have implicated GABHS in the development of com-mon childhood neuropsychiatric disorders. In addition, there is evi-dence that early antibiotic therapy may be useful in treating symptoms of GABHS. As a result, appropriate diagnosis and treatment of these infections is imperative.

Incidence of GABHS pharyngitis has not been estimated on the basis of population-based data. Nevertheless, "strep throat" is well recognized as a common disease among children and adolescents. Incidence peaks during winter and spring and is more common in cooler, temperate climates. Close, interpersonal contact in schools, military quarters, dormitories, and families with several children appears to be a risk factor for the disease.

Transmission of GABHS is believed to occur through droplet spread. Individuals are most infectious early in the course of disease, and risk of contagion depends on the inoculum size and virulence of the infecting strain. Incubation period is usually between 1 and 4 days. After starting antimicrobial therapy, most physicians will allow affected children to return to school within 36 to 48 hours. The role of individuals colonized with GABHS in the spread of the disease is uncertain, although data suggest that carriers rarely spread the disease to close contacts.

Streptococci are gram-positive, catalase-negative cocci characterized by their growth in long chains or pairs in culture. These organisms are traditionally classified into 18 groups with letter designations (Lancefield groups) on the basis of the antigenic carbohydrate component of their cell walls. While GABHS is isolated from most patients with streptococcal pharyngitis, group C, G, and B streptococci may also occasionally cause this disorder. Further subclassification of streptococci is made based on their ability to lyse sheep red blood cells in culture; beta-hemolytic strains cause hemolysis associated with a clear zone surrounding their colonies, while alpha-hemolytic strains cause partial hemolysis, and gamma-hemolytic strains cause no hemolysis. *Alpha-hemolytic strains are normal flora of the oral cavity and pharynx and should not be confused with the more pathogenic beta-hemolytic strains.*

The primary determinant of streptococcal pathogenicity is an antigenically distinct protein known as the M protein. This molecule is found within the fimbriae, which are fingerlike projections from the cell wall of the organism that facilitate adherence to pharyngeal and tonsillar epithelium. More than 120 M serotypes are known. The M protein allows *Streptococcus* to resist phagocytosis in the absence of type-specific antibody. In the immunocompetent host, synthesis of type-specific anti-M and other antibodies confers long-term serotype-specific immunity to the particular strain in question. In laboratory-produced penicillin-resistant strains of GABHS, M protein is absent, thereby rendering these strains more vulnerable to phagocytosis. This finding may help to explain why there have been no naturally occurring penicillin-resistant GABHS isolated in more than 70 years of penicillin use.

Group A beta-hemolytic streptococci are capable of elaborating at least 20 extracellular substances that affect host tissue. Among the most important are streptolysin O, an oxygen-labile hemolysin, and streptolysin S, an oxygen-stable hemolysin, which lyse erythrocytes and damage other cells such as myocardial cells. Streptolysin O is antigenic, while streptolysin S is not. Group A beta-hemolytic streptococci also produce 3 erythrogenic or pyrogenic toxins (A, B, and C) whose activity is similar to that of bacterial endotoxin. Other agents of significance include exotoxin A, which may be associated with toxic shock syndrome, and bacteriocins, which destroy other gram-positive organisms. Spread of infection may be facilitated by a variety of enzymes elaborated by GABHS, which attack fibrin and hyaluronic acid.

Signs and symptoms of GABHS pharyngotonsillitis are acute in onset, usually characterized by high fever, odynophagia, headache, and abdominal pain. However, presentation may vary from mild sore throat and malaise (30%–50% of cases) to high fever, nausea and vomiting, and dehydration (10%). Pharyngeal and tonsillar mucosa are typically erythematous and occasionally edematous, with exudate present in 50% to 90% of cases. Cervical adenopathy is also common and is seen in 30% to 60% of cases. Most patients improve spontaneously in 3 to 5 days, unless otitis media, sinusitis, or peritonsillar abscess occurs secondarily.

The risk of rheumatic fever following GABHS infection of the pharynx is approximately 0.3% in endemic situations and 3% under epidemic circumstances. A single episode of rheumatic fever places an individual at high risk for recurrence following additional episodes of GABHS pharyngitis. Acute glomerulonephritis occurs as a sequela in 10% to 15% of patients infected with nephritogenic strains. In patients who develop these sequelae, there is usually a latent period of 1 to 3 weeks.

Pediatric autoimmune neuropsychiatric disorder associated with group A streptococcal infection (PANDAS) has been described as a selective immunopathy similar to Sydenham chorea in which the response to streptococcal infection leads to dysfunction in the basal ganglia, resulting in tic, obsessive-compulsive, and affective disorders. Classically, behaviors are abrupt in onset and must have some temporal relationship to infection by GABHS. Clinical improvement has been reported among some patients treated with antibiotics, particularly as prophylaxis against recurrence. However, a cause-and-effect association of PANDAS with GABHS infection has yet to be established. Many experts believe that as has been observed with other stressors, infection of any kind may provoke the neuropsychiatric phenomena.

Early diagnosis of streptococcal pharyngitis has been a priority in management of the disease, primarily because of the risk of renal and cardiac sequelae. A number of authors have studied the predictive value of various combinations of signs and symptoms in an effort to distinguish streptococcal from non-streptococcal pharyngitis; however, none of these has been particularly reliable. Taken together, these studies demonstrate a false-negative rate of about 50% and a false-positive rate of 75%. Adenopathy, fever, and pharyngeal exudate have the highest predictive value for a positive culture and rise in anti-streptolysin O (ASO) titer, and absence of these findings in the presence of cough, rhinorrhea, hoarseness, or conjunctivitis most reliably predicts a negative culture, or positive culture without rise in ASO.

Most clinicians advocate throat culture as the gold standard to determine appropriate treatment for GABHS. However, tonsils, tonsillar crypts, or posterior pharyngeal wall must be swabbed for greatest accuracy. Tests for rapid detection of group-specific carbohydrate simplify the decision to treat at the time of the office visit and often eliminate the need for additional post-visit communication. However, while these tests have demonstrated a specificity of greater than 95%, their sensitivity is generally in the 70% to 90% range. As a result, many clinicians advocate throat culture for children with suspected streptococcal disease and negative rapid strep tests. Rapid antigen detection is usually more expensive than throat culture, and this technique must still be interpreted with care, given the high incidence of posttreatment carriers. Studies also suggest possible clinician bias in interpretation of the test.

Carriage of GABHS may be defined as a positive culture for the organism in the absence of a rise in ASO convalescent titer or absence of symptoms. The prevalence of GABHS carriers has been estimated at anywhere from 5% to 50% depending on the time of year and location; however, this figure is sometimes overestimated because of use of antibiotics that occasionally interfere with rise in ASO titer. Carriers are at low risk to transmit GABHS or to develop symptoms or sequelae of the disease. The importance of this condition is in the distinction of true acute streptococcal pharyngitis from non-streptococcal sore throat in a carrier. When this distinction is important, a baseline convalescent ASO titer should be drawn. A subsequent positive test may be defined as a twofold dilution increase in titer between acute and convalescent serum, or any single value above 333 Todd units in children. However, a low titer does not rule out acute infection, and a high titer may represent infection in the distant past. As a result, the American Academy of

Pediatrics and Infectious Diseases Society of America currently recommend that testing for GABHS should not be performed in children with conjunctivitis, cough, hoarseness, coryza, diarrhea, oral ulcerations, or other clinical manifestations highly suggestive of viral infection. Furthermore, it is critical that patients referred for potential tonsillectomy for "recurrent strep" be ruled out as carriers before they are considered candidates for surgery.

Although most upper respiratory infections by GABHS resolve without treatment, studies suggest that antimicrobial therapy prevents suppurative and nonsuppurative sequelae including rheumatic fever and may also hasten clinical improvement. Treatment is therefore indicated for most patients with positive rapid tests for the group A antigen. When the test result is negative or not available, one may treat for a few days while formal throat cultures are incubating.

Group A beta-hemolytic streptococcus is sensitive to a number of antibiotics, including penicillins, cephalosporins, macrolides, and clindamycin. Expert panels have designated penicillin the drug of choice in managing GABHS because of its track record of safety, efficacy, and narrow spectrum. To date, no strains of GABHS acquired in vivo have demonstrated penicillin resistance or increased minimum inhibitory concentrations in vitro. Beginning in the 1980s, several studies reported a decrease in bacteriologic control rates, attributed primarily to inoculum effects and increased tolerance to penicillin. Whether cephalosporins may achieve greater eradication of GABHS than penicillin remains controversial.

Depot benzathine penicillin G is still advocated by the American Heart Association for primary treatment of GABHS pharyngitis; however, a 10-day course of penicillin orally is the most widely prescribed regimen. Twice-daily dosing by the enteral route yields results similar to those obtained with 4-times-a-day dosing. Courses of shorter duration are associated with bacteriologic relapse and are less efficacious in prevention of rheumatic fever. Amoxicillin appears to have efficacy equal to that of penicillin. In poorly compliant or penicillin-allergic patients, azithromycin dosed once daily for 5 days may be a reasonable alternative. Erythromycin is now used less commonly than in the past because of its gastrointestinal side effects.

Most patients with positive culture results following treatment are GABHS carriers; these individuals need not be retreated if their symptoms have resolved. For patients in whom complete bacteriologic clearance is desirable, such as those with a family member with a history of rheumatic fever, a course of clindamycin or a second course of penicillin combined with rifampin may yield increased success. In patients with recurrent symptoms, serotyping may aid in distinguishing bacterial persistence from recurrence. There are no data available about the use of antibiotic prophylaxis in these patients, and in such cases tonsillectomy may sometimes be advantageous.

During antimicrobial therapy, patients must be monitored carefully for fluid intake, pain control, and impending suppurative complications such as peritonsillar abscess. Small children may become dehydrated rapidly and may require hospitalization for administration of fluids intravenously.

Pearls

1. Symptoms of group A beta-hemolytic streptococcus (GABHS) infection resolve without treatment; the purpose of antimicrobial therapy is prevention of suppurative and nonsuppurative sequelae.

2. No naturally occurring penicillin-resistant GABHS have been identified.

3. Patients with recurrent sore throat need not be cultured if symptoms are otherwise suggestive of viral illness.

4. The importance of identifying GABHS carriers is in distinguishing their likely viral sore throats from true acute streptococcal infection.

5. Carriers rarely spread GABHS to close contacts, and there is no evidence that the disease is spread by pets or toothbrushes.

6. Asymptomatic patients with positive culture results following treatment need not be retreated.

INFECTIOUS MONONUCLEOSIS, EPSTEIN-BARR VIRAL INFECTION, AND POSTTRANSPLANTATION LYMPHOPROLIFERATIVE DISORDER

Pharyngitis is one of the hallmarks of infectious mononucleosis, a disorder associated with primary infection by EBV. The universality of exposure to EBV is demonstrated by studies in populations around the world in which 80% to 95% of adults have exhibited serologic reactivity to EBV antigens. However, while primary infection by EBV occurs during the second and third decade in developed nations and regions of high socioeconomic status, young children may still be exposed, especially in developing countries and regions of low socioeconomic status. When the virus is acquired at a younger age, symptoms are generally less severe.

Incidence of infectious mononucleosis in the United States is approximately 1 per 50,000 to 100,000 per year, but increases to about 100 per 100,000 among adolescents and young adults. Infected individuals transmit EBV by way of saliva exchanged during kissing or other close contact.

Epstein-Barr virus is a member of the herpesvirus family that preferentially infects and transforms human B lymphocytes. The virus enters the cell by attaching to a receptor designed for proteins of the complement chain, and its genetic material is transported by vesicles to the nucleus, where it dwells as a plasmid and maintains a latent state of replication. An incubation period of 2 to 7 weeks follows initial exposure, during which EBV induces a proliferation of infected B cells. This process is subsequently countered by a potent cellular immune response, characterized by the appearance of atypical lymphocytes (most likely T lymphocytes responding to the B-cell infection) in the blood. The number of infected circulating B cells is reduced during this 4- to 6-week period.

Infectious mononucleosis is characterized by a prodrome of malaise and fatigue, followed by acute onset of fever and sore throat. Physical examination typically reveals enlarged, erythematous palatine tonsils, in most cases with yellow-white exudate on the surface and within the crypts. Cervical adenopathy is present in nearly all patients, and involvement of the posterior cervical nodes often helps distinguish EBV infection from that by streptococcus or other organisms. Between the second and fourth weeks of illness, approximately 50% of patients develop splenomegaly, and 30% to 50% develop hepatomegaly. Rash, palatal petechiae, and abdominal pain may also be present in some cases. Fever and pharyngitis generally subside within about 2 weeks, while adenopathy, organomegaly, and malaise may last as long as 6 weeks.

Diagnosis of infectious mononucleosis can usually be made on the basis of clinical presentation, absolute lymphocytosis, presence of atypical lymphocytes in the peripheral smear, and detection of Paul-Bunnell heterophil antibodies. The latter is the basis of monospot assays, which screen for agglutination of horse erythrocytes. Children younger than 5 years may not develop a detectable heterophil antibody titer; in these patients, it is possible to determine titers of IgG antibodies to the viral capsid antigen, as well as antibodies to the early antigen complex. Antibodies to EBV nuclear antigen appear late in the course of disease (Table 9-1). In most cases, rest, fluids, and analgesics are adequate to manage symptoms of infectious mononucleosis. In more symptomatic patients, particularly those with respiratory compromise caused by severe tonsillar enlargement and those with hematologic or neurologic complications, a course of systemic steroids may hasten resolution of acute symptoms. Placement of a nasopharyngeal trumpet or endotracheal intubation may be necessary on rare occasions when complete airway obstruction is imminent. Antibiotics may be useful in cases of concomitant group A beta-hemolytic pharyngotonsillitis; however, ampicillin use is known to induce a rash in this setting.

The use of antiviral agents in infectious mononucleosis has yielded disappointing results. In clinical trials, acyclovir reduced viral shedding in the pharynx but demonstrated little efficacy in the treatment of symptoms. Other agents have exhibited greater in vitro effect than acyclovir but have yet to be tested clinically.

Exposure to EBV has been implicated in the development of post-transplantation lymphoproliferative disorder (PTLD). Children who have received bone marrow and solid organ transplants may develop abnormal proliferation of lymphoid cells in the setting of immunosuppression; approximately 80% of affected individuals have a history of

Table 9-1. Expected Results of Serologic Testing for Epstein-Barr Virus

	Never Been EBV Infected	EBV Infected Now	EBV Infected in Past
Antiviral capsid antigen	Negative	Positive	Positive
Anti–Epstein-Barr nuclear antigen	Negative	Negative	Positive

Abbreviation: EBV, Epstein-Barr virus.

EBV infection. Epstein-Barr virus seronegative transplant recipients may develop acute EBV infection from environmental exposure or from the EBV seropositive donor once they become immunosuppressed. Clinical presentation is variable and can mimic graft-versus-host disease, graft rejection, or more conventional infections. Signs and symptoms may resemble an infectious mononucleosis–like illness or an extra-nodal tumor, commonly involving the gut, brain, or transplanted organ. Mononucleosis-like presentations typically occur in children within the first year after transplant and are often associated with primary EBV infection after transfer of donor virus from the grafted organ. Extra-nodal tumors are more common among EBV-seropositive recipients several years after transplant. Studies have shown that young age at the time of transplant and EBV seronegativity conferred increased risk of adenotonsillar hyperplasia, which may be a precursor to PTLD. A higher incidence of PTLD has also been demonstrated with use of more potent immunosuppressive agents.

Initial management involves reduction of immunosuppression with care to preserve the transplanted organ. Patients who do not tolerate or respond to reduction of immunosuppression require more aggressive therapy and often have a poorer prognosis. Additional treatments include antivirals such as acyclovir and ganciclovir, antibody therapy, interferon, chemotherapy, and radiation therapy, with varying results. Prognosis is poor with mortality rates as high as 50% to 90%. Novel forms of immunotherapy have been tested in PTLD, including antibody and cell-mediated approaches.

Pearls

1. Children younger than 5 years may not develop a detectable heterophil antibody titer and should therefore have serologic testing for Epstein-Barr viral capsid antigen and early antigen.

2. Patients with a history of organ transplantation who develop tonsil enlargement should be evaluated for posttransplantation lymphoproliferative disorder, a condition linked to Epstein-Barr virus infection.

PERITONSILLAR INFECTION

Peritonsillar infection may present as cellulitis or abscess (PTA). Most cases are thought to represent a suppurative complication of tonsil infection. Peritonsillar infection occurs more commonly in adolescents and young adults than in young children. Affected patients present with symptoms of sore throat, odynophagia, fever, voice change, and otalgia. Common physical findings include fever, drooling, trismus, muffled "hot potato" voice, and pharyngeal asymmetry with inferior and medial displacement of the tonsil. Radiographic evaluation is usually not necessary but may be useful in young or uncooperative children or equivocal cases. Although some authors have found intraoral ultrasound to be useful in adults, computed tomography with contrast remains the imaging modality of choice in children.

While patients with peritonsillar cellulitis may be treated with antibiotics alone, most abscesses require removal of the pus as definitive therapy. Evacuation of PTA can be managed by needle aspiration, incision and drainage, or immediate (quinsy) tonsillectomy with nearly equivalent efficacy. In very young or poorly cooperative patients, or in those in whom an abscess has been inadequately drained, tonsillectomy is curative and essentially eliminates any chance of recurrence.

Abscess cultures usually reveal a polymicrobial infection, often containing gram-positive organisms and anaerobes. Appropriate antimicrobial therapy in the emergency department or office setting would include initial parenteral administration of penicillin with or without metronidazole, clindamycin, or ampicillin-sulbactam. Options for oral therapy include amoxicillin-clavulanate, penicillin, and clindamycin, although children may resist taking the latter due to its taste. Intravenous hydration should also be considered for those individuals who have not been able to take liquids orally.

The efficacy of tonsillectomy in the prevention of recurrent PTA has not been compared with that of watchful waiting in a prospective, controlled trial. In the only large retrospective cohort investigation on the subject, Kronenberg et al studied 290 patients and demonstrated an increased rate of recurrent PTA among those who also had recurrent tonsillitis. A later study by the same group showed no difference in recurrent PTA based on prior history of tonsillitis but included only 38 patients. Other case series suggest that recurrence may be predicted based on a history of 2 to 3 episodes of acute tonsillitis in the year prior to the initial episode; such a history has been elicited in 15% to 30% of patients with PTA. Based on available evidence, it has been suggested that routine elective or quinsy tonsillectomy is not indicated for patients who present with their first PTA. However, if a patient is a candidate for elective tonsillectomy for other reasons (eg, 2 to 3 tonsillitis events in the previous 12 months), it seems rational to perform a quinsy tonsillectomy for treatment or to proceed with planned elective tonsillectomy after successful abscess drainage.

> **Pearls**
>
> 1. Quinsy, or urgent, tonsillectomy should be considered for patients with peritonsillar abscess (PTA) whose abscesses cannot be drained in an ambulatory setting.
>
> 2. Tonsillectomy after PTA management is a consideration for patients who have had 2 to 3 episodes of tonsillitis in the previous year.

CHRONIC TONSILLITIS

Chronic tonsillitis is poorly defined in the literature but may be the appropriate terminology for sore throat of at least 3 months' duration accompanied by physical findings of tonsillar inflammation. Affected individuals may report symptoms of chronic sore throat, halitosis, or debris or concretions in the tonsil crypts known as tonsilloliths, in which the presence of biofilms has been implicated. Affected patients may also have persisting cervical adenopathy. Throat culture results in such cases are usually negative. Although there exist no clinical trials to help guide medical management of such patients, tonsillectomy is a reasonable consideration for those patients who do not respond to improved oropharyngeal hygiene and aggressive antibiotic therapy.

RECURRENT TONSILLITIS AND TONSILLECTOMY

When tonsils have been recurrently or chronically infected, the controlled process of antigen transport and presentation is altered because of shedding of the transporting M cells from the tonsil epithelium. As a result, tonsillar lymphocytes can theoretically become overwhelmed with persistent antigenic stimulation, rendering them unable to respond to antigens or function adequately in local protection or reinforcement of the upper respiratory secretory immune system. Furthermore, direct influx of antigens disproportionately expands the population of mature B-cell clones and as a result, fewer early memory B cells go on to become J-chain positive IgA immunocytes. There would therefore appear to be a therapeutic advantage to removing recurrently or chronically diseased tonsils. The surgeon should bear in mind, however, that tonsillectomy and adenoidectomy procedures remove a source of immunocompetent cells, and some studies demonstrate minor alterations of immunoglobulin concentrations in adjacent tissues following tonsillectomy.

Cultures from deeper tissues of recurrently infected tonsils frequently reveal unusual pathogens including *Staphylococcus aureus*, *H influenzae*, *Actinomycetes*, *Chlamydia*, *Mycoplasma*, and anaerobes; however, it remains unclear whether such cultures truly represent the offending organisms. Several studies suggest that bacteria in biofilms may be more important in recurrent tonsillitis than their planktonic counterparts.

Recurrent sore throat of a noninfectious nature is a hallmark of periodic fever, aphthous stomatitis, pharyngitis, and adenopathy (PFAPA), or Marshall syndrome. This disorder occurs primarily in children younger than 5 years and usually lasts more than 5 days and recurs at regular intervals of 3 to 6 weeks. Systemic steroids and cimetidine have demonstrated efficacy in controlling the events. Two small, randomized, controlled trials demonstrated that tonsillectomy was effective for treating PFAPA, but children in the control groups also showed improvement. Tonsillectomy may be considered based on frequency of illness, severity of infection, and child's response to medical management.

Appropriate medical and surgical management of children with recurrent infectious pharyngotonsillitis depends on accurate documentation of the cause and severity of individual episodes as well as frequency of the events. The clinician should record for each event a subjective assessment of the patient's severity of illness; physical findings including body temperature, pharyngeal or tonsillar erythema, tonsil size, tonsillar exudate, and cervical adenopathy (presence, size, and tenderness); and the results of microbiologic testing for GABHS. A summary of the documentation should be made available to the consultant to aid in medical decision-making about potential surgical intervention. In children with recurrent sore throat whose test results for GABHS are repeatedly positive, it may be desirable to rule out streptococcal carriage concurrent with viral infection, as carriers are unlikely to transmit GABHS or develop suppurative complications or nonsuppurative sequelae of the disease such as acute rheumatic fever. Supportive documentation in children who meet criteria for tonsillectomy may include absence from school, spread of infection within the family, and family history of rheumatic heart disease or glomerulonephritis.

In all randomized, controlled trials of tonsillectomy for infection, sore throat with each event was a necessary entrance criterion, and in most of these trials sore throat was the primary outcome studied. As a result, no claim can be made that tonsillectomy is indicated for children whose constellation of symptoms does not include sore throat, even when GABHS can be cultured from the throat. These studies also suggest that patients whose events are less severe or well documented do not gain sufficient benefit from tonsillectomy to justify the risk and morbidity of the procedure; in such patients, tonsillectomy should be considered only after a period of observation during which documentation of additional events may be made.

Children with frequent recurrences of throat infection over a period of several months demonstrate high rates of spontaneous resolution. As a result, an observation period of at least 12 months is generally recommended prior to consideration of tonsillectomy. In rare cases, early surgery may reasonably be considered for severely affected patients, such as those with histories of hospitalization for recurrent severe infections, rheumatic heart disease in the family, or numerous repeat infections in a single household (ping-pong spread), or those with complications of infection such as PTA or Lemierre syndrome (thrombophlebitis of the internal jugular vein).

Observation of patients is also a reasonable management strategy in children who have had frequent recurrences of pharyngotonsillitis for more than one year. In several studies, children who have not had tonsillectomies demonstrated spontaneous improvement during the follow-up period, often with patients no longer meeting the original criteria for study entry. Additional information about the natural history of recurrent pharyngotonsillitis is found in case series describing outcomes for patients on wait-list tonsillectomy; many children who were reevaluated after months on such lists no longer met criteria for surgery.

Tonsillectomy has been suggested for centuries as a means of controlling recurrent infection of the throat. However, clinical trials investigating the efficacy of tonsillectomy have had a high risk of bias because of poorly defined entrance criteria, nonrandom selection of operated subjects, exclusion of severely affected patients, or reliance on caregivers for postoperative data collection. In the most frequently cited and meticulous trial, Paradise and colleagues included patients only if their episodes of throat infection met strict criteria as outlined in Table 9-2. The key findings of the study were as follows:

- A mean rate reduction of 1.9 episodes of sore throat per year among children with tonsillectomies during the first year of follow-up compared with controls. However, sore throat associated with performance of the surgery (which would otherwise count as one episode) was excluded from the data. In the control group, patients also improved compared with their preenrollment frequency of infection, experiencing a mean of only 3.1 annual events. Differences between groups were reduced in the second year and not significant by the third year of follow-up.

- For episodes of *moderate or severe* throat infection, the control group experienced 1.2 episodes compared with 0.1 in the surgical group. Rate reductions diminished over the subsequent 2 years of follow-up and were not significant in the third year.

- Mean days with sore throat in the first 12 months were not statistically different between the 2 groups but included a predictable period of sore throat postoperatively.

Table 9-2. Paradise Criteria for Tonsillectomy in Recurrent Tonsillitis	
Criterion	**Definition**
Frequency of sore throat events	7 or more episodes in the preceding year, OR 5 or more episodes in each of the preceding 2 years, OR 3 or more episodes in each of the preceding 3 years
Clinical features (one required in addition to sore throat)	Temperature >38.3°C, OR Cervical lymphadenopathy (tender lymph nodes or >2 cm), OR Tonsillar exudate, OR Positive culture for GABHS
Treatment	Antibiotics are administered at appropriate dose for proven or suspected episodes of GABHS.
Documentation	Each episode and its qualifying characteristics are synchronously documented in the medical record, OR In cases of insufficient documentation, 2 subsequent episodes of throat infection are observed by the clinician with frequency and clinical features consistent with the initial history.

Abbreviation: GABHS, group A beta-hemolytic streptococcus.

From Baugh RF, Archer SM, Mitchell RB, et al. Clinical practice guideline: tonsillectomy in children. *Otolaryngol Head Neck Surg.* 2011;144(1 Suppl):S1–S30. Reprinted by permission of SAGE Publications.

In a subsequent study by the same authors, entrance criteria were relaxed, with less rigorous criteria for the number of episodes, clinical features required, and documentation (ie, 4 to 6 episodes in the last year or 3 to 4 episodes per year in the last 2 years). In the 2 arms of the study (tonsillectomy or adenotonsillectomy vs control, and adenotonsillectomy vs control), patients undergoing surgery experienced rate reductions of 0.8 and 1.7 episodes per year, respectively, in the first year. For episodes of moderate or severe sore throat, control subjects in the 2 arms of the study combined experienced 0.3 episodes per year overall, compared with 0.1 episodes per year in subjects undergoing surgery. Mean days with sore throat in the first 12 months were not statistically different in either arm of the study. Investigators concluded that the modest benefit conferred by tonsillectomy in children moderately affected with recurrent throat infection did not justify inherent risks, morbidity, and cost of the surgery.

A randomized, controlled trial comparing tonsillectomy with watchful waiting in children aged 2 to 8 years examined temperature above 38.0°C for at least 1 day as the primary outcome measure. During a mean follow-up of 22 months, children in the tonsillectomy group had 0.2 fewer episodes of fever per person year; from 6 to 24 months there was no difference between the groups. The surgical group also demonstrated, per person year, mild reductions in throat infections (0.2), sore throats (0.6), days with sore throat (5.9), and upper respiratory tract infections (0.5).

Pooled data from these studies were also analyzed in a Cochrane systematic review. Patients undergoing tonsillectomy experienced 1.4 fewer episodes of sore throat in the first year compared with the control group; however, the "cost" of this reduction was 1.0 episodes of sore throat in the immediate postoperative period. Another systematic review suggested a 43% overall reduction in sore throat events. The number needed to treat with tonsillectomy to prevent 1 sore throat per month for the first year after surgery was 11. A third systematic review that included 13 randomized, controlled trials and non-randomized, controlled studies on the efficacy of tonsillectomy in children reported pooled estimated risk differences favoring tonsillectomy over observation of 1.2 fewer episodes of sore throat, 2.8 fewer days of school absence, and 0.5 fewer episodes of upper respiratory infection per person-year.

Despite modest advantages conferred by tonsillectomy for sore throat, studies of quality of life universally suggest a significant improvement in patients undergoing the procedure. Only 2 of these studies enrolled children exclusively, and both reported improved scores in nearly all subscales. However, both also had numerous methodologic flaws including enrollment of patients with "chronic tonsillitis" without definition based on signs and symptoms, absence of a control group, low response rates with potential selection bias, poor follow-up, and caregiver collection of data.

A recent guideline on tonsillectomy suggests that tonsillectomy for severely affected children with recurrent throat infection should be considered an option. Families of patients who meet appropriate criteria for tonsillectomy must weigh modest anticipated benefits of tonsillectomy for this indication against the natural history of resolution and risk of surgical morbidity and complications.

Pearls

1. Recurrent tonsillitis may result from abnormal antigen processing due to repeated infectious insults to the tonsil epithelium.

2. Tonsillectomy should be considered an option in the management of recurrent acute tonsillitis meeting the strict criteria of frequency, severity, and documentation listed in Table 9-2.

3. No claim can be made that tonsillectomy is indicated for children whose constellation of symptoms does not include sore throat, even when GABHS can be cultured from the throat.

RECURRENT AND CHRONIC ADENOIDITIS

Disorders characterized in children as adenoiditis, rhinosinusitis, and nasopharyngitis are not easily distinguished from one another on the basis of symptoms. Most individuals in whom diagnosis is made present with nasal stuffiness, mucopurulent rhinorrhea, chronic cough, halitosis, and "snorting" or "gagging" on mucus throughout the day. Diagnosis of recurrent or chronic adenoiditis was based in one study on 3 or more months of chronic or recurrent nasal discharge associated with persistent or recurrent otitis media. In another, the disorder was characterized by a constellation of findings including mucopurulent exudates on the adenoid surface with or without inflammation, recurrent fever or cold with persistent cough or serous otitis, and enlargement of posterior tonsillar lymph nodes. However, there are no established criteria for making this diagnosis or differentiating it from viral upper respiratory illness or acute sinusitis.

In chronic or recurrent nasopharyngitis, persistence of disease may be caused by colonization by pathogenic bacteria. *H influenzae, Streptococcus pneumoniae, Streptococcus pyogenes,* and *S aureus* are commonly found in adenoid cultures and tissue samples among children so affected. Rates of drug-resistant bacteria may be higher among patients with chronic or recurrent infection. Furthermore, molecular typing of paired bacterial isolates from the adenoid and lateral nasal wall in children undergoing adenoidectomy demonstrates a high degree of correlation, and sinonasal symptom scores appear to correlate with quantitative bacteriology of the adenoid core and not with adenoid size. Several studies have demonstrated bacterial biofilm formation in the adenoid; however, it is not clear if this is more common in persistent and recurrent nasopharyngitis than in obstructive adenoid hyperplasia. In some patients, sinonasal infection is more likely caused by stasis of secretions secondary to obstructive adenoid tissue rather than bacterial factors, although the two may certainly be related. Gastroesophageal reflux has not been established as a cause of chronic adenoid inflammation.

Data suggest that adenoidectomy may be useful in management of children with persistent and recurrent sinonasal complaints, although systematic review indicates evidence is currently inadequate to firmly establish efficacy. Most clinicians favor adenoidectomy prior to consideration of endoscopic sinus surgery. The study by Weinberg et al suggests that children with recurrent acute symptoms may have greater benefit from adenoidectomy than those with more chronic sinonasal disease.

> **Pearl:** Adenoidectomy is a reasonable alternative to repeated pharmacotherapy and endoscopic sinus surgery in patients with well-documented recurrent or chronic sinonasal illness.

OTITIS MEDIA AND ADENOIDITIS

Proximity of the adenoid pad to the eustachian tube has prompted a number of clinicians to study potential benefits of adenoidectomy and adenotonsillectomy in the management of otitis media. The effect of the adenoid on the eustachian tube is likely one of regional inflammation or infection rather than one of direct compression.

Since 1980, there has been substantial evidence that adenoidectomy and perhaps adenotonsillectomy have a role in the management of recurrent acute and chronic otitis media. However, some studies report results to the contrary, at least for recurrent acute otitis media. Benefit may be greatest for those children in whom the adenoid pad abuts the eustachian tube; however, such children can be identified only by preoperative nasopharyngoscopy.

Based on available data, it is reasonable that adenoidectomy be considered along with the first set of tubes if the child has significant symptoms of nasal obstruction or recurrent rhinorrhea, or when a second set of tubes is necessary, particularly for chronic middle ear effusion. Children with tympanostomy tubes who develop otorrhea refractory to management with topical or systemic antibiotics may also reasonably be considered candidates for adenoidectomy. In children with a history of cleft palate, the procedure should be performed only when the otitis is relentless; in such cases, an inferior strip of adenoid should be preserved to avoid velopharyngeal insufficiency. Tonsillectomy with adenoidectomy carries additional morbidity and has less support in the literature. Tonsillectomy is a reasonable additional procedure when indications such as airway obstruction or recurrent pharyngitis are also present.

> **Pearl:** Adenoidectomy may be considered for the indication of chronic otitis media
> - With the first set of tubes if the child has significant symptoms of nasal obstruction or recurrent rhinorrhea
> - When a second set of tubes is necessary, particularly for chronic middle ear effusion
> - For children with refractory tympanostomy tube otorrhea

■ Hyperplasia of Tonsils and Adenoid

UPPER AIRWAY OBSTRUCTION AND SLEEP-RELATED BREATHING DISORDERS

When lymphoid tissue occupies a disproportionate amount of space in the pharynx, the upper airway becomes compromised. The condition can be exacerbated by other anatomic conditions, such as those seen in obesity, achondroplasia, mucopolysaccharidoses, or craniofacial syndromes, or by dynamic collapse such as occurs in the supine position and under conditions of diminished neuromuscular tone such as sleep, Down syndrome, and cerebral palsy.

Hyperplasia of the tonsils and adenoid in children is commonly associated with pharyngeal obstruction. During the daytime, children with an enlarged adenoid demonstrate mouth breathing, rhinorrhea, and hyponasal speech, while those with tonsil hyperplasia may exhibit a muffled, "hot potato" voice. However, the obstruction is even more apparent during sleep, when relaxation of pharyngeal musculature exacerbates resistance to airflow. Affected children often snore loudly with intermittent audible gasps, sternal retractions, and paradoxical motion of the chest. Attempts to overcome obstruction by increasing respiratory effort often exaggerate collapse of the airway, resulting in a paradoxical increase in resistance to airflow. The physiologic sequelae may include hypoxemia, hypercapnia, and acidosis, which in turn signal central and peripheral chemoreceptors and baroreceptors to initiate pharyngeal dilation and arousals. Poor-quality sleep may result, and affected children often demonstrate daytime tiredness or hyperactivity as well as behavioral problems. Collectively, disturbances in sleep caused by obstruction are known as sleep-related breathing disorders (SRBD).

Sleep-related breathing disorders comprise a spectrum of obstructive breathing maladies. Children affected by upper airway resistance syndrome (UARS) demonstrate symptoms of snoring, mouth breathing, and sleep pauses without apnea or hypopnea. The hallmark of UARS is a significant elevation in respiratory effort-related arousals resulting in daytime fatigue but not sleepiness. Insomnia and somatic complaints are also common. More severely affected patients may have obstructive hypopnea syndrome or obstructive sleep apnea syndrome (OSAS). Untreated patients may, over time, develop cor pulmonale, right ventricular hypertrophy, congestive heart failure, alveolar hypoventilation, pulmonary hypertension, pulmonary edema, or failure to thrive and are at risk for permanent neurologic damage and even death. While the prevalence of OSAS in the pediatric population is 1% to 4%, as many as 10% of children have primary snoring.

Physical examination of children with SRBD should include assessment of the patient's weight and body mass index, as well as auscultation of the patient's heart and lungs. A complete examination of the head and neck is critical, with special attention to potential nonlymphoid sites of obstruction, including hypoplasia of the midface and mandible and nasopharyngeal or choanal pathology. Patients with adenoid enlargement often present with adenoid facies (open mouth, flat midface, dark discoloration under the eyes).

Tonsil size is best determined in a neutral state (ie, without the child gagging on a tongue depressor) to accurately estimate the volume of the pharynx they occupy. Tonsil hyperplasia is graded visually, most commonly using a scale of 1 to 4, as demonstrated in Figure 9-1. However, studies suggest that tonsil size as estimated by this scale does not always correlate with polysomnographic results.

In the primary care setting, evaluation of adenoid size is best accomplished using lateral neck radiographs to assess the anteroposterior dimension of the adenoid; however, correlation between

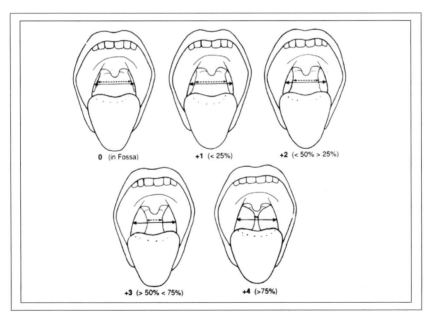

Figure 9-1. Assessment tool for tonsil size. Percentages represent portion of transverse dimension of airway occupied by tonsil tissue. From Brodsky L. Modern assessment of tonsils and adenoids. *Pediatr Clin North Am.* 1989;36(6): 1551–1569, with permission from Elsevier.

radiographically enlarged adenoid tissue and sleep apnea is lacking. In addition, results and interpretation are technique-sensitive, requiring an experienced radiology technician to achieve appropriate penetration and direct lateral projection without palate elevation. Another disadvantage is the exposure, though limited, to external beam radiation. Direct visualization can also be performed by fiber-optic endoscopy in the otolaryngologist's office.

Hyperplasia of the tonsils and adenoid increases the likelihood of airway obstruction; consequently, most otolaryngologists will perform an adenotonsillectomy when clinical history correlates well with clinical findings of adenotonsillar hyperplasia. However, the severity of obstruction during sleep often cannot be determined by static examination in the office setting, with clinical evaluation yielding a success rate of only 25% to 75% in predicting who has OSAS. As a result, the gold standard for diagnosis and quantification of SRBD is full-night polysomnography. Polysomnography objectively correlates ventilatory abnormalities with physiologic changes including electroencephalogram and electrocardiogram changes, limb movement, and body position. The study also determines sleep onset latency, sleep efficiency, and sleep staging. An obstructive apnea is defined as a greater than 90% drop in signal amplitude of airflow for greater than 90% of the entire event, compared with the pre-event baseline amplitude, with continued chest wall and abdominal movement, for a duration of at least 2 breaths. A hypopnea is always obstructive and is defined as a greater than 50% drop in airflow signal amplitude compared with the pre-event baseline amplitude for at least 90% of the duration of the event; the event must last at least 2 missed breaths and should be associated with an arousal, awakening, or greater than 3% desaturation. Severity is generally quantified based on the obstructive apnea hypopnea index (OAHI). The OAHI is the total number of obstructive apneas and hypopneas divided by the total duration of sleep in hours. Although there is no consensus on the definition of OSAS in children, an OAHI of less than or equal to 1 is considered within normal limits. An OAHI of 1 to 5 is very mildly increased; 5 to 10 is mildly increased; 10 to 15 is moderately increased; and greater than 15 is severely abnormal. Unfortunately, polysomnography is expensive, time-consuming, and often unavailable. Other techniques of assessment, such as audiotaping, videotaping, and home and abbreviated polysomnography, may be helpful but are far less accurate.

The systemic effects of SRBD are protean. Studies suggest that children with even mild OSAS demonstrate a morning blood pressure surge, and those with OAHI greater than 5 show increased blood pressure load and 24-hour ambulatory blood pressure, leading to cardiac hypertrophy. An association with enuresis has also been demonstrated in up to 50% of children with SRBD. The mechanism by which this occurs is not established, but theories include alterations in normal arousal and self-alerting mechanisms, hormonal changes (lower levels of antidiuretic hormone), and increased intra-abdominal pressure.

In behavioral studies, children with SRBD demonstrate significantly higher prevalence rates of problematic behaviors, including internalized (eg, withdrawal, shyness, anxiety) and externalized (eg, emotional lability, impulsivity, hyperactivity, aggressiveness, oppositional personality, somatic complaints, social problems) behaviors, compared with controls. The strongest, most consistent associations are for externalizing, hyperactive-type behaviors. Even children with primary snoring and OAHI less than 5 have been found to perform worse than controls on measures related to attention, social problems, and anxious or depressive symptoms, as well as overall cognitive abilities and some language and visuospatial functions. As a result, the polysomnographic level at which intervention should be considered for children with SRBD and problem behaviors remains unclear.

Neurocognitive impairment is also noted in children with SRBD and appears to be more severe in children with OSAS than in those with primary snoring. It has been suggested that such impairment may result from hypoxemia-induced dysfunction of the frontal lobe. Verbal abilities and language scores are also reduced in children with severe OSAS or severe hypoxemia, but data yield conflicting results of the effect of less severe forms of SRBD on such skills. Several studies have established a lower level of school performance among children with SRBD, and children with poor academic performance are also more likely to demonstrate sleep disturbances.

TONSIL AND ADENOID SURGERY FOR AIRWAY OBSTRUCTION

There are few randomized studies of the efficacy of tonsillectomy and adenoidectomy for SRBD in children; most investigations have been observational studies or systematic reviews of observational studies. Most have concluded that adenotonsillectomy should be considered first-line therapy for SRBD, providing the patient has at least mild adenotonsillar hyperplasia. Outcomes appear to improve regardless of the measure used. Polysomnographic improvement may be anticipated in 20% to 90%, depending on the criteria used to define OSAS and patient population studied. Among obese children with OSAS,

Pearls

1. Tonsil size does not always correlate with severity of airway obstructive as determined by polysomnography.

2. The primary care practitioner can assess adenoid size by ordering a soft tissue lateral radiograph of the adenoid pad.

3. Polysomnography is most useful

   a) When the degree of lymphoid hyperplasia does not correlate with the severity of presenting symptoms

   b) When accurate assessment of the degree of obstruction is imperative

   c) In the evaluation for continuous positive airway pressure in patients who have undergone adenotonsillectomy or may not be good candidates for surgery

although adenotonsillectomy improves quality of life and severity of obstruction, most patients have residual sleep disorder or airway obstruction. Children with allergies and craniofacial, neuromuscular, and genetic disorders are also known to be at high risk for persistent postoperative OSAS. Such patients are also at greater risk for postoperative complications, including early respiratory embarrassment, residual airway obstruction, and velopharyngeal insufficiency among those with cleft palate.

Children with tonsillar disease (including those with throat infections or SRBD) have been shown to score significantly lower than their healthy counterparts in several quality-of-life subscales, including general health, physical functioning, behavior, bodily pain, and caregiver effect. However, dramatic improvements in quality-of-life scores have been achieved following adenotonsillectomy in a number of studies, with follow-up as long as 3 years after surgery. Improvement reported by caregivers in most studies occurred irrespective of the severity of OSAS and without complete resolution of OSAS. Children with SRBD also have a significantly higher rate of health care utilization and cost, mostly because of complicated respiratory tract infections, requiring greater use of antibiotics and a 40% higher rate of hospital visits. In those children who subsequently underwent adenotonsillectomy, total health care costs were reduced by one-third, a change not observed among untreated control patients.

A reduction in problem behaviors and cognitive impairment in patients with SRBD has been reported following adenoidectomy or tonsillectomy. As an example, Mitchell and Kelly showed dramatic improvement in externalizing and internalizing behaviors in children with OSAS following adenotonsillectomy that were seen to persist up to 18 months after surgery and were independent of factors such as gender, age, ethnicity, parental education, and parental income. Interestingly, severity of problem behaviors in children with OSAS, as well as improvements after adenotonsillectomy, appear to be similar regardless of severity of sleep disorder. These results suggest that a diagnosis of SRBD should be entertained in children with behavioral problems and that these children may experience sustained benefits in behavior after adenotonsillectomy. Documentation of behavioral problems may affect the decision to undertake surgical therapy especially in children with mild OSAS.

Cognitive improvements following adenotonsillectomy have been demonstrated in several studies. As an example, Gozal found a 6- to 9-fold increase in the expected incidence of OSAS among first grade children who ranked in the lowest 10th percentile of their class. A significant improvement in academic performance followed adenotonsillectomy and resolution of OSAS; however, in some children, long-term residual deficits persisted even after treatment. As with behavior, caregivers of children with cognitive impairment or poor academic performance should be questioned about symptoms of SRBD, and surgery should be considered even in those cases deemed mild based on polysomnography.

Studies suggest that enuresis in children with SRBD resolves or improves in the majority of children after adenotonsillectomy. One study found that 61% of children no longer had enuresis and 23% had a decrease in bed-wetting after surgical therapy for SRBD. Other studies that have followed children beyond 1 year have reported similar results, with resolution rate increasing proportionally as time following surgery increases.

Pearls

1. Adenotonsillectomy is effective in reducing physiological, behavioral, and cognitive sequelae in patients with lymphoid hyperplasia and sleep apnea.

2. Some patients, especially those who are obese, develop recurrent obstructive apnea after tonsillectomy; the primary care practitioner should inquire about recurrent symptoms at subsequent well-child visits.

■ Malignancy of Tonsils or Adenoid

Pharyngeal malignancy, most notably lymphoma, may present as asymmetric tonsil hyperplasia. However, the vast majority of children with apparent tonsil asymmetry more commonly have asymmetric effacement of the tonsils by tonsillar pillars or benign asymmetry of the tonsils. In a series of children with unilateral tonsil enlargement, Berkowitz and Mahadevan observed that all patients with lymphoma experienced enlargement of the tonsil within a 6-week period prior to diagnosis, and most had additional signs and symptoms distinguishing their disease from benign tonsil hyperplasia, such as adenopathy greater than 3 cm, dysphagia, night sweats, and fevers. However, Dolev and Daniel reported that among 6 children identified with palatine tonsil lymphoma, all 6 presented at their first visit with no symptoms. In studies including adults, incidence of malignancy is low, and patients identified with tonsil malignancy have presented with symptoms. As a result, most children with tonsil asymmetry who do not also have symptoms of obstruction are not likely candidates for tonsillectomy. However, children with asymptomatic tonsil asymmetry should be followed for several months to monitor for symptoms suggestive of a malignant process.

Pearl: Children with tonsil asymmetry are generally not candidates for tonsillectomy unless they have symptoms of obstruction or symptoms or findings suggestive of a malignant process.

■ Other Tonsil and Adenoid Disorders

SPEECH IMPAIRMENT AND DYSPHAGIA

Hyperplasia of tonsil or adenoid tissue commonly results in decreased nasal airflow causing hyponasal or muffled speech. Language and articulation are not affected except in unusual patients with hypernasal speech due to impaired velopharyngeal closure secondary to tonsil enlargement. Rarely, severe enlargement of the tonsils or adenoid may cause dysphagia because of impairment of the pharyngeal phase of swallowing. Such patients will usually have greater difficulty swallowing solids than liquids. When tonsil hyperplasia interferes with velopharyngeal closure, dysphagia is greater for liquids and characterized by nasal regurgitation. In patients with adenoid hyperplasia, swallowing difficulties are more commonly related to poor coordination of breathing and swallowing. Dysphagia associated with failure to thrive and speech impairment due to unintelligible speech may be considered reasonable indications for adenotonsillectomy.

ABNORMAL DENTOFACIAL GROWTH

It has been postulated that chronic nasal obstruction from adeno-tonsillar hyperplasia may predispose some children to abnormalities of dentofacial growth. In such individuals, it is theorized that downward growth of the mandible and repositioning of the tongue compensates for the absence of nasal airflow by creating a larger oral airway. This results, in turn, in an increased vertical facial dimension and increased gonial angle. Absence of contact between the tongue and palate causes a high and narrow palatal vault and a secondary posterior dental crossbite.

Medical and dental literature in this area has been extensively reviewed by Klein and by Smith and Gonzalez and continues to be an area of interest in orthodontic research. Though there is clearly a correlation between chronic nasal obstruction and long face syndrome, a cause-and-effect relationship has never been established in humans. Differences in study outcomes in animal models and humans are the result of inadequate means of determining the ratio of nasal breathing to mouth breathing; absence of normative data addressing nasal volume and resistance by age, sex, and body weight; and inadequate length of follow-up. Although some data suggest that abnormalities of dentofacial growth in patients with adenotonsillar hyperplasia may be reversible, alterations may be minimal. Additional studies looking at more variables over a longer period of follow-up are necessary. In the interim, it behooves the otolaryngologist to evaluate children referred for adenotonsillectomy for orthodontic indications on a case-by-case basis and to consider the procedure only for those with significant adenotonsillar hyperplasia.

HALITOSIS

Halitosis may result from food debris and bacteria retained within crypts of the tonsils and adenoid. However, although bad breath is often cited as an indication of adenotonsillectomy, a wide variety of other causes, including periodontal disease, debris of the tongue or lingual tonsils, sinonasal infection or foreign body, and gastroesophageal reflux, should also be entertained. There are no clinical trials to support adenotonsillectomy for this indication.

HEMORRHAGIC TONSILLITIS

Recurrent bleeding from prominent tonsil vessels may be controlled by cautery in most cooperative patients. However, patients who experience recurrence or cannot cooperate in the office setting may require tonsillectomy if bleeding becomes a nuisance or causes a significant reduction in hemoglobin or hematocrit.

■ Tonsillectomy and Adenoidectomy

Tonsillectomy and adenoidectomy remain among the most commonly performed operations in children. Between 1915 and the 1960s, these were the most frequently performed surgical procedures in the United States. Traditionally, their popularity resulted from a desire to control recurrent infection for which there was no appropriate medical therapy. Later, the focus of infection theory was the primary indication for surgery, which assumed that localized infections in these tissues could lead to systemic disease in other parts of the body.

Over the last 3 decades, clinical trials and systematic reviews have demonstrated that tonsillectomy and adenoidectomy have only modest efficacy in relieving recurrent or persistent upper respiratory infections and middle ear disorders. However, during the same period there has been a greater awareness of the role of tonsil and adenoid hyperplasia in upper airway obstruction resulting in SRBD. As a result, incidence rates of tonsillectomy in the United States have significantly increased in the past 35 years, with SRBD being the primary indication for surgery. In

1970, the tonsillectomy rate was 126 procedures per 100,000 population, compared with 153 procedures per 100,000 in 2005. Coinciding with this has been a shift in indications for surgery from relief of recurrent infection to treatment of obstructive symptoms. In 1970, roughly 88% of tonsillectomies were done for infection indications, while approximately 23% were performed for this reason in 2005.

Primary care practitioners considering referral for tonsil or adenoid surgery must weigh the possibility that harm will result. Unfortunately, accurate statistics on mortality and morbidity in large patient populations are not readily available. Post-adenotonsillectomy complications are divided into perioperative, immediate postoperative, and delayed postoperative periods. Perioperative complications include hemorrhage; intubation trauma causing laryngeal injury, laryngospasm, or laryngeal edema; respiratory compromise or cardiac arrest; aspiration; malignant hyperthermia; and trauma to the teeth, pharyngeal wall, soft palate, or lips. Burns of the oral commissure are the most common complication for which litigation occurs after tonsillectomy. Hemorrhage, infections, postoperative pain, edema and hematoma of the uvula, and pulmonary complications are common immediate postoperative complications, while postoperative scarring of the soft palate or nasopharyngeal stenosis and tonsillar regrowth or remnant are delayed complications.

Hemorrhage, primary (within 24 hours of surgery) or secondary (more than 24 hours after surgery), is the most common serious complication of adenotonsillar surgery and is more likely to result from tonsillectomy than adenoidectomy. In published reports, rate of primary hemorrhage from tonsillectomy has ranged from 0.2% to 2.2% and rate of secondary hemorrhage from 0.1% to 3%. Fever is an accepted complication in the first 36 hours but will increase insensible water loss and predispose to dehydration. Parents need to be forewarned to maintain adequate hydration and should be given specific hydration goals as part of their discharge instructions. Dehydration may also result from nausea or vomiting secondary to anesthesia as well as swallowed blood and decreased oral intake secondary to pain. Younger children are especially prone as they are less cooperative and have less volume reserve. Mortality from tonsillectomy is estimated at 1 per 16,000 to 35,000 tonsillectomies, with about one-third attributable to primary bleeding and the majority related to anesthetic mishaps.

The surgeon or a surrogate must have postoperative contact with patients or their caregivers to ensure there have been no postoperative complications. This may be accomplished at an office visit or by telephone assessment 2 to 8 weeks after surgery. Caregivers should be questioned about resolution of obstruction (if present preoperatively), return to normal diet, and evidence of velopharyngeal insufficiency (excessive air escape with speech). Conversely, patients may develop recurrent obstruction or stenosis of the operated area months or years after the surgery; such patients have usually been discharged from the surgeon's care, and it is incumbent on the primary care professional to inquire about obstructive symptoms at follow-up visits.

Although some studies demonstrate minor alterations of immuno-globulin concentrations in the serum and adjacent tissues following tonsillectomy, there are no studies to date that demonstrate a significant clinical effect of tonsillectomy on the immune system. Heightened risk of poliomyelitis, which was an important deterrent to surgery before the advent of an effective vaccine and for which an immunologic basis was later elucidated, is no longer of practical concern in this era of virtually universal immunization. Finally, concern that tonsillectomy might predispose to the development of Hodgkin disease appears to have been dispelled by later epidemiologic investigations. Although it remains possible that the removal of immunologically active tonsils and adenoid will someday prove to undermine resistance to disease of some sort, the likelihood at present seems small.

> **Pearl:** There are no studies to date that demonstrate significant clinical effect of tonsillectomy on the immune system.

■ Selected References

Agren K, Nordlander B, Linder-Aronsson S, Zettergren-Wijk L, Svanborg E. Children with nocturnal upper airway obstruction: postoperative orthodontic and respiratory improvement. *Acta Otolaryngol.* 1998;118(4):581–587

Ali NJ, Pitson D, Stradling JR. Sleep disordered breathing: effects of adenotonsillectomy on behaviour and psychological functioning. *Eur J Pediatr.* 1996;155(1):56–62

Ali NJ, Pitson DJ, Stradling JR. Snoring, sleep disturbance, and behaviour in 4-5 year olds. *Arch Dis Child.* 1993;68(3):360–366

Al-Mazrou KA, Al-Khattaf AS. Adherent biofilms in adenotonsillar diseases in children. *Arch Otolaryngol Head Neck Surg.* 2008;134(1):20–23

American Academy of Pediatrics. Group A streptococcal infections. In: Pickering LK, Baker CJ, Kimberlin DW, Long SS, eds. *Red Book: 2009 Report of the Committee on Infectious Diseases.* 28th ed. Elk Grove Village, IL: American Academy of Pediatrics; 2009:616–628

American Academy of Pediatrics Section on Pediatric Pulmonology, Subcommittee on Obstructive Sleep Apnea Syndrome. Clinical practice guideline: diagnosis and management of childhood obstructive sleep apnea syndrome. *Pediatrics.* 2002;109(4):704–712

Amin R, Somers VK, McConnell K, et al. Activity-adjusted 24-hour ambulatory blood pressure and cardiac remodeling in children with sleep disordered breathing. *Hypertension.* 2008;51(1):84–91

Amin RS, Kimball TR, Bean JA, et al. Left ventricular hypertrophy and abnormal ventricular geometry in children and adolescents with obstructive sleep apnea. *Am J Respir Crit Care Med.* 2002;165(10):1395–1399

Andersson J, Britton S, Ernberg I, et al. Effect of acyclovir on infectious mononucleosis: a double-blind, placebo-controlled study. *J Infect Dis.* 1986;153(2):283–290

Avior G, Fishman G, Leor A, Sivan Y, Kaysar N, Derowe A. The effect of tonsillectomy and adenoidectomy on inattention and impulsivity as measured by the Test of Variables of Attention (TOVA) in children with obstructive sleep apnea syndrome. *Otolaryngol Head Neck Surg.* 2004;131(4):367–371

Aydil U, Ieri E, Kizil Y, Bodur S, Ceylan A, Uslu S. Obstructive upper airway problems and primary enuresis nocturna relationship in pediatric patients: reciprocal study. *J Otolaryngol Head Neck Surg.* 2008;37(2):235–239

Baldassari CM, Mitchell RB, Schubert C, Rudnick EF. Pediatric obstructive sleep apnea and quality of life: a meta-analysis. *Otolaryngol Head Neck Surg.* 2008;138(3):265–273

Basha S, Bialowas C, Ende K, Szeremeta W. Effectiveness of adenotonsillectomy in the resolution of nocturnal enuresis secondary to obstructive sleep apnea. *Laryngoscope.* 2005;115(6):1101–1103

Baugh RF, Archer SM, Mitchell RB, et al. Clinical practice guideline: tonsillectomy in children. *Otolaryngol Head Neck Surg.* 2011;144(1 Suppl):S1–S30

Beebe DW. Neurobehavioral morbidity associated with disordered breathing during sleep in children: a comprehensive review. *Sleep.* 2006;29(9):1115–1134

Beebe DW, Gozal D. Obstructive sleep apnea and the prefrontal cortex: towards a comprehensive model linking nocturnal upper airway obstruction to daytime cognitive and behavioral deficits. *J Sleep Res.* 2002;11(1):1–16

Berkowitz RG, Mahadevan M. Unilateral tonsillar enlargement and tonsillar lymphoma in children. *Ann Otol Rhinol Laryngol.* 1999;108(9):876–879

Bernstein JM, Dryja D, Murphy TF. Molecular typing of paired bacterial isolates from the adenoid and lateral wall of the nose in children undergoing adenoidectomy: implications in acute rhinosinusitis. *Otolaryngol Head Neck Surg.* 2001;125(6):593–597

Bhattacharjee R, Kheirandish-Gozal L, Spruyt K, et al. Adenotonsillectomy outcomes in treatment of obstructive sleep apnea in children: a multicenter retrospective study. *Am J Respir Crit Care Med.* 2010;182(5):676–683

Bisno AL, Gerber MA, Gwaltney JM Jr, Kaplan EL, Schwartz RH. Diagnosis and management of group A streptococcal pharyngitis: a practice guideline. Infectious Diseases Society of America. *Clin Infect Dis.* 1997;25(3):574–583

Bisno AL, Gerber MA, Gwaltney JM Jr, Kaplan EL, Schwartz RH; Infectious Diseases Society of America. Practice guidelines for the diagnosis and management of group A streptococcal pharyngitis. *Clin Infect Dis.* 2002;35(2):113–125

Blaivas M, Theodoro D, Duggal S. Ultrasound-guided drainage of peritonsillar abscess by the emergency physician. *Am J Emerg Med.* 2003;21(2):155–158

Blakley BW, Magit AE. The role of tonsillectomy in reducing recurrent pharyngitis: a systematic review. *Otolaryngol Head Neck Surg.* 2009;140(3):291–297

Bluestone CD, Klein JO. *Otitis Media in Infants and Children.* Philadelphia, PA: WB Saunders Co; 1995:215–223

Blunden S, Lushington K, Kennedy D. Cognitive and behavioural performance in children with sleep-related obstructive breathing disorders. *Sleep Med Rev.* 2001;5(6):447–461

Blunden S, Lushington K, Kennedy D, Martin J, Dawson D. Behavior and neurocognitive performance in children aged 5-10 years who snore compared to controls. *J Clin Exp Neuropsychol.* 2000;22(5):554–568

Böck A, Popp W, Herkner KR. Tonsillectomy and the immune system: a long-term follow up comparison between tonsillectomized and non-tonsillectomized children. *Eur Arch Otorhinolaryngol.* 1994;251(7):423–427

Boston M, McCook J, Burke B, Derkay C. Incidence of and risk factors for additional tympanostomy tube insertion in children. *Arch Otolaryngol Head Neck Surg.* 2003;129(3):293–296

Brandtzaeg P. Immune functions and immunopathology of palatine and nasopharyngeal tonsils. In: Bernstein JM, Ogra PL, eds. *Immunology of the Ear.* New York, NY: Raven Press; 1987:63–106

Brodsky L. Modern assessment of tonsils and adenoids. *Pediatr Clin North Am.* 1989;36(6):1551–1569

Brodsky L, Koch RJ. Bacteriology and immunology of normal and diseased adenoids in children. *Arch Otolaryngol Head Neck Surg.* 1993;119(8):821–829

Brook I, Shah K. Bacteriology of adenoids and tonsils in children with recurrent adenotonsillitis. *Ann Otol Rhinol Laryngol.* 2001;110(9):844–848

Brook I, Shah K, Jackson W. Microbiology of healthy and diseased adenoids. *Laryngoscope.* 2000;110(6):994–999

Brooks LJ, Stephens BM, Bacevice AM. Adenoid size is related to severity but not the number of episodes of obstructive apnea in children. *J Pediatr.* 1998;132(4):682–686

Brooks LJ, Topol HI. Enuresis in children with sleep apnea. *J Pediatr.* 2003;142(5):515–518

Burk CD, Miller L, Handler SD, Cohen AR. Preoperative history and coagulation screening in children undergoing tonsillectomy. *Pediatrics.* 1992;89(4 Pt 2):691–695

Burton MJ, Glasziou PP. Tonsillectomy or adeno-tonsillectomy versus non-surgical treatment for chronic/recurrent acute tonsillitis. *Cochrane Database Syst Rev.* 2009;1: CD001802

Canter RJ, Rogers J. Tonsillectomy: home after 24 hours? *J Laryngol Otol.* 1985;99(2):177–178

Capper JW, Randall C. Postoperative haemorrhage in tonsillectomy and adenoidectomy in children. *J Laryngol Otol.* 1984;98(4):363–365

Casey JR, Pichichero ME. Meta-analysis of cephalosporin versus penicillin treatment of group A streptococcal tonsillopharyngitis in children. *Pediatrics.* 2004;113(4):866–882

Cherry JD. Pharyngitis. In: Feigin RD, Cherry JD, eds. *Textbook of Pediatric Infectious Diseases.* 4th ed. Philadelphia, PA: WB Saunders Co; 1998:148–156

Chervin RD, Dillon JE, Bassetti C, Ganoczy DA, Pituch KJ. Symptoms of sleep disorders, inattention, and hyperactivity in children. *Sleep.* 1997;20(12):1185–1192

Chervin RD, Ruzicka DL, Giordani BJ, et al. Sleep-disordered breathing, behavior, and cognition in children before and after adenotonsillectomy. *Pediatrics.* 2006;117(4):e769–e778

Chole RA, Faddis BT. Anatomical evidence of microbial biofilms in tonsillar tissues: a possible mechanism to explain chronicity. *Arch Otolaryngol Head Neck Surg.* 2003;129(6):634–636

Cinar U, Vural C, Cakir B, Topuz E, Karaman MI, Turgut S. Nocturnal enuresis and upper airway obstruction. *Int J Pediatr Otorhinolaryngol.* 2001;59(2):115–118

Colclasure JB, Graham SS. Complications of outpatient tonsillectomy and adenoidectomy: a review of 3,340 cases. *Ear Nose Throat J.* 1990;69(3):155–160

Colen TY, Seidman C, Weedon J, Goldstein NA. Effect of intracapsular tonsillectomy on quality of life for children with obstructive sleep-disordered breathing. *Arch Otolaryngol Head Neck Surg.* 2008;134(2):124–127

Constantin E, Kermack A, Nixon GM, Tidmarsh L, Ducharme FM, Brouillette RT. Adenotonsillectomy improves sleep, breathing, and quality of life but not behavior. *J Pediatr.* 2007;150(5):540–546

Coticchia J, Zuliani G, Coleman C, et al. Biofilm surface area in the pediatric nasopharynx: chronic rhinosinusitis vs obstructive sleep apnea. *Arch Otolaryngol Head Neck Surg.* 2007;133(2):110–114

Coyte PC, Croxford R, McIsaac W, Feldman W, Friedberg J. The role of adjuvant adenoidectomy and tonsillectomy in the outcome of the insertion of tympanostomy tubes. *N Engl J Med.* 2001;344(16):1188–1195

Cullen KA, Hall MJ, Golosinskiy A. Ambulatory surgery in the United States, 2006. *Natl Health Stat Report.* 2009;11:1–25

Dajani A, Taubert K, Ferrieri P, Peter G, Shulman S; Committee on Rheumatic Fever, Endocarditis, and Kawasaki Disease of the Council on Cardiovascular Disease in the Young, American Heart Association. Treatment of acute streptococcal pharyngitis and prevention of rheumatic fever: a statement for health professionals. *Pediatrics.* 1995;96(4):758–764

De Serres LM, Derkay C, Sie K, et al. Impact of adenotonsillectomy on quality of life in children with obstructive sleep disorders. *Arch Otolaryngol Head Neck Surg.* 2002;128(5):489–496

Del Mar CB, Glasziou PP, Spinks AB. Antibiotics for sore throat. *Cochrane Database Syst Rev.* 2006;4:CD000023

Díez-Montiel A, de Diego JI, Prim MP, Martín-Martínez MA, Pérez-Fernández E, Rabanal I. Quality of life after surgical treatment of children with obstructive sleep apnea: long-term results. *Int J Pediatr Otorhinolaryngol.* 2006;70(9):1575–1579

Dolev Y, Daniel SJ. The presence of unilateral tonsillar enlargement in patients diagnosed with palatine tonsil lymphoma: experience at a tertiary care pediatric hospital. *Int J Pediatr Otorhinolaryngol.* 2008;72(1):9–12

Donn AS, Giles ML. Do children waiting for tonsillectomy grow out of their tonsillitis? *N Z Med J.* 1991;104(910):161–162

Erickson BK, Larson DR, St Sauver JL, Meverden RA, Orvidas LJ. Changes in incidence and indications of tonsillectomy and adenotonsillectomy, 1970-2005. *Otolaryngol Head Neck Surg.* 2009;140(6):894–901

Ericsson E, Lundeborg I, Hultcrantz E. Child behavior and quality of life before and after tonsillotomy versus tonsillectomy. *Int J Pediatr Otorhinolaryngol.* 2009;73(9):1254–1262

Fearon M, Bannatyne RM, Fearon BW, Turner A, Cheung R. Differential bacteriology in adenoid disease. *J Otolaryngol.* 1992;21(6):434–436

Feder HM, Salazar JC. A clinical review of 105 patients with PFAPA (a periodic fever syndrome). *Acta Paediatr.* 2010;99(2):178–184

Fekete-Szabo G, Berenyi I, Gabriella K, Urban E, Nagy E. Aerobic and anaerobic bacteriology of chronic adenoid disease in children. *Int J Pediatr Otorhinolaryngol.* 2010;74(11):1217–1220

Fernbach SK, Brouillette RT, Riggs TW, Hunt CE. Radiologic evaluation of adenoids and tonsils in children with obstructive sleep apnea: plain films and fluoroscopy. *Pediatr Radiol.* 1983;13(5):258–265

Finkelstein Y, Nachmani A, Ophir D. The functional role of the tonsils in speech. *Arch Otolaryngol Head Neck Surg.* 1994;120(8):846–851

Firoozi F, Batniji R, Aslan AR, Longhurst PA, Kogan BA. Resolution of diurnal incontinence and nocturnal enuresis after adenotonsillectomy in children. *J Urol.* 2006;175(5):1885–1888

Flanary VA. Long-term effect of adenotonsillectomy on quality of life in pediatric patients. *Laryngoscope.* 2003;113(10):1639–1644

Fox R, Temple M, Owens D, Short A, Tomkinson A. Does tonsillectomy lead to improved outcomes over and above the effect of time? A longitudinal study. *J Laryngol Otol.* 2008;122(11):1197–1200

Freeland AP, Curley JW. The consequences of delay in tonsil surgery. *Otolaryngol Clin North Am.* 1987;20(2):405–408

Friday GA Jr, Paradise JL, Rabin BS, Colborn DK, Taylor FH. Serum immunoglobulin changes in relation to tonsil and adenoid surgery. *Ann Allergy.* 1992;69(3):225–230

Friedman BC, Hendeles-Amitai A, Kozimsky E, et al. Adenotonsillectomy improves neurocognitive function in children with obstructive sleep apnea syndrome. *Sleep.* 2003;26(8):999–1005

Friedman NR, Mitchell RB, Pereira KD, Younis RT, Lazar RH. Peritonsillar abscess in early childhood. Presentation and management. *Arch Otolaryngol Head Neck Surg.* 1997;123(6):630–632

Galli J, Ardito F, Calò L, et al. Recurrent upper airway infections and bacterial biofilms. *J Laryngol Otol.* 2007;121(4):341–344

Galli J, Calò L, Ardito F, et al. Biofilm formation by *Haemophilus influenzae* isolated from adeno-tonsil tissue samples, and its role in recurrent adenotonsillitis. *Acta Otorhinolaryngol Ital.* 2007;27(3):134–138

Garavello W, Romagnoli M, Gaini RM. Effectiveness of adenotonsillectomy in PFAPA syndrome: a randomized study. *J Pediatr.* 2009;155(2):250–253

Garetz SL. Behavior, cognition, and quality of life after adenotonsillectomy for pediatric sleep-disordered breathing: summary of the literature. *Otolaryngol Head Neck Surg.* 2008;138(1 Suppl):S19–S26

Gates GA, Avery CA, Prihoda TJ. Effect of adenoidectomy upon children with chronic otitis media with effusion. *Laryngoscope.* 1988;98(1):58–63

Gates GA, Avery CA, Prihoda TJ, Cooper JC Jr. Effectiveness of adenoidectomy and tympanostomy tubes in the treatment of chronic otitis media with effusion. *N Engl J Med.* 1987;317(23):1444–1451

Georgalas C, Thomas K, Owens C, Abramovich S, Lack G. Medical treatment for rhinosinusitis associated with adenoidal hypertrophy in children: an evaluation of clinical response and changes on magnetic resonance imaging. *Ann Otol Rhinol Laryngol.* 2005;114(8):638–644

Gerber MA. Diagnosis and treatment of pharyngitis in children. *Pediatr Clin North Am.* 2005;52(3):729–747

Gerber MA, Shulman ST. Rapid diagnosis of pharyngitis caused by group A streptococci. *Clin Microbiol Rev.* 2004;17(3):571–580

Gerber MA, Spadaccini LJ, Wright LL, Deutsch L, Kaplan EL. Twice-daily penicillin in the treatment of streptococcal pharyngitis. *Am J Dis Child.* 1985;139(11):1145–1148

Goldstein NA, Fatima M, Campbell TF, Rosenfeld RM. Child behavior and quality of life before and after tonsillectomy and adenoidectomy. *Arch Otolaryngol Head Neck Surg.* 2002;128(7):770–775

Goldstein NA, Post JC, Rosenfeld RM, Campbell TF. Impact of tonsillectomy and adenoidectomy on child behavior. *Arch Otolaryngol Head Neck Surg.* 2000;126(4):494–498

Goldstein NA, Stewart MG, Witsell DL, et al. Quality of life after tonsillectomy in children with recurrent tonsillitis. *Otolaryngol Head Neck Surg.* 2008;138(1 Suppl):S9–S16

Gozal D. Sleep-disordered breathing and school performance in children. *Pediatrics.* 1998;102(3 Pt 1):616–620

Guilleminault C, Korobkin R, Winkle R. A review of 50 children with obstructive sleep apnea syndrome. *Lung.* 1981;159(5):275–287

Guilleminault C, Pelayo R, Leger D, Clerk A, Bocian RC. Recognition of sleep-disordered breathing in children. *Pediatrics.* 1996;98(5):871–882

Guilleminault C, Winkle R, Korobkin R, Simmons B. Children and nocturnal snoring: evaluation of the effects of sleep related respiratory resistive load and daytime functioning. *Eur J Pediatr.* 1982;139(3):165–171

Gul M, Okur E, Ciragil P, Yildirim I, Aral M, Akif Kilic M. The comparison of tonsillar surface and corte cultures in recurrent tonsillitis. *Am J Otolaryngol.* 2007;28(3):173–176

Hammarén-Malmi S, Saxen H, Tarkkanen J, Mattila PS. Adenoidectomy does not significantly reduce the incidence of otitis media in conjunction with the insertion of tympanostomy tubes in children who are younger than 4 years: a randomized trial. *Pediatrics.* 2005;116(1):185–189

Harley EH. Asymmetric tonsil size in children. *Arch Otolaryngol Head Neck Surg.* 2002;128(7):767–769

Henle W, Henle G. Epidemiologic aspects of Epstein-Barr virus (EBV)-associated diseases. *Ann N Y Acad Sci.* 1980;354:326–331

Herzon FS, Harris P. Mosher Award thesis. Peritonsillar abscess: incidence, current management practices, and a proposal for treatment guidelines. *Laryngoscope*. 1995;105(8 Pt 3 Suppl 74):1–17

Herzon FS, Nicklaus P. Pediatric peritonsillar abscess: management guidelines. *Curr Probl Pediatr*. 1998;26(8):270–278

Holm S, Henning C, Grahn E, Lomberg H, Staley H. Is penicillin the appropriate treatment for recurrent tonsillopharyngitis? Results from a comparative randomized blind study of cefuroxime axetil and phenoxymethylpenicillin in children. The Swedish Study Group. *Scand J Infect Dis*. 1995;27(3):221–228

Howard NS, Brietzke SE. Pediatric tonsil size: objective vs subjective measurements correlated to overnight polysomnogram. *Otolaryngol Head Neck Surg*. 2009;140(5):675–681

Iber C, Ancoli-Israel S, Chesson AL, Quan SF. *The AASM Manual for the Scoring of Sleep and Associated Events: Rules, Terminology, and Technical Specifications*. Westchester, IL: American Academy of Sleep Medicine; 2007

Isaacson G, Parikh T. Developmental anatomy of the tonsil and its implications for intracapsular tonsillectomy. *Int J Pediatr Otorhinolaryngol*. 2008;72(1):89–96

Jain A, Sahni JK. Polysomnographic studies in children undergoing adenoidectomy and/or tonsillectomy. *J Laryngol Otol*. 2002;116(9):711–715

Johnson RF, Stewart MG, Wright CC. An evidence-based review of the treatment of peritonsillar abscess. *Otolaryngol Head Neck Surg*. 2003;128(3):332–343

Johnson SK, Johnson RE. Tonsillectomy history in Hodgkin's disease. *N Engl J Med*. 1972;287(22):1122–1125

Jung KY, Lim HH, Choi G, Choi JO. Age-related changes of IgA immunocytes and serum and salivary IgA after tonsillectomy. *Acta Otolaryngol Suppl*. 1996;523:115–119

Kadhim AL, Spilsbury K, Semmens JB, Coates HL, Lannigan FJ. Adenoidectomy for middle ear effusion: a study of 50,000 children over 24 years. *Laryngoscope*. 2007;117(3):427–433

Kania RE, Lamers GE, Vonk MJ, et al. Demonstration of bacterial cells and glycocalyx in biofilms on human tonsils. *Arch Otolaryngol Head Neck Surg*. 2007;133(2):115–121

Kaplan EL, Gerber MA. Group A streptococcal infections. In: Feigin RD, Cherry JD, eds. *Textbook of Pediatric Infectious Diseases*. 4th ed. Philadelphia, PA: WB Saunders Co; 1998:1076–1088

Kaplan EL, Johnson DR. Unexplained reduced microbiological efficacy of intramuscular benzathine penicillin G and of oral penicillin V in eradication of group A streptococci from children with acute pharyngitis. *Pediatrics*. 2001;108(5):1180–1186

Kaygusuz I, Gödekmerdan A, Karlidag T, et al. Early stage impacts of tonsillectomy on immune functions of children. *Int J Pediatr Otorhinolaryngol*. 2003;67(12):1311–1315

Klein JC. Nasal respiratory function and craniofacial growth. *Arch Otolaryngol Head Neck Surg*. 1986;112(8):843–849

Kline JA, Runge JW. Streptococcal pharyngitis: a review of pathophysiology, diagnosis, and management. *J Emerg Med*. 1994;12(5):665–680

Koivunen P, Uhari M, Luotonen J, et al. Adenoidectomy versus chemoprophylaxis and placebo for recurrent acute otitis media in children aged under 2 years: randomized controlled trial. *BMJ*. 2004;328(7438):487

Krober MS, Bass JW, Michels GN. Streptococcal pharyngitis. Placebo-controlled double-blind evaluation of clinical response to penicillin therapy. *JAMA.* 1985;253(9):1271–1274

Kronenberg J, Wolf M, Leventon G. Peritonsillar abscess: recurrence rate and the indication for tonsillectomy. *Am J Otolaryngol.* 1987;8(2):82–84

Kummer AW, Billmire DA, Myer CM 3rd. Hypertrophic tonsils: the effect on resonance and velopharyngeal closure. *Plast Reconstr Surg.* 1993;91(4):608–611

LaCasce AS. Post-transplant lymphoproliferative disorders. *Oncologist.* 2006;11(6):674–680

Laurikainen E, Erkinjuntti M, Alihanka J, Rikalainen H, Suonpää J. Radiological parameters of the bony nasopharynx and the adenotonsillar size compared with sleep apnea episodes in children. *Int J Pediatr Otorhinolaryngol.* 1987;12(3):303–310

Lee D, Rosenfeld RM. Adenoid bacteriology and sinonasal symptoms in children. *Otolaryngol Head Neck Surg.* 1997;116(3):301–307

Lewin DS, Rosen RC, England SJ, Dahl RE. Preliminary evidence of behavioral and cognitive sequelae of obstructive sleep apnea in children. *Sleep Med.* 2002;3(1):5–13

Li HY, Huang YS, Chen NH, Fang TJ, Lee LA. Impact of adenotonsillectomy on behavior in children with sleep-disordered breathing. *Laryngoscope.* 2006;116(7):1142–1147

Macsween KF, Crawford DH. Epstein-Barr virus-recent advances. *Lancet Infect Dis.* 2003;3(3):131–140

Markowitz M, Gerber MA, Kaplan EL. Treatment of streptococcal pharyngotonsillitis: reports of penicillin's demise are premature. *J Pediatr.* 1993;123(5):679–685

Maryn Y, Van Lierde K, De Bodt M, Van Cauwenberge P. The effects of adenoidectomy and tonsillectomy on speech and nasal resonance. *Folia Phoniatr Logop.* 2004;56(3):182–191

Maw AR. Age and adenoid size in relation to adenoidectomy in otitis media with effusion. *Am J Otolaryngol.* 1985;6(3):245–248

Maw AR. Chronic otitis media with effusion (glue ear) and adenotonsillectomy: prospective randomised controlled study. *Br Med J (Clin Res Ed).* 1983;287(6405):1586–1588

Maw R, Bawden R. Spontaneous resolution of severe chronic glue ear in children and the effect of adenoidectomy, tonsillectomy, and insertion of ventilation tubes (grommets). *BMJ.* 1993;306(6880):756–760

Maw AR, Herod F. Otoscopic, impedance, and audiometric findings in glue ear treated by adenoidectomy and tonsillectomy. A prospective randomised study. *Lancet.* 1986;1(8495):1399–1402

McClay JE. Resistant bacteria in the adenoids: a preliminary report. *Arch Otolaryngol Head Neck Surg.* 2000;126(5):625–629

Mitchell RB, Boss EF. Pediatric obstructive sleep apnea in obese and normal-weight children: impact of adenotonsillectomy on quality-of-life and behavior. *Dev Neuropsychol.* 2009;34(5):650–661

Mitchell RB, Kelly J. Adenotonsillectomy for obstructive sleep apnea in obese children. *Otolaryngol Head Neck Surg.* 2004;131(1):104–108

Mitchell RB, Kelly J. Behavioral changes in children with mild sleep-disordered breathing or obstructive sleep apnea after adenotonsillectomy. *Laryngoscope.* 2007;117(9):1685–1688

Mitchell RB, Kelly J. Child behavior after adenotonsillectomy for obstructive sleep apnea syndrome. *Laryngoscope.* 2005;115(11):2051–2055

Mitchell RB, Kelly J. Long-term changes in behavior after adenotonsillectomy for obstructive sleep apnea syndrome in children. *Otolaryngol Head Neck Surg.* 2006;134(3):374–378

Mitchell RB, Kelly J. Outcome of adenotonsillectomy for obstructive sleep apnea in obese and normal-weight children. *Otolaryngol Head Neck Surg.* 2007;137(1):43–48

Mitchell RB, Kelly J. Outcome of adenotonsillectomy for severe obstructive sleep apnea in children. *Int J Pediatr Otorhinolaryngol.* 2004;68(11):1375–1379

Mitchell RB, Kelly J. Quality of life after adenotonsillectomy for SDB in children. *Otolaryngol Head Neck Surg.* 2005;133(4):569–572

Mitchell RB, Kelly J, Call E, Yao N. Long-term changes in quality of life after surgery for pediatric obstructive sleep apnea. *Arch Otolaryngol Head Neck Surg.* 2004;130(4):409–412

Mitchell RB, Kelly J, Call E, Yao N. Quality of life after adenotonsillectomy for obstructive sleep apnea in children. *Arch Otolaryngol Head Neck Surg.* 2004;130(2):190–194

Mitchell RB, Pereira KD, Friedman NR. Sleep-disordered breathing in children: survey of current practice. *Laryngoscope.* 2006;116(6):956–958

Montgomery-Downs HE, Crabtree VM, Gozal D. Cognition, sleep and respiration in at-risk children treated for obstructive sleep apnoea. *Eur Resp J.* 2005;25(2):336–342

Nave H, Gebert A, Pabst R. Morphology and immunology of the human palatine tonsil. *Anat Embryol (Berl).* 2001;204(5):367–373

Nguyen LH, Manoukian JJ, Yoskovitch A, Al-Sebeih KH. Adenoidectomy: selection criteria for surgical cases of otitis media. *Laryngoscope.* 2004;114(5):863–866

Nieminen P, Tolonen U, Löppönen H. Snoring and obstructive sleep apnea in children: a 6-month follow-up study. *Arch Otolaryngol Head Neck Surg.* 2000;126(4):481–486

O'Brien LM, Mervis CB, Holbrook CR, et al. Neurobehavioral correlates of sleep-disordered breathing in children. *J Sleep Res.* 2004;13(2):165–172

O'Brien LM, Mervis CB, Holbrook CR, et al. Neurobehavioral implications of habitual snoring in children. *Pediatrics.* 2004;114(1):44–49

O'Brien LM, Tauman R, Gozal D. Sleep pressure correlates of cognitive and behavioural morbidity in snoring children. *Sleep.* 2004;27(2):279–282

Ogra PL. Effect of tonsillectomy and adenoidectomy on nasopharyngeal antibody response to poliovirus. *N Engl J Med.* 1971;284(2):59–64

Oomen KP, Rovers MM, van den Akker EH, van Staaij BK, Hoes AW, Schilder AG. Effect of adenoidectomy on middle ear status in children. *Laryngoscope.* 2005;115(4):731–734

Owens JA. Neurocognitive and behavioral impact of sleep disordered breathing in children. *Pediatr Pulmonol.* 2009;44(5):417–422

Paradise JL, Bluestone CD, Bachman RZ, et al. History of recurrent sore throat as an indication for tonsillectomy. Predictive limitations of histories that are undocumented. *N Engl J Med.* 1978;298(8):409–413

Paradise JL, Bluestone CD, Colborn DK, Bernard BS, Rockette HE, Kurs-Lasky M. Tonsillectomy and adenotonsillectomy for recurrent throat infection in moderately affected children. *Pediatrics*. 2002;110(1):7–15

Paradise JL, Bluestone CD, Colborn DK, et al. Adenoidectomy and adenotonsillectomy for recurrent acute otitis media: parallel randomized clinical trials in children not previously treated with tympanostomy tubes. *JAMA*. 1999;282(10):945–953

Paradise JL, Bluestone CD, Rogers KD, et al. Efficacy of adenoidectomy for recurrent otitis media in children previously treated with tympanostomy-tube placement. Results of parallel randomized and nonrandomized trials. *JAMA*. 1990;263(15):2066–2073

Paulussen C, Claes J, Claes G, Jorissen M. Adenoids and tonsils, indications for surgery and immunological consequences of surgery. *Acta Otorhinolaryngol Belg.* 2000;54(3):403–408

Pichichero ME, Casey JR, Mayes T, et al. Penicillin failure in streptococcal tonsillopharyngitis: causes and remedies. *Pediatr Infect Dis J.* 2000;19(9):917–923

Plotkin SA. Infectious mononucleosis. In: Behrman RE, Kliegman RM, Nelson WE, eds. *Nelson's Textbook of Pediatrics*. 14th ed. Philadelphia, PA: WB Saunders Co; 1992:805–808

Powell SM, Tremlett M, Bosman DA. Quality of life of children with sleep-disordered breathing treated with adenotonsillectomy. *J Laryngol Otol*. 2011;125(2):193–198

Pratt LW. Tonsillectomy and adenoidectomy: mortality and morbidity. *Trans Am Acad Ophthalmol Otolaryngol*. 1970;74(6):1146–1154

Prim MP, de Diego JI, Larrauri M, Diaz C, Sastre N, Gavilan J. Spontaneous resolution of recurrent tonsillitis in pediatric patients on the surgical waiting list. *Int J Pediatr Otorhinolaryngol*. 2002;65(1):35–38

Puttasiddaiah P, Kumar M, Gopalan P, Browning ST. Tonsillectomy and biopsy for asymptomatic asymmetric tonsillar enlargement: are we right? *J Otolaryngol*. 2007;36(3):161–163

Randolph MF, Gerber MA, DeMeo KK, Wright L. Effect of antibiotic therapy on the clinical course of streptococcal pharyngitis. *J Pediatr*. 1985;106(6):870–875

Renko M, Salo E, Putto-Laurila A, et al. A randomized, controlled trial of tonsillectomy in periodic fever, aphthous stomatitis, pharyngitis, and adenitis syndrome. *J Pediatr*. 2007;151(3):289–292

Richards W, Ferdman RM. Prolonged morbidity due to delays in the diagnosis and treatment of obstructive sleep apnea in children. *Clin Pediatr (Phila)*. 2000;39(2):103–108

Richardson MA. Sore throat, tonsillitis, and adenoiditis. *Med Clin North Am.* 1999;83(1):75–83

Rosen CL, Storfer-Isser A, Taylor HG, Kirchner HL, Emancipator JL, Redline S. Increased behavioral morbidity in school-aged children with sleep-disordered breathing. *Pediatrics*. 2004;114(6):1640–1648

Rosenfeld RM. Pilot study of outcomes in pediatric rhinosinusitis. *Arch Otolaryngol Head Neck Surg*. 1995;121(7):729–736

Schwentner I, Schmutzhard J, Schwentner C, Abraham I, Höfer S, Sprinzl GM. The impact of adenotonsillectomy on children's quality of life. *Clin Otolaryngol*. 2008;33(1):56–59

Scott PM, Loftus WK, Kew J, Ahuja A, Yue V, van Hasselt CA. Diagnosis of peritonsillar infections: a prospective study of ultrasound, computerized tomography and clinical diagnosis. *J Laryngol Otol.* 1999;113(3):229–232

Shapiro NL, Strocker AM, Bhattacharyya N. Risk factors for adenotonsillar hypertrophy in children following solid organ transplantation. *Int J Pediatr Otorhinolaryngol.* 2003;67(2):151–155

Shin KS, Cho SH, Kim KR, et al. The role of adenoids in pediatric rhinosinusitis. *Int J Pediatr Otolaryngol.* 2008;72(11):1643–1650

Shulman ST. Pediatric autoimmune neuropsychiatric disorders associated with streptococci (PANDAS): update. *Curr Opin Pediatr.* 2009;21(1):127–130

Shulman ST, Gerber MA. So what's wrong with penicillin for strep throat? [Commentary] *Pediatrics.* 2004;113(6):1816–1819

Shulman ST, Tanz RR, Gerber MA. Streptococcal pharyngitis. In: Stevens DL, Kaplan EL, eds. *Streptococcal Infections.* New York, NY: Oxford University Press; 2000:76–101

Siegel G, Linse R, Macheleidt S. Factors of tonsillar involution: age-dependent changes in B-cell activation and Langerhans' cell density. *Arch Otorhinolaryngol.* 1982;236(3):261–269

Simonsen AR, Duncavage JA, Becker SS. A review of malpractice cases after tonsillectomy and adenoidectomy. *Int J Pediatr Otorhinolaryngol.* 2010;74(9):977–979

Smith RM, Gonzalez C. The relationship between nasal obstruction and craniofacial growth. *Pediatr Clin North Am.* 1989;36(6):1423–1434

Stewart MG, Glaze DG, Friedman EM, Smith EO, Bautista M. Quality of life and sleep study findings after adenotonsillectomy in children with obstructive sleep apnea. *Arch Otolaryngol Head Neck Surg.* 2005;131(4):308–314

Stillerman M. Comparison of oral cephalosporins with penicillin therapy for group A streptococcal pharyngitis. *Pediatr Infect Dis.* 1986;5(6):649–654

Stoodley P, Debeer D, Longwell M, et al. Tonsillolith: not just a stone but a living biofilm. *Otolaryngol Head Neck Surg.* 2009;141(3):316–321

Stradling JR, Thomas G, Warley AR, Williams P, Freeland A. Effect of adenotonsillectomy on nocturnal hypoxaemia, sleep disturbance, and symptoms in snoring children. *Lancet.* 1990;335(8684):249–253

Suen JS, Arnold JE, Brooks LJ. Adenotonsillectomy for treatment of obstructive sleep apnea in children. *Arch Otolaryngol Head Neck Surg.* 1995;121(5):525–530

Sumaya CV. Epstein-Barr virus. In: Feigin RD, Cherry JD, eds. *Textbook of Pediatric Infectious Diseases.* 4th ed. Philadelphia, PA: WB Saunders Co; 1998:1751–1764

Sunkaraneni VS, Jones SE, Prasai A, Fish BM. Is unilateral tonsillar enlargement alone an indication for tonsillectomy? *J Laryngol Otol.* 2006;120(7):E21

Swedo SE, Leonard HL, Garvey M, et al. Pediatric autoimmune neuropsychiatric disorders associated with streptococcal infections: clinical description of the first 50 cases. *Am J Psychiatry.* 1998;155(2):264–271

Syms MJ, Birkmire-Peters DP, Holtel MR. Incidence of carcinoma in incidental tonsil asymmetry. *Laryngoscope.* 2000;110(11):1807–1810

Takahashi H, Honjo I, Fujita A, Kurata K. Effects of adenoidectomy on sinusitis. *Acta Otorhinolaryngol Belg.* 1997;51(2):85–87

Tanz RR, Shulman ST. Pharyngitis. In: Long SS, Pickering LK, Prober CG, eds. *Principles and Practice of Pediatric Infectious Diseases.* 2nd ed. Philadelphia, PA: Churchill-Livingstone; 2005:176–185

Tarasiuk A, Greenberg-Dotan S, Simon-Tuval T, et al. Elevated morbidity and health care use in children with obstructive sleep apnea syndrome. *Am J Respir Crit Care Med.* 2007;175(1):55–61

Tauman R, Gulliver TE, Krishna J, et al. Persistence of obstructive sleep apnea syndrome in children after adenotonsillectomy. *J Pediatr.* 2006;149(6):803–808

Tran KD, Nguyen CD, Weedon J, Goldstein NA. Child behavior and quality of life in pediatric obstructive sleep apnea. *Arch Otolaryngol Head Neck Surg.* 2005;131(1):52–57

Tuncer U, Aydogan B, Soylu L, Simsek M, Akcali C, Kucukcan A. Chronic rhinosinusitis and adenoid hypertrophy in children. *Am J Otolaryngol.* 2004;25(1):5–10

Ungkanont K, Damrongsak S. Effect of adenoidectomy in children with complex problems of rhinosinusitis and associated diseases. *Int J Pediatr Otorhinolaryngol.* 2004;68(4):447–451

Urschitz MS, Wolff J, Sokollik C, et al. Nocturnal arterial oxygen satura-tion and academic performance in a community sample of children. *Pediatrics.* 2005;115(2):e204–e209

Valera FC, Travitzki LV, Mattar SE, Matsumoto MA, Elias AM, Anselmo-Lima WT. Muscular, functional and orthodontic changes in pre school children with enlarged adenoids and tonsils. *Int J Pediatr Otorhinolaryngol.* 2003;67(7):761–770

van den Aardweg MT, Schilder AG, Herkert E, Boonacker CW, Rovers MM. Adenoidectomy for recurrent or chronic nasal symptoms in children. *Cochrane Database Syst Rev.* 2010;1:CD008282

van der Horst C, Joncas J, Ahronheim G, et al. Lack of effect of peroral acyclovir for the treatment of acute infectious mononucleosis. *J Infect Dis.* 1991;164(4):788–792

Van Staaij BK, Van Den Akker EH, De Haas Van Dorsser EH, Fleer A, Hoes AW, Schilder AG. Does the tonsillar surface flora differ in children with and without tonsillar disease? *Acta Otololaryngol.* 2003;123(7):873–878

van Staaij BK, van den Akker EH, Rovers MM, Hordijk GJ, Hoes AW, Schilder AG. Effectiveness of adenotonsillectomy in children with mild symptoms of throat infections or adenotonsillar hypertrophy: open, randomised controlled trial. *BMJ.* 2004;329(7467):651

van Staaij BK, van den Akker EH, van der Heijden GJ, Schilder AG, Hoes AW. Adenotonsillectomy for upper respiratory infections: evidence based? *Arch Dis Child.* 2005;90(1):19–25

Vandenberg SJ, Heatley DG. Efficacy of adenoidectomy in relieving symptoms of chronic sinusitis in children. *Arch Otolaryngol Head Neck Surg.* 1997;123(7):675–678

Vianna NJ, Greenwald P, Davies JN. Tonsillectomy and Hodgkin's disease: the lymphoid tissue barrier. *Lancet.* 1971;1(7696):431–432

Weinberg EA, Brodsky L, Brody A, Pizzuto M, Stiner H. Clinical classification as a guide to treatment of sinusitis in children. *Laryngoscope.* 1997;107(2):241–246

Weissbach A, Leiberman A, Tarasiuk A, Goldbart A, Tal A. Adenotonsillectomy improves enuresis in children with obstructive sleep apnea syndrome. *Int J Pediatr Otorhinolaryngol.* 2006;70(8):1351–1356

Weissbluth M, Davis AT, Poncher J, Reiff J. Signs of airway obstruction during sleep and behavioral, developmental, and academic problems. *J Dev Behav Pediatr.* 1983;4(2):119–121

Windfuhr JP, Chen YS. Incidence of post-tonsillectomy hemorrhage in children and adults: a study of 4,848 patients. *Ear Nose Throat J.* 2002;81(9):626–628, 630, 632

Windfuhr JP, Chen YS, Remmert S. Hemorrhage following tonsillectomy and adenoidectomy in 15,218 patients. *Otolaryngol Head Neck Surg.* 2005;132(2):281–286

Winther B, Gross BC, Hendley JO, Early SV. Location of bacterial biofilm in the mucus overlying the adenoid by light microscopy. *Arch Otolaryngol Head Neck Surg.* 2009;135(12):1239–1245

Wolf M, Kronenberg J, Kessler A, Modan M, Leventon G. Peritonsillar abscess in children and its indication for tonsillectomy. *Int J Pediatr Otorhinolaryngol.* 1988;16(2):113–117

Wood B, Wong YK, Theodoridis CG. Paediatricians look at children awaiting adenotonsillectomy. *Lancet.* 1972;2(7778):645–647

Woolford TJ, Ahmed A, Willatt DJ, Rothera MP. Spontaneous resolution of tonsillitis in children on the waiting list for tonsillectomy. *Clin Otolaryngol Allied Sci.* 2000;25(5):428–430

World Health Organization. *Rheumatic Fever and Rheumatic Heart Disease.* Geneva, Switzerland: World Health Organization; 1988. Technical Report Series No. 764

Ye J, Liu H, Zhang GH, et al. Outcome of adenotonsillectomy for obstructive sleep apnea syndrome in children. *Ann Otol Rhinol Laryngol.* 2010;119(8):506–513

CHAPTER 10

Pediatric Oropharyngeal Trauma

David L. Mandell, MD

■ Introduction

Injuries to the oropharynx of children are thought to be quite commonplace. Many such injuries may not be witnessed or brought to medical attention because of absence of any major symptoms. However, when oropharyngeal trauma is associated with bleeding, pain, or dysphagia, a caregiver is usually prompted to seek medical attention. Prophylactic antibiotics are often recommended in cases in which the oropharyngeal mucosa has been lacerated. Most cases of oropharyngeal trauma in children heal with no lasting damage to the patient, usually without the need for surgical closure.

Although recovery from oropharyngeal trauma is usually uneventful, there have been rare cases reported in which children have developed neurologic complications (eg, stroke, death) following such injuries, presumably because of occult internal carotid artery injury. Unfortunately, there is currently no definitive mechanism by which medical providers can try to predict which children with oropharyngeal trauma might go on to develop these catastrophic neurologic complications. One way to attempt to assess the carotid artery is to obtain an imaging study, although it is not agreed on as to which study should be obtained (computed tomography [CT], CT angiogram, magnetic resonance angiogram [MRA], or no study at all), and even within institutions where imaging is obtained, there is considerable variability in which patients are actually imaged.

> **Pearl:** Although most cases of pediatric oropharyngeal trauma heal rapidly and without complications, rare instances of internal carotid injury and delayed onset of severe neurologic sequelae have been reported.

■ Epidemiology

Oropharyngeal injury in children occurs at an average age of 3.5 years. One theory why toddlers comprise the highest risk group for oropharyngeal injury is that they tend to run and fall with objects in their mouths. As with most types of trauma, males are more affected than females and are 1.5 to 5.5 times more likely to experience oropharyngeal trauma, possibly because of generally more aggressive behavior. The most common objects that cause such injury are pens, pencils, musical instruments, pipes, tubes, toys, and sticks. Other offending objects may include toothbrushes, straws, and lollipops. In approximately 5% of cases of pediatric oropharyngeal trauma that present to medical attention, the object that caused the trauma is not witnessed and is unknown. Approximately 18 such injuries per year have been reported at a large tertiary care pediatric hospital.

> **Pearl:** Pediatric oropharyngeal injury is most common in male toddlers, who often run and fall with toys and other objects in their mouths.

■ Presenting Symptoms

The median amount of time that elapses from oropharyngeal injury to presentation to a health care practitioner is 3 hours. Most of these children will have expectorated 5 to 20 mL of blood prior to their arrival in the emergency department (ED). Some patients will complain of pain or odynophagia, although most will be asymptomatic by the time they are seen by a medical practitioner. Typically there are no neurologic symptoms at time of presentation. If the patient complains of headache, blurred vision, or nausea, or if the parent or guardian describes the child as being unusually irritable, the clinician should be suspicious of a potential neurovascular injury and initiate the appropriate imaging study.

> **Pearl:** Although bleeding after oropharyngeal trauma is the most common factor that prompts parents to bring their children for medical attention, by the time most of these children are seen, they are usually entirely asymptomatic.

■ Physical Examination

Hemodynamic stability is the norm on initial physical examination of children presenting with oropharyngeal trauma. Although younger children and those who are mentally disabled may resist oropharyngeal examination, visualization of the site of potential injury is essential and may require use of parental-assisted restraint of the child, a tongue depressor, and a headlight, with suction available to clear away oropharyngeal secretions. On oropharyngeal examination, the site of injury involves the lateral oropharynx in 70% to 81% of injuries, with the remainder occurring in the midline. It has been reported by some (but not all) authors that the left side of the oropharynx is involved more than the right side, theoretically because of the predominance of right-handedness among the general population (ie, children are running while their right hand is placing the offending object in their oral cavities).

The appearance of oropharyngeal injury can range from mild bruising with no mucosal disruption, to a large avulsed tissue flap with a fistula into the nasopharynx, or great vessel exposure. A grading scale has been developed to help standardize the description of injuries. Grade I injuries consist of ecchymosis without mucosal penetration (7% of cases). Grade II injuries are puncture wounds or lacerations measuring 1 cm or less (64% of cases). Grade III injuries are lacerations greater than 1 cm or with an oronasal fistula or avulsed tissue flap (29% of cases). The foreign body itself has been noted to be present, protruding from the oropharyngeal wound, in approximately 2% of cases that present to a physician.

Signs of neurologic dysfunction are usually absent. However, the clinician should still closely assess for drowsiness and listlessness, irritability, confused speech, vision changes, vomiting, and arm or leg weakness. Also, auscultation for a carotid bruit should be performed, and the clinician should assess for any external neck swelling.

> **Pearl:** Clear visualization of the site of injury is recommended, and severity of the injury appearance can be graded for descriptive purposes.

■ Diagnostic Imaging

Because of the rarity of neurologic sequelae, there is some debate about whether imaging studies should be routinely obtained to look for potential carotid artery injury in children with otherwise benign-appearing oropharyngeal traumatic injury. The potential benefit of imaging is that if early intimal damage to the internal carotid artery can somehow be identified, anti-coagulation therapy can be instituted, thus potentially decreasing the likelihood of thrombus formation and propagation and development of neurologic sequelae. Imaging is less likely to be required for midline traumatic palatal injuries because injuries in this location are less likely to injure the great vessels (ie, a wound at the hard palate–soft palate junction). Lateral oropharyngeal lesions are thought to be associated with higher risk of causing complications.

One increasingly popular mechanism for assessing potential internal carotid injury from pediatric oropharyngeal trauma is the use of CT with intravenous (IV) contrast. Although clinicians may be more tempted to order a radiographic study in cases in which the size and appearance of the wound is more severe, it should be cautioned that the mechanism of carotid injury in this scenario is from arterial compression, not penetration, so even grade I injuries (no mucosal penetration) can lead to a carotid intimal tear and subsequent thrombosis. Computed tomography images can be reconstructed to create a CT angiogram, and MRAs may also be used, although MRA studies cost more, take longer to perform (and thus are more likely to require sedation in young children), and may not be as readily available in the typical ED setting.

When pooling the data from the largest, most recently published series of children with oropharyngeal trauma, 89 of 358 total patients underwent CT scan. Among those 89 patients who underwent a CT scan, 2 cases (2.2%) were found to have intimal disruption of the internal carotid artery, which was then confirmed with conventional angiography; the patients were treated expectantly with aspirin. In addition, 1 case (1.1%) was found to have a carotid artery "spasm," and another case was found to have a soft tissue hematoma adjacent to the internal carotid artery with no direct association with the artery on follow-up conventional angiogram. Thus, among all recent large series in the literature (including all patients, even those who weren't scanned), the likelihood of discovering a true intimal carotid artery injury in the setting of pediatric oropharyngeal trauma is 2 out of 358 (0.6%), and the likelihood of developing neurologic sequelae for all patients in all these series combined was 0.0%.

> **Pearl:** If an imaging study is performed to assess the status of the carotid artery in the setting of pediatric oropharyngeal trauma, the likelihood of finding a true intimal arterial tear is approximately 2.2%. Most routine pediatric oropharyngeal trauma cases in the literature, however, have not undergone scanning.

■ Treatment Options

SURGICAL CLOSURE

Most traumatic oropharyngeal injuries heal well spontaneously. Surgical closure is performed in only 4% to 8% of all cases. Patients who are more likely to require surgical closure are those with large avulsion flaps, those with an impaled foreign body still present in the wound, and those rare patients in whom open neck exploration might be needed for great vessel access in the event of significant bleeding on foreign body extraction (figures 10-1 and 10-2).

PROPHYLACTIC ANTIBIOTICS

Prophylactic antibiotics are reportedly used in up to 88% of cases. Typically, a dose of IV antibiotics is given while the patient is in the ED, followed by post-discharge oral antibiotics. The antibiotics should cover gram-positive organisms and anaerobes; one reasonable choice is IV ampicillin-sulbactam followed by oral amoxicillin-clavulanate.

HOSPITAL ADMISSION AND OBSERVATION

Most patients stay in the hospital less than 24 hours, and many are discharged home from the ED. Hospitalization with longer admissions may be required for those patients who are younger than 1 year; who are mentally disabled (in whom assessment of changes in mental status may be more difficult); with poor oral intake, infection, or pneumomediastinum; who are undergoing a child abuse workup or have unsafe home situations; and who are recovering from surgical palatal repair. Neurologic complications are rare; when they do occur, there is often a delay of up to several days until symptom onset, such that overnight

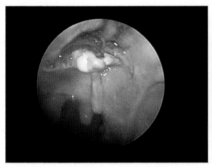

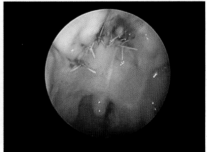

Figure 10-1. Acute penetrating injury of the oropharynx in a child.

Figure 10-2. Surgical repair of the pediatric oropharyngeal traumatic wound.

admission for observation may provide a false sense of security and is generally not recommended. When discharged home, patients should be given similar instructions as those given to minor head trauma patients. Parents are asked to closely monitor for any neurologic signs or symptoms for a few more days, with a follow-up outpatient office visit within a week.

> **Pearl:** Most oropharyngeal wounds heal well without surgery; prophylactic antibiotics are often given if the mucosa of the oropharynx has been penetrated; and most children may be discharged home without hospital admission. Admitting the child overnight may provide a false sense of security because if neurologic symptoms are to develop, they can occur up to several days later.

■ Natural History and Prognosis

All but the most dramatic avulsed tissue flaps tend to heal spontaneously within 1 to 2 weeks without surgical closure, and symptoms such as pain and dysphagia are usually short-lived. As innocuous as this type of trauma may appear, there is still the potential for devastating neurologic sequelae to occur if there has been any injury to the internal carotid artery. Such complications are fortunately quite rare. In fact, when compiling data from the largest cases series of pediatric oropharyngeal trauma over the past 2 decades, not a single case with neurologic complications was noted in a total of 358 cases. In addition, no specific clinical factors have been identified to help predict which of these patients may be more at risk for developing neurologic complications.

Scattered throughout the medical literature are rare case reports of children developing neurologic signs and symptoms such as hemiparesis, hemiplegia, seizure, coma, and even death following lateral oropharyngeal trauma that initially seemed unassuming and benign. In these cases, it is believed that the foreign body doesn't actually puncture the internal carotid artery but rather briefly compresses it against internal bony structures such as the skull base and the first 2 to 3 cervical vertebrae. As a result, the internal carotid artery can develop an intimal tear with subsequent gradual development of a mural thrombus. The thrombus can eventually lead to luminal occlusion, although in children, this event alone is usually not enough to cause overt neurologic symptoms due to adequate circle of Willis collateral circulation. In some cases, the thrombus can propagate distally, growing to occlude the middle or anterior cerebral arteries, at which point cerebral infarction can occur. It can take up to 60 hours for such a thrombus to form and propagate distally, thus likely accounting for the so-called lucid period during which patients appear asymptomatic prior to onset of neurologic signs and symptoms.

Thus, when it comes to pediatric oropharyngeal trauma, a high level of suspicion has to be maintained regarding the potential for delayed onset of neurologic complications. Currently, the most efficient type of evaluation to attempt to detect early internal carotid artery appears to be a contrast CT scan of the neck. However, because of the rarity of arterial injury, imaging does not appear to be used for most cases in the literature, and routine use of imaging cannot be emphatically recommended.

> **Pearl:** The natural history of pediatric oropharyngeal trauma is almost always very favorable with no lasting adverse effects, but the rare possibility of intimal disruption of the internal carotid artery with delayed onset of neurologic signs and symptoms should be kept in mind.

■ Selected References

Brietzke SE, Jones DT. Pediatric oropharyngeal trauma: what is the role of CT scan? *Int J Pediatr Otorhinolaryngol.* 2005;69(5):669–679

Hellmann JR, Shott SR, Gootee MJ. Impalement injuries of the palate in children: review of 131 cases. *Int J Pediatr Otorhinolaryngol.* 1993;26(2):157–163

Hengerer AS, DeGroot TR, Rivers RJ Jr, Pettee DS. Internal carotid artery thrombosis following soft palate injuries: a case report and review of 16 cases. *Laryngoscope.* 1984;94(12 Pt 1):1571–1575

Marom T, Russo E, Ben-Yehuda Y, Roth Y. Oropharyngeal injuries in children. *Pediatr Emerg Care.* 2007;23(12):914–918

Pierrot S, Bernardeschi D, Morrisseau-Durand MP, Manach Y, Couloigner V. Dissection of the internal carotid artery following trauma of the soft palate in children. *Ann Otol Rhinol Laryngol.* 2006;115(5):323–329

Radkowski D, McGill TJ, Healy GB, Jones DT. Penetrating trauma of the oropharynx in children. *Laryngoscope.* 1993;103(9):991–994

Ratcliff DJ, Okada PJ, Murray AD. Evaluation of pediatric lateral oropharyngeal trauma. *Otolaryngol Head Neck Surg.* 2003;128(6):783–787

Schoem SR, Choi SS, Zalzal GH, Grundfast KM. Management of oropharyngeal trauma in children. *Arch Otolaryngol Head Neck Surg.* 1997;123(12):1267–1270

Soose RJ, Simons JP, Mandell DL. Evaluation and management of pediatric oropharyngeal trauma. *Arch Otolaryngol Head Neck Surg.* 2006;132(4):446–451

Suskind DL, Tavill MA, Keller JL, Austin MB. Management of the carotid artery following penetrating injuries of the soft palate. *Int J Pediatr Otorhinolaryngol.* 1997;39(1):41–49

Zonfrillo MR, Roy AD, Walsh SA. Management of pediatric penetrating oropharyngeal trauma. *Pediatr Emerg Care.* 2008;24(3):172–175

CHAPTER 11

Cleft Lip and Palate

Patrick D. Munson, MD, and Charles M. Bower, MD

Introduction

Orofacial clefting is the most common congenital craniofacial mal-formation. Although most clefts are isolated anomalies, cleft lip and palate (CL/P) may be associated with other malformations or defined syndromes. The pediatrician is essential in the initial diagnosis of a child with CL/P and the continued coordinated care. Because most CL/Ps are diagnosed prenatally or soon postnatally, the pediatrician's role can be invaluable when dealing with issues such as feeding, developmental delays, behavior problems, and recurrent infections. Following identification of a child with a cleft, referral to a CL/P multidisciplinary team is essential. Caring for clefts requires experienced professionals from multiple specialties and often several surgeries over a span of years to optimize patient outcomes. The American Cleft Palate-Craniofacial Association (ACPA) recommends referral to credentialed teams in which care is delivered by professionals with a sufficient number of patients per year to ensure optimal care.

One in 800 children are born with a cleft lip or palate, which means pediatricians will likely encounter these children throughout their career. A recent survey of primary care physicians (PCPs) indicated that they currently treated a mean of 1.1 children with clefts. Additionally, 87% of those PCPs gave appropriate referrals to a tertiary center within 2 weeks of birth. Despite this experience, 67% desired a medical update concerning clefts. The goal of this review is to provide a firm foundation for understanding the diagnosis and presenting symptoms of clefts and the appropriate time line for medical and surgical management.

Epidemiology

Cleft lip and palate is the most common congenital facial malforma-tion. In the United States, 1 in 800 babies are born with a cleft lip or palate. Cleft lip and palate is more common in boys, and cleft palate alone is more common in girls. The incidence of CL/P varies by ethnicity—American Indians, 3.7 per 1,000 live births; Chinese, 2.0 per 1,000; whites, 1.7 per 1,000; and blacks, 0.4 per 1,000. Previous reports indicate the breakdown of cleft type as CL/P, 35%; isolated cleft lip, 26%; and isolated cleft palate, 39%.

Clefts are typically isolated defects, related to several genetic and environmental factors. Most CL/P occurs in children with no family history of CL/P. Only a small percentage of defects have been attributed to a known environmental teratogenic agent, eg, sodium valproate. Approximately 20% to 25% of children with clefts will have an associated malformation. Anomalies of the craniofacial, skeletal/extremity, and cardiovascular systems can occur. Clefting is associated with more than 400 syndromes, including velocardiofacial syndrome (22q11 deletion), Stickler syndrome, van der Woude syndrome, Kabuki syndrome, trisomy 13 (Patau syndrome), trisomy 18 (Edwards syndrome), and Pierre Robin sequence. Children with clefts should be properly examined to detect anomalies. Consultation with a geneticist is appropriate.

> **Pearl:** While a cleft lip or palate is usually an isolated anomaly, the clinician should be alert for examination findings consistent with associated syndromes.

■ Presenting Symptoms

An embryologic understanding of cleft development provides the anatomic basis for symptom presentation. The location and severity of the cleft will predict associated clinical manifestations that the care provider should be aware of. Starting at 5 weeks of gestation, the embryonic midfacial structures are organized from the 5 facial prominences. The maxillary processes from each side of the face grow toward each other until they meet and fuse in front of the medial nasal passages, forming the upper lip (Figure 11-1). The frontonasal process develops into the primary palate and primary nasal septum. The inner aspect of the maxillary process on each side develops into palatine shelves, which fuse in the midline forming the secondary palate. A CL/P deformity results from an interruption of fusion of the prominences and subsequent failure of mesoderm ingrowth. Thus, an isolated cleft lip, an isolated cleft palate, or a combined CL/P may form depending on the disruption in embryonic development.

The initial presentation in children with clefts is an anatomic malformation found on physical examination. While often discovered at an initial postnatal examination, an increasing number of clefts are detected on prenatal ultrasonography. Unilateral, bilateral, and midline CL/P may be detected using prenatal ultrasound. Ultrasound has been used for 30 years, with enhanced detection based on classification schemes and technologic improvement. A systematic review of the literature in 2010 revealed that 2-D ultrasound screening for CL/P has relatively low detection rate but is associated with few false-positive

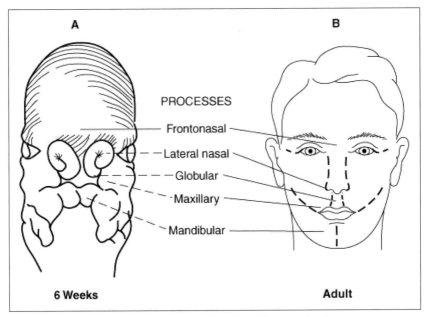

Figure 11-1. Embryologic fusion of the facial prominences leads to normal facial development. From Lalwani AK. *Current Diagnosis & Treatment in Otolaryngology—Head & Neck Surgery.* 2nd ed. New York, NY: McGraw-Hill; 2008. Reprinted by permission of The McGraw-Hill Companies.

results. Three-dimensional ultrasound, however, achieved a 90% detection rate for cleft lip and variably lower rate for cleft palate. With continued experience, caregivers will likely see a rise in clefts diagnosed prenatally, especially cleft lip.

Despite improvements in prenatal ultrasound detection, CL/P typically is discovered on postnatal examination. A cleft lip usually is obvious, and an appropriate palatal examination will demonstrate most clefts of the palate. Occasionally, submucous cleft palates (ie, secondary palate intact but muscles not joined properly) will present late with failure to thrive or even later with speech problems. During the initial examination, concomitant feeding issues become the central presenting symptom. While most children with an isolated cleft lip have little difficulty with feeding, children with a cleft palate often require significant assistance. This is because of significant problems generating negative intraoral pressure, creating difficulty with breastfeeding and bottle-feeding. Reduced efficiency of nutritive sucking can lead to lengthy feeding times, the ingestion of excessive amounts of air, and fatigue for babies and parents. Moreover, it may be difficult for the baby to stabilize the nipple in the mouth because the opposing palatal tissue surface for tongue compression is absent. How to overcome these feeding deficiencies will be covered in the treatment section of this chapter.

> **Pearl:** Increasing numbers of clefts are detected on prenatal ultrasound, with the remainder detected by proper physical examination at birth.

■ Physical Examination Findings

A complete initial physical examination in a child with a cleft serves as a bridge to further appropriate diagnostic and therapeutic interventions. As with any newborn seen for the first time, Apgar scores, vital signs, and weight should be obtained. Respiratory distress may specifically be present in children with Pierre Robin sequence and require airway evaluation and management for obstruction. Pierre Robin sequence is a condition involving a combination of micrognathia (small mandible) and glossoptosis (protruding tongue), often with a cleft of the secondary palate. In these children, prone position, nasal airway, or intubation may be necessary to support the airway. After confirming the child is stable, a more though examination may ensue.

The upper lip should be examined and classified as unilateral or bilateral and as complete or incomplete. In a complete unilateral cleft lip, the orbicularis oris sphincter is interrupted and muscle fibers turn upward at the cleft to insert partly onto its margin, while other fibers extend to the anterior nasal spine and alar base of the nose. In an incomplete cleft lip, the orbicularis is also interrupted, but often a bridge of skin and mucosa spans the cleft (Figure 11-2A). In a complete bilateral cleft lip, there is no functional orbicularis muscle in the central soft tissue (prolabium) (Figure 11-2B). The nose is also disrupted by the cleft with septal deviation and displaced lower lateral nasal cartilage leading to a slumped nasal contour on the side of the cleft (Figure 11-2C). The gumline (alveolar ridge) and palate should then be inspected for a cleft. Complete cleft palates (unilateral or bilateral) affect the primary and secondary palate (Figure 11-3). Incomplete cleft palates may involve a variable amount of the soft and hard palate. Submucous cleft palates may present with only a bifid uvula, a muscular diastasis of the soft palate in the midline (zona pellucida), or a

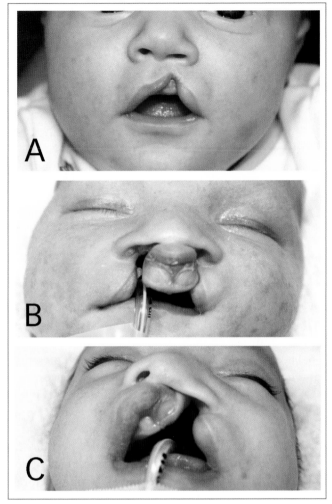

Figure 11-2. The variable presentations of cleft lip. A, Left incomplete cleft lip. B, Bilateral cleft lip. C, Left complete cleft lip.

V-shaped notch at the junction of the hard and soft palate. The posterior palatal muscles form the velum, a muscular sling that acts to lengthen the soft palate and narrow the pharynx. In a cleft palate, this musculature is unable to join in the midline and abnormally inserts at the posterior edge of the hard palate. This disruption helps to explain the feeding, speech, and eustachian tube dysfunction present in children with cleft palate.

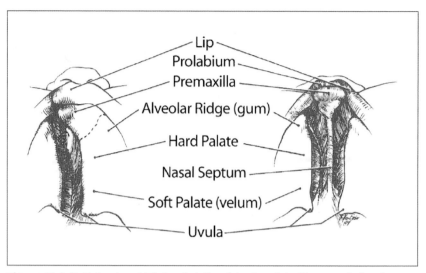

Figure 11-3. Unilateral and bilateral cleft palate. Reprinted by permission from Cleft Palate Foundation.

The ears should be examined and assessed for otitis media with effusion (OME) via pneumatic otoscopy. There exists a high rate of eustachian tube dysfunction in children with cleft palate. Children with cleft palate are highly susceptible to OME, which presents at an early age and has a prolonged course and high rate of recurrence.

Because the prognosis for children with isolated clefts is good, whereas the prognosis for those children with associated anomalies is variable, a complete craniofacial, cardiopulmonary, and extremity examination should also be performed. Pits of the lower lip are seen in van der Woude syndrome. Pierre Robin sequence in a child with a flat nasal bridge and myopia typifies Stickler syndrome. Velocardiofacial syndrome presents variably with cleft palate, velopharyngeal insufficiency (VPI), cardiac anomalies, unusual facial appearance, and learning difficulties. Children with Treacher Collins syndrome often demonstrate auricular anomalies, midfacial hypoplasia, down-slanting palpebral fissures, and cleft palate. There are many more syndromes associated with CL/P, and genetic consultation is appropriate for further diagnostic workup and parental counseling.

> **Pearl:** The disruption of the normal palatal muscular anatomy seen in cleft palates explains the feeding, speech, and otologic difficulties that arise.

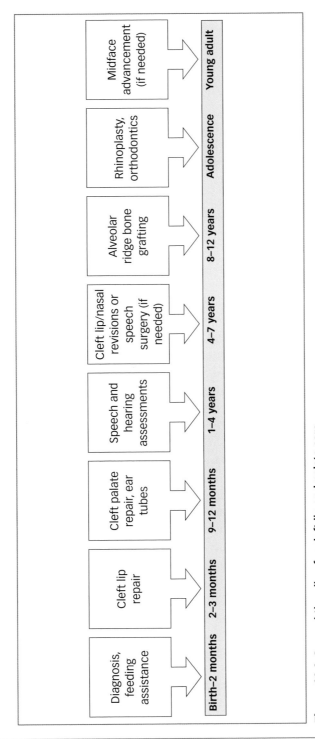

Figure 11-4. General time line for cleft lip and palate care.

■ Diagnosis

The diagnosis of CL/P is usually via prenatal ultrasound or in the early postnatal period. If detected on prenatal ultrasound, a prenatal consultation with a cleft team is appropriate. Parents of babies with clefts are often shocked and confused. To cope with these feelings, they find it very useful to have a prenatal meeting with the cleft team who will be caring for their child after birth. Following birth, a previously undiagnosed cleft is typically recognized on initial physical examination. A diagnosis of CL/P following birth is equally traumatic to parents, with similar feelings of bereavement and loss while the family copes with all the typical issues of having a new baby. Occasionally, small posterior or submucous cleft palates may initially go unrecognized. These babies may present as failing to thrive or be slow feeders and unable to breast-feed. To ensure diagnosis, it is important to examine inside the mouth with a tongue depressor and palpate the palate.

Proper physical diagnosis will lead to appropriate classification of the cleft. The ACPA introduced a complex classification in 1962, and many more have been introduced since that time. While these are important for the cleft team and to monitor specific patient outcomes, they are not critical for effective caregiver and provider communication. A more straightforward scheme stratifies patients into 3 categories: cleft lip (including alveolus), CL/P, and isolated cleft palates as far forward as the incisive foramen. The description should also indicate whether the cleft is unilateral or bilateral in nature. Simplifying the classification allows for improved communication between the pediatrician and cleft team, as well as informing parents about their child's diagnosis.

In addition to the diagnostic aspects of the physical examination in identifying the classification of CL/P, assessment of hearing is important. Universal newborn hearing screening should identify those children with moderate to severe hearing loss early. The increased incidence of OME, glue ear, and conductive hearing loss in cleft palate patients has long been recognized. Because OME occurs essentially in all cleft palate patients, early recognition, treatment, and audiologic follow-up are crucial. Although not initially diagnosed because of potential impairments in velopharyngeal function and hearing, speech development should be assessed early. Children with cleft palate who are at risk can be identified at 18 months of age on 98% of occasions by a cleft-trained speech pathologist.

> **Pearls:** A simple classification for clefts includes isolated cleft lip, isolated cleft palate, and cleft lip and palate. The cleft should be further described as unilateral or bilateral.

■ Treatment Options

Children with CL/P will often require an ongoing treatment plan spanning from birth into late adolescence. This treatment follows a sequence of staged surgical procedures associated with rehabilitative speech, orthodontic measures, and attention to psychosocial needs. The pediatrician is often a pivotal person in the care coordination of the child with CL/P. If a child with a cleft is born, it is important that parents have the opportunity to meet with a cleft team member soon after diagnosis for accurate information (Box 11-1). When a newborn is found to have a CL/P, most parents initially experience shock, denial, sadness, anger, and anxiety before they are able to bond with their baby. Early interaction with a cleft team can reassure parents and address their fears. Members of a cleft team typically include a cleft surgeon, audiologist, speech pathologist, dentist/orthodontist, social worker, otolaryngologist, oral maxillofacial surgeon, geneticist, psychologist, pediatrician, nutritionist, and patient care coordinator.

When a neonate is born with a cleft (especially cleft palate), initial treatment should focus on feeding. Although babies with clefts may require modifications in feeding practices prior to surgical closure of the defect, few changes in dietary recommendations are necessary. A feeding assessment should ideally be carried out by a feeding specialist (eg, speech pathologist) within 24 hours of the birth. A variety of specific nipples and bottles are specially designed to assist a child with

---

Box 11-1. Topic Areas to Discuss With Parents of Newborns With Cleft Lip or Palate

♦ Explain that the cleft is not their fault.
♦ Use proper medical terminology (ie, cleft lip or palate).
♦ Demonstrate normal aspects of the physical examination.
♦ Discuss feeding difficulties and demonstrate feeding techniques.
♦ Reassure that the child is not in pain.
♦ Discuss and arrange cleft team consultation.
♦ Reassure parents that cleft lip or palate is correctable with surgery.

a cleft palate to effectively feed. No single device is superior to others, and the feeding specialist can aid the parents or caregivers in determining what works best for their child. Common names of feeders used in the United States include the Haberman feeder, Mead Johnson Cleft Palate Nurser, and Pigeon Nipple. Most children can obtain an adequate number of calories strictly on oral feeding. Close follow-up is required after hospital discharge to ensure adequate weight gain. Alterations to increased calories in the formula or substitution of assisted devices may be required if there is poor weight gain. A nutritionist can be a valuable resource in treating feeding difficulties.

Depending on the anomaly, children with CL/P will follow a general time line of surgical interventions throughout their first 20 years of life (Figure 11-4). The cleft surgeon, under the recommendations of the cleft team, performs the initial surgeries. If a cleft lip is present it is typically repaired at 2 to 3 months of age. A generally quoted parameter for surgery is the rule of 10s: the child is older than 10 weeks, weighs more than 10 lb, and has a hemoglobin greater than 10 g/dL. Occasionally, if the cleft lip is wide, techniques will first be used to narrow the cleft gap. These include lip taping, nasal alveolar molding, or lip adhesion. After the cleft lip repair, children are often placed in soft arm restraints to limit digital trauma to the surgical site.

Cleft palate repair is usually around 9 to 12 months of age to allow sufficient palatal and maxillary growth for the repair and to minimize subsequent growth problems but before the child develops speech. Surgery involves the palate muscles being detached and moved from their abnormal lateral insertion to reform a more normally functioning sling across the midline. Nasal and oral mucosal flaps are joined in the midline to prevent oronasal communication. Patients are admitted postoperatively, often with a stitch in the tongue placed in case of airway obstruction (so as not to use an oral airway). The infant's oxygen saturation is monitored overnight, and the patient can usually be discharged the following day if taking adequate nutrition by mouth. Avoiding bottles, pacifiers, and straws minimizes sucking motion, which could potentially disrupt the palate repair. Arm restraints are again used to avoid digital trauma to the palate.

Eustachian tube dysfunction is extremely common in children with cleft palate because of the altered muscle position of the palate and anomalies of the eustachian tube. Close medical and audiologic follow-up during the first 5 years of life ensures detection of significant hearing loss. The American Academy of Pediatrics (AAP) clinical practice guideline on OME places children with cleft palate in an at-risk group for development delays. Consideration for early placement of ventilation ear tubes is thus recommended. A recent study provides evidence that most children with cleft palate have reduced hearing levels unless ventilation tubes have been inserted. Most ventilation tubes are placed at the time of cleft palate repair, although some will be placed earlier at the time of cleft lip repair. The role of the audiologist and otolaryngologist is to continue to monitor hearing and eustachian tube function when patients return to the cleft team.

After the initial surgical repairs of the clefts and placement of ear tubes, patients are typically followed every 9 to 12 months with the cleft team. A hearing and speech assessment at those visits will determine any deficits. From 18 months on, the patient will be regularly monitored for speech development and proper function of the palate. The specific structural deficiencies of a cleft palate can impose articulatory constraints on speech development. These include VPI, residual clefts or fistula after initial repair, nasal obstruction, and dental/occlusal anomalies. An estimated two-thirds of children with cleft palate repairs are recommended to receive speech therapy. Often, speech therapy will be all that is required to overcome articulation problems. Velopharyngeal insufficiency is characterized by hypernasal resonance, weak pressure consonants, or nasal emission accompanying pressure-consonant production. A dysfunctional palate with incomplete closure of the velopharyngeal sphincter can lead to VPI. Approximately 5% to 30% of children will require secondary speech surgery following cleft palate repair due to VPI. Most surgeons will accomplish the repair with a pharyngeal flap or sphincter pharyngoplasty, essentially narrowing the nasopharyngeal inlet. The goal is eliminating velopharyngeal dysfunction without creating obstructive sleep apnea, which is a known side effect of the operations. The role of the speech pathologist on a cleft team is to identify and recommend appropriate treatment.

Dental, orthodontic, and oral-maxillofacial physicians play an important role in the care of a child with a cleft of the palate or alveolus. Children with CL/P may have missing or extra teeth. They have an increased incidence of tooth decay, so earlier cleanings and preventive dental care are important. While the child has mixed dentition (7–10 years of age) and prior to eruption of the cleft canine, the cleft alveolus is typically closed with a bone graft. The bone graft is obtained from autologous cancellous bone from the iliac crest. Formal orthodontics can then proceed to improve dental occlusion. Occasionally, cleft patients will develop midface retrusion because of impaired maxillary growth after CL/P repair. The need for maxillary advancement surgery to bring the midface forward occurs in about 5% to 25% of CL/P patients. The oral-maxillofacial surgeon or cleft surgeon on the cleft team performs this surgery.

Children with cleft lip deformities often have underlying nasal deformities caused by the altered anatomy. To improve appearance and function of the nose, most cleft surgeons will perform septorhinoplasty for correction. A primary rhinoplasty is often carried out at the time of cleft lip repair. Further nasal tip work may be performed to achieve symmetry with other future surgeries. A definitive secondary septorhinoplasty that includes improving septal and bony abnormalities is reserved until adolescence. This ensures that nasal development is not interrupted and an appropriate-sized nose has formed. Revisions of cleft lip (to improve lip scar) and palate (close fistulas) can also be combined with these secondary procedures if necessary.

> **Pearl:** Early referral to a cleft team can ensure the proper stepwise treatment plan necessary for children with clefts.

■ Natural History and Prognosis

The natural history of an unrepaired CL/P is that of continued facial deformity, speech and feeding difficulties, and ear problems into adulthood. Studies of young adults with unoperated CL/P demonstrate less facial growth restriction than in those with early repair. Treating the facial disfigurement and speech and feeding impairments far outweighs any potential midface growth restriction challenges. Based on refinements of technique and successful outcomes, the question has not been whether to repair but the appropriate timing of surgery.

Regarding cleft lip repair, studies have shown that neonatal surgery does not provide better results or any psychological benefit for parents. In addition, permitting the child to grow and tolerate surgery at 3 months of age allows the parents time to get to know their child and adjust to the appearance of the cleft. Children who cope well later in life are those whose parents are psychologically well-adjusted to the CL/P.

Following cleft lip surgery at 2 to 3 months, the timing of cleft palate repair must be decided. Early studies have definitively proven that a child has a better chance of normal speech if the cleft palate is repaired early. Unfortunately, surgery to the bony cleft alveolus and palate has been shown to interfere with maxillary growth. Despite this paradox, evidence exists that good facial growth and good speech can be achieved following closure of the palate, in a single stage before 1 year of age—thus, the selection of a 9- to 12-month window for closure of the cleft palate. If cleft palate repair is delayed, speech development will be worse. Even following these parameters, 20% to 30% of children will require prolonged intense speech therapy or secondary speech surgery because of articulation errors and VPI.

The natural otologic history of children with cleft palate is that of OME and eustachian tube dysfunction. Prospective trials in which myringotomy has been undertaken routinely at the same time as cleft repair demonstrate an incidence of 92%, as compared with a prevalence of 20% in children without cleft palate. Eustachian tube function improves in older children with cleft palates, and after the age of 6 years there is likely to be resolution of OME. Otologic examination in older children with cleft palate should evaluate for tympanic membrane perforations, persistent OME, and cholesteatoma. Referral to an otolaryngologist is appropriate if suspicious of these disorders.

By following an appropriate surgical and intervention time line in children with CL/P, excellent results are obtained. Early referral to a cleft team will place the child under the umbrella of many trained professionals. Their common goal is to attain as much normalcy for the child with CL/P as possible, and the reported outcome studies demonstrate that this is achievable.

■ Ankyloglossia

INTRODUCTION

Ankyloglossia, commonly known as tongue-tie, is a congenital oral anomaly characterized by an abnormally short lingual frenulum. The extent to which ankyloglossia results in clinical symptoms and the appropriate treatment of this condition have long been a subject of controversy. In the 18th century, there are reports recommending clipping the lingual frenulum in tongue-tied infants to facilitate breastfeeding. Many midwives during this period would divide the lingual frenulum of all babies with their fingernails. Current opinion ranges from the belief that ankyloglossia only rarely interferes with feeding, speech, and mechanical dysfunction of the tongue to enthusiastic support for frenotomy, especially in babies. Part of the disparity is that the definition of ankyloglossia is not standardized, and there is wide variation of opinion about its clinical significance and optimal management.

This section discusses the presentation and examination of a child with ankyloglossia and reviews the literature for evidence-based treatment and outcomes.

EPIDEMIOLOGY

The reported incidence of ankyloglossia ranges from 1% to 5%. Messner et al screened 1,041 newborns and found 50 with ankyloglossia (4.8%). Most affected neonates were graded as having mild ankyloglossia with thin frenula. They found a male-to-female ration of 2.6:1. Other studies have noted a male predominance but no racial predilection. As the AAP recommends breastfeeding, there may be a rise in detection of ankyloglossia for babies whose parents follow those guidelines.

> **Pearl:** The incidence of ankyloglossia ranges from 1% to 5% in newborns.

PRESENTING SYMPTOMS

Symptoms caused by ankyloglossia ultimately result from impaired tongue mobility. This impairment may be associated with breastfeeding difficulty (eg, poor latch, maternal nipple pain), speech difficulty (articulation), social embarrassment, or mechanical problems. Most women with babies affected by tongue-tie are able to breastfeed without difficulty. However, breastfeeding problems are more frequent among babies with ankyloglossia than without (25% versus 3%). Feeding issues are characterized by nipple pain lasting longer than 6 weeks, difficulty with latching, poor weight gain, and even failure to thrive.

The older child with ankyloglossia may present with articulation problems. The disorder does not prevent vocalization or delay the onset of speech. Speech sounds that may be affected include sibilants and lingual sounds (t, d, z, s, th, n, and l). Preteens and adolescents with ankyloglossia may present with mechanical problems due to tongue mobility deficit. This may include difficulty with oral hygiene, licking ice cream, kissing, licking lips, local discomfort, and playing a wind instrument.

> **Pearl:** In babies with ankyloglossia, early symptoms will center on feeding difficulties, whereas speech and social issues affect older children.

PHYSICAL EXAMINATION FINDINGS

Ankyloglossia features a congenitally shortened lingual frenulum or a highly attached genioglossus muscle that restricts tongue movement (Figure 11-5A). Physical examination features include a short frenulum inserting at or near the tip of the tongue, a notched or heart-shaped tongue when protruded, difficulty lifting the tongue to the upper dental alveolus, inability to protrude the tongue more than 1 to 2 mm past the lower central incisors, or impaired side-to-side movement. The oral cavity and tongue should be visually and manually inspected for these deficiencies. Placement of a tongue blade along the undersurface of the tongue permits ideal visualization of the frenulum insertion. In the

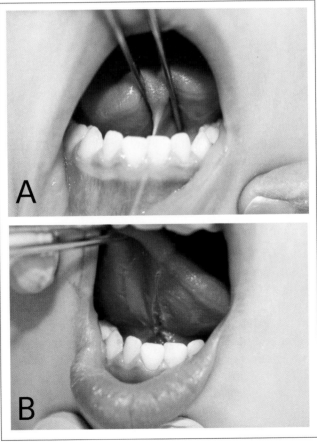

Figure 11-5. A, Ankyloglossia with tethered anterior lingual frenulum. **B,** Following division and suture closure (frenuloplasty).

infant, breastfeeding difficulties can be monitored for poor latch or nipple pain. In older children, articulation difficulty should be assessed for lingual sounds. Tongue mobility can also be assessed objectively to gauge impairment or mechanical problems. Tongue protrusion can be measured by recording maximal extension (in mm) of the tongue tip past the lower dentition. Tongue elevation can be assessed by measuring the maximal interincisal distance (in mm) that the patient can achieve while maintaining the tongue tip in contact with the posterior surface of the upper central incisor teeth.

> **Pearl:** Lifting the tongue with a gloved finger or tongue depressor can aid the physical evaluation of ankyloglossia.

DIAGNOSIS

The diagnosis of ankyloglossia is relatively straightforward and based on the anatomic findings of a shortened and tethered lingual frenulum. Clinically significant ankyloglossia includes the symptoms covered in the previous section: breastfeeding difficulties, speech articulation deficits, mechanical problems, and social embarrassment. Differential diagnosis would include a tethered frenulum from previous trauma or surgery with subsequent scarring leading to restricted lingual movement.

TREATMENT OPTIONS

Opinions and practice regarding ankyloglossia vary among pediatricians, lactation consultants, otolaryngologists, and speech pathologists, often with no clear consensus. This may be related to the lack of a uniformly accepted standard for diagnosis. By defining the parameters to include the physical examination findings of a shortened or tethered lingual frenulum in the setting of clinical sequelae, a more consistent plan of treatment may be followed.

The most prevalent segment of the ankyloglossia population is the infant with breastfeeding difficulty. While some postulate that progressive stretching and use of the frenulum leads to spontaneous elongation, this has not been substantiated in prospective studies. In an infant with suspicion of tongue-tie and early feeding difficulty, consultation with a lactation specialist or speech pathologist may help the child compensate. The other viable option is the surgical division of the frenulum. Referral to a physician trained in this surgery is appropriate.

The goal of surgical division of the frenulum is to increase the mobility of the tongue. Surgical options include frenotomy or frenuloplasty. Frenotomy is a simple release or cutting of the frenulum. Neonatal frenotomy is a straightforward procedure that can be safely accomplished in the office setting at the time of consultation. Local anesthesia can aid pain control but is not mandatory. The infant is typically restrained for safety and to assess the mouth. The tongue is elevated and divided with scissors near the lingual undersurface of the tongue to avoid the submandibular ducts. Clipping of the frenulum rarely leads to significant bleeding and can be controlled with gauze or pressure. Acetaminophen may be used for pain control but is often not required. The infant may immediately resume breastfeeding without restriction.

Frenuloplasty is division of the frenulum with plastic repair (Figure 11-5B). This is reserved for thick frenula, older children, those prone to scar formation, or revision cases. In frenuloplasty, the frenulum is similarly divided with scissors or cautery as in frenotomy. The surround mucosa, however, is then closed with absorbable sutures to prevent recurrence of tethering. In severe cases, a V-Y advancement, Z-plasty, or buccal mucosal graft may be required. With either surgical option, treatment is effective with few side effects, minimal postoperative discomfort, and low recurrence rates.

> **Pearl:** Frenotomy and frenuloplasty are safe surgical options with minimal morbidity in the management of ankyloglossia.

NATURAL HISTORY AND PROGNOSIS

Most babies born with ankyloglossia have mild cases and may even go unnoticed. Clinically significant problems caused by the tongue restriction are unlikely to self-resolve. Fortunately, frenotomy is reliable, safe, and effective. Additionally, large series detailing frenotomy have been published, often without any complications. A prospective trial compared babies with ankyloglossia and feeding problems who were randomly assigned to 48 hours of lactation support or immediate frenotomy. Feeding difficulty improved in all the babies who received frenotomy but in only one of the babies who received intense support.

Geddes et al showed that for breastfeeding babies who were experiencing feeding difficulties, frenotomy improved tongue movement and nipple distortion, as imaged by ultrasound. Improved milk intake, milk transfer, attachment, and maternal nipple pain were also improved. Moreover, comparison of weight gain (based on percentile increases) consistently improved in those affected by ankyloglossia following frenotomy. Finally, for older children with articulation errors, mechanical symptoms, or social embarrassment related to tongue mobility impairment, frenuloplasty is an effective solution.

The overall prognosis is excellent for the infant or child with ankyloglossia, with treatment reserved for those symptomatic because of their anatomic defect. Frenotomy and frenuloplasty are immediate and effective surgical options, with minimal morbidity.

■ Selected References

American Academy of Family Physicians, American Academy of Otolaryngology-Head and Neck Surgery, American Academy of Pediatrics Subcommittee on Otitis Media With Effusion. Clinical practice guideline: otitis media with effusion. *Pediatrics.* 2004;113(5):1412–1429

Atkinson M. Surgical management of otitis media with effusion in children—NICE guideline: what paediatricians need to know. *Arch Dis Child Educ Pract Ed.* 2009;94(4):115–117

Ballard JL, Auer CE, Khoury JC. Ankyloglossia: assessment, incidence, and effect of frenuloplasty on the breastfeeding dyad. *Pediatrics.* 2002;110(5):e63

Bender PL. Genetics of cleft lip and palate. *J Pediatr Nurs.* 2000;15(4):242–249

Bluestone CD. Eustachian tube obstruction in the infant with cleft palate. *Ann Oto Rhino Laryngol.* 1978;80(Suppl 2):1–30

Boyne PJ, Sands NR. Secondary bone grafting of residual alveolar and palate clefts. *J Oral Surg.* 1972;30(2):87–92

Broen PA, Moller KT, Carlstrom J, Doyle SS, Devers M, Keenan KM. Comparison of the hearing histories of children with and without cleft palate. *Cleft Palate Craniofac J.* 1996;33(2):127–133

Coy K, Speltz ML, Jones K. Facial appearance and attachment in infants with orofacial clefts: a replication. *Cleft Palate Craniofac J.* 2002;39(1):66–72

Dalston RM. Communication skills of children with cleft lip and palate: a status report. In: Bardach J, Morris HL, eds. *Multidisciplinary Management of Cleft Lip and Palate.* Philadelphia, PA: Saunders; 746–749

Fraser GR, Calnan JS. Cleft lip and palate: seasonal incidence, birth weight, birth rank, sex, site, associated malformations and parental age. A statistical survey. *Arch Dis Child.* 1961;36:420–423

Geddes DT, Langton DB, Gollow I, Jacobs LA, Hartmann PE, Simmer K. Frenulotomy for breastfeeding infants with ankyloglossia: effect on milk removal and sucking mechanism as imaged by ultrasound. *Pediatrics.* 2008;122(1):e188–e194

Grow JL, Lehman JA. A local perspective on the initial management of children with cleft lip and palate by primary care physicians. *Cleft Palate Craniofac J.* 2002;39(5): 535–540

Hogan M, Westcott C, Griffiths M. Randomized, controlled trial of division of tongue-tie in infants with feeding problems. *J Paediatr Child Health.* 2005;41(5-6):246–250

Horton CE, Crawford HH, Adamson JE, Ashbell TS. Tongue-tie. *Cleft Palate J.* 1969;6:8–23

Jorgenson RJ, Shapiro SD, Salinas CF, Levin LS. Intraoral findings and anomalies in neonates. *Pediatrics.* 1982;69(5):577–582

Kaufman FL. Managing the cleft lip and palate patient. *Pediatr Clin North Am.* 1991; 38(5):1127–1147

Lalakea ML, Messner AH. Ankyloglossia: does it matter? *Pediatr Clin North Am.* 2003; 50(2):381–397

Lalakea ML, Messner AH. Ankyloglossia: the adolescent and adult perspective. *Otolarygol Head Neck Surg.* 2003;128(5):746–752

Lees M. Genetics of cleft lip and palate. In: Watson Ach, Sell DA, Grunwell P, eds. *Management of Cleft Lip and Palate.* London, England: Whurr; 2001

Maarse W, Bergé SJ, Pistorius L, et al. Diagnostic accuracy of transabdominal ultrasound in detecting prenatal cleft lip and palate: a systematic review. *Ultrasound Obstet Gynecol.* 2010;35(4):495–502

Messner AH, Lalakea ML. Ankyloglossia: controversies in management. *Int J Pediatr Otorhinolaryngol.* 2000;54(2-3):123–131

Messner AH, Lalakea ML, Aby J, Macmahon J, Blair E. Ankyloglossia: incidence and associated feeding difficulties. *Arch Otolaryngol Head Neck Surg.* 2000;126(1):36–39

Milerad J, Larson O, Hagberg C, Ideberg M. Associated malformations with cleft lip and palate: a prospective, population-based study. *Pediatrics.* 1997;100(2 Pt 1):180–186

Noar JH. Questionnaire survey of attitudes and concerns of parents with cleft lip and palates and their parents. *Cleft Palate Craniofac J.* 1991;28(3):279–284

Nyberg DA, Sickler Gk, Hegge FN, Kramer DJ, Kropp RJ. Fetal cleft lip with and without cleft palate: US classification and correlation with outcome. *Radiology.* 1995;195(3):677–684

Paradise JL, Bluestone CD, Felder H. The universality of otitis media in 50 infants with cleft palate. *Pediatrics.* 1969;44(1):35–42

Randall P, LaRossa DD, Fakhraee SM, Cohen MA. Cleft palate closure at 3 to 7 months of age: a preliminary report. *Plast Reconstr Surg.* 1983;71(5):624–628

Redford-Badwal DA, Mabry K, Frassinelli JD. Impact of cleft lip and/or palate on nutritional health and oral-motor development. *Dent Clin North Am.* 2003;47(2):305–317

Robinson PJ, Lodge S, Jones BM, Walker CC, Grant HR. The effect of palate repair on otitis media with effusion. *Plast Reconstr Surg.* 1992;89(4):640–645

Senders CW, Peterson EC, Hendrickx AG, Cukierski MA. Development of the upper lip. *Arch Facial Plast Surg.* 2003;5(1):16–25

Slade P, Emerson DJ, Freedlander E. A longitudinal comparison of the psychological impact on mothers of neonatal and 3 month repair of cleft lip. *Br J Plast Surg.* 1999; 52(1):1–5

Strauss RP, Sharp MC, Lorch SC, Kachalia B. Physicians and the communication of "bad news": parent experiences of being informed of their child's cleft lip and/or palate. *Pediatrics.* 1995;96(1 Pt 1):82–89

Suslak L, Desposito F. Infants with cleft lip/cleft palate. *Pediatr Rev.* 1988;9(10):331–334

Vanderas AP. Incidence of cleft lip, cleft palate, and cleft lip and palate among races: a review. *Cleft Palate J.* 1987;24(3):216–225

Williams WN, Waldron CM. Assessment of lingual function when ankyloglossia (tongue-tie) is suspected. *J Am Dent Assoc.* 1985;110(3):353–356

Young JL, O'Riordan M, Goldstein JA, Robin NH. What information do parents of newborns with cleft lip, palate, or both want to know? *Cleft Palate Craniofac J.* 2001;38(1):55–58

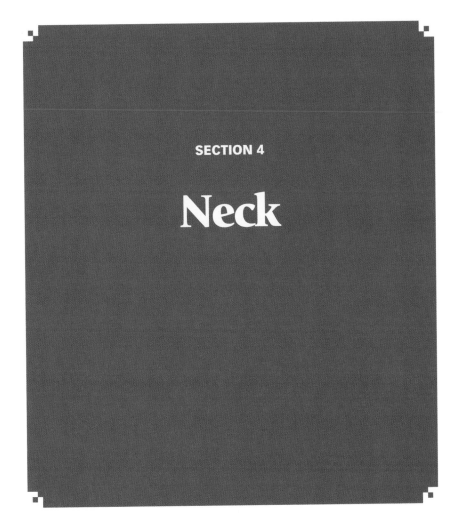

SECTION 4

Neck

CHAPTER 12

Neck Masses and Adenopathy

Randall A. Bly, MD, and Sanjay R. Parikh, MD

■ Introduction

Neck masses in children represent a variety of pathologies, encompassing many possible etiologies, ranging from congenital to infectious to neoplastic. Masses can be present anywhere in the head and neck with varying rates of growth and age of onset. Initial assessment must include evaluation of the airway because compression can occur with some masses. Infectious masses may present with septicemia and the patient may be acutely ill. Certainly in these cases urgent treatment should be initiated, typically with referral to an emergency department and otolaryngology consultation.

In general, differential diagnosis favors infectious and congenital etiologies because of the rarity of neoplasms in the pediatric population. Palpable cervical lymphadenitis is common and prevalent in nearly half of all healthy children. Fortunately, in most cases these represent benign processes. However, a level of suspicion must be maintained for cases in which history, physical examination, or imaging are concerning. In many of these cases, additional workup or biopsy may be necessary.

To formulate differential diagnosis and begin treatment, it is helpful for the clinician to classify the mass by its clinical presentation and history. A useful way to organize the neck mass is by location, whether it is midline or lateral on the neck (Figure 12-1). In general, midline neck masses will represent congenital etiology. Any mass that is not located near the anterior midline is referred to as lateral, including masses that arise in the posterior neck. Lateral neck masses are more variable in their etiology, but infectious is the most likely cause. When combined with clinical history and examination, differential diagnosis can be made to guide the workup of neck masses in children.

> **Pearl:** Midline neck masses are more likely to be caused by congenital malformations, whereas lateral neck masses are often seen with infectious etiologies.

■ Epidemiology

The most common presentation of masses in the neck is cervical adenopathy. A study in Sweden demonstrated that up to 45% of healthy schoolchildren had palpable cervical lymphadenopathy on examination. When symptomatic patients who are seeking treatment for cervical

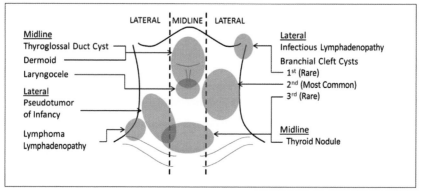

Figure 12-1. Typical location regions for common midline and lateral pediatric neck masses. There is significant variability in the location for many etiologies. Infectious lymphadenopathy can occur anywhere but is more likely to be located in the lateral neck. Lymphoma lymphadenopathy may present anywhere in the neck but typically laterally in the posterior triangle. *Note:* Region locations drawn for clarity in labeling and can occur on the left or right side (slight left- or right-sided propensities for certain congenital etiologies not necessarily depicted).

lymphadenopathy are studied, up to 75% of cases are due to reactive lymph nodes caused by bacterial or viral infections. In most of these cases, neck masses were located in the lateral neck.

Congenital etiologies such as thyroglossal duct cysts, branchial cleft cysts, and lymphatic malformations have been reported to represent 12% to 22% of all neck masses in multiple studies.

Neoplastic processes such as lymphoma, sarcoma, or metastatic lesions account for less than 8% of neck masses in the pediatric population.

■ Presenting Symptoms

Masses can present in a variety of ways—painless lumps noted incidentally or acute, painful, erythematous masses in the neck. Cervical adenopathy can be discrete or diffuse with or without local inflammation. Detailed clinical history about the mass or masses should be obtained. Additional information such as tuberculosis exposure, prior bacille Calmette-Guérin (BCG) vaccine, or cat exposure can be helpful. Abscesses can occur anywhere in the head and neck, superficial and deep.

Congenital etiologies may present with infectious symptoms. A tender midline neck mass in a patient with fevers and localized erythema may represent a previously subclinical thyroglossal duct cyst or dermoid cyst that has become acutely infected.

Because of the wide variety of pathology that can manifest as neck masses, presenting symptoms discussed as follows relate to the specific diagnosis.

■ Physical Examination Findings

Careful attention should be paid to vital signs, including growth curve to assess trends in weight loss. This is particularly important in more chronic processes. Neck masses are characterized by location, quality, size, and appearance.

In young children, many neck masses can be seen with simple visual inspection if the patient looks up toward the ceiling. This will stretch the skin, bring the larynx forward, and especially help to reveal midline masses (Figure 12-2). Palpation with the pads of the index and middle fingers are best to appreciate subtle masses underlying the skin. Palpation of all regions of the neck can discover a diffuse process that a patient initially thought was a single mass. In these cases especially, an examination of lymph node regions outside the neck is important, including supraclavicular, axillary, and inguinal lymph node groups.

A thorough head and neck examination is essential, including testing of cranial nerves. For example, a rare first branchial cleft cyst presents as a mass near the angle of the mandible, but a sinus tract may also be seen in the external auditory canal on otoscopy. This provides important clues about etiology. A mass in a similar location over the parotid gland may be associated with peritonsillar swelling and may represent a mass in the deep lobe of the parotid. In addition, there are systemic inflammatory etiologies that cause cervical adenopathy. Thus,

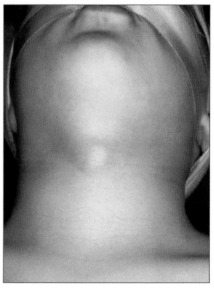

Figure 12-2. Midline neck mass in a 14-year-old boy confirmed to be a thyroglossal duct cyst on pathology after Sistrunk procedure.

a complete history and physical examination can help elucidate these challenging diagnoses.

■ Differential Diagnosis of Midline Neck Masses

THYROGLOSSAL DUCT CYSTS

Thyroglossal duct cysts represent nearly 75% of all midline neck masses in children. These cysts are remnants of the embryologic descent of the thyroid gland, which begins at the foramen caecum at the base of the tongue. In nearly 70% of cases, initial presentation is a midline, nontender neck mass at the level of the thyroid cartilage. About 20% of the time it will present with an infection. Ultrasound is the diagnostic imaging modality of choice. It can often confirm the diagnosis as well as confirm that the thyroid gland is normal appearing.

Ectopic thyroid tissue is present within the cyst in 1% to 2% of cases. There is no definitive evidence, but in general there is no need for radioisotope scanning if ultrasound shows a normal thyroid gland in its anatomic position lower in the neck. In those cases, it is also useful to obtain thyroid function tests.

Treatment options are observation versus surgical removal via the Sistrunk procedure, which also removes a portion of the hyoid bone and the tract that extends into the base of tongue. Recurrence rate is extremely high if only the cyst is removed. If a patient presents with an infected cyst, antibiotic therapy is best initial management and a Sistrunk procedure should be considered when inflammation has reduced. Performing a simple incision and drainage on an acutely infected cyst may cause scarring and make the Sistrunk procedure more challenging and increase the risk of recurrence. Regardless, this may be necessary for infections that are refractory to medical therapy. Typically, if the mass is bothersome or has been infected, it is recommended that it be surgically removed to prevent future problems.

> **Pearl:** An acutely inflamed thyroglossal duct cyst is best managed with medical therapy to avoid scarring. This will improve outcome of a complete resection later when there is less inflammation.

DERMOID CYSTS

Dermoid cysts are part of a spectrum of benign neoplasms. They are composed of ectoderm and mesoderm tissue and are the most common type. Only 7% of all dermoid cysts occur in the head and neck, and the periorbital region is the most common location. Other locations include nasal tip and neck, and they are often found near the midline.

Dermoid cysts in the neck present similarly to thyroglossal duct cysts with palpable mass, frequently with noted recent change and firm consistency. Unlike thyroglossal duct cysts, dermoid cysts generally present with progressive indolent growth and no history of fluctuating size. Ultrasound may not be able to discern between the two. Treatment is complete surgical resection, but observation is an option if the patient is asymptomatic and the mass is small. Acute infectious episodes should be managed medically with antibiotics and consideration for surgical excision when acute infection has resolved.

Other lesions in the spectrum are rare and include *teratoid tumors* (contains poorly differentiated ectoderm, mesoderm, and endoderm), *true teratomas* (contains well-differentiated tissue from all 3 layers), and *epignathus,* in which identifiable fetal organs may be seen such as limbs within the mass. These tumors may be very large and present at birth. Some may cause airway obstruction. When possible, complete surgical resection is the best treatment option.

THYROID AND PARATHYROID MASSES

Thyroid and parathyroid masses are rare in the pediatric population. Thyroid nodules occur in 0.05% to 1.8% of children, and it is estimated that malignant thyroid disease occurs in fewer than 2 per 100,000 children per year. On examination, there is often a visible and palpable mass that moves in conjunction with the larynx during swallowing. Thyroid function tests, calcium levels, and ultrasound should be ordered for initial evaluation. For lesions greater than 1 cm, tissue biopsy should be obtained to rule out malignancy (Figure 12-3).

There is some evidence to support obtaining a fine-needle aspiration (FNA) biopsy, but there is no general consensus recommendation. In a recent study of 30 pediatric patients undergoing FNA biopsy, there was 1 false-negative result and 5 that were inconclusive. If the patient and family have already decided on surgical excision, or if general anesthesia is needed for FNA, there may be limited utility in obtaining the test in these instances. Conversely, when FNA reveals a cystic lesion with no atypical cells, this study may obviate the need for surgical intervention.

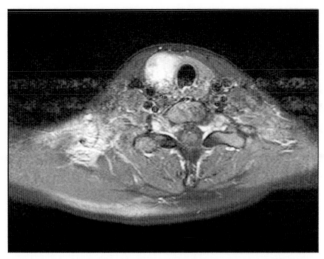

Figure 12-3. Axial T1-weighted magnetic resonance imaging with contrast in a 15-year-old girl with a right thyroid lobe mass who underwent total thyroidectomy after suspicious fine-needle biopsy suggested papillary carcinoma, which was confirmed on final pathology.

The decision to perform FNA is best discussed individually with the patient and family and can be incorporated into the ultrasound assessment by an appropriately trained radiologist.

Thyroid lobectomy is performed when open surgery is required for a tissue diagnosis. When a malignant diagnosis is confirmed, total thyroidectomy with or without nodal dissection of the neck is indicated depending on the pathology. In cases of multiple endocrine neoplasia type 2A, total thyroidectomy is recommended before age 5 years to prevent medullary thyroid carcinoma.

Parathyroid masses are exceedingly rare. Only 7 cases of parathyroid carcinoma are recorded in the literature, and they may not even present with palpable neck mass.

INFANTILE HEMANGIOMAS

Infantile hemangiomas are the most common benign neoplasm of childhood, affecting up to 10% of children in the first 12 months of life. They can occur anywhere in the body, but the most common location is the central portion of the face. These characteristically present in the first few months of life with a proliferative stage and then a variable involution phase after approximately 12 months of age. In recent years, propanolol therapy has become the mainstay treatment for symptomatic or cosmetically significant lesions. Surgery is indicated for certain large lesions or those in close proximity to the orbit. Children should be referred to an institution where multidisciplinary evaluation can occur with a surgeon, cardiologist, and radiologist familiar with the pathology. Vascular malformations are discussed in Chapter 22.

LARYNGOCELES

Laryngoceles are rare and caused by outpouchings of the saccule of the larynx. They can present as a midline neck mass if herniation extends beyond thyroid cartilage. They may protrude through the thyrohyoid membrane, palpable just above thyroid cartilage. If outpouching is internal, infants or children may present with stridor and airway obstruction. Ultrasound and computed tomography (CT) may help delineate the extent of the mass. Flexible or direct laryngoscopy should be performed to assess for internal components. Surgical resection is the recommended treatment.

■ Differential Diagnosis of Lateral Neck Masses

Infectious etiologies are the most common cause of lateral neck masses in the pediatric population. Studies have demonstrated that nearly half of healthy children have a palpable neck mass on examination. Indeed, many cases are benign, self-limiting, and a seemingly normal process in children. The most common locations involved are the submandibular and deep cervical lymph nodes, as these drain most of the cervical lymphatics. Pharyngeal, dental, and scalp infections are sources that lead to reactive cervical lymphadenopathy. Based on clinical presentation, these neck masses can be further divided into acute and chronic categories.

Congenital etiologies are the next most frequently encountered lateral neck masses. Malignancies and inflammatory syndromes are less common but represent a broad spectrum of causes.

In many cases of cervical lymphadenopathy in healthy patients with no associated symptoms or clinical findings, it is not necessary to determine definitive diagnosis if the patient can be closely followed clinically. In most such cases, biopsy will return a diagnosis of reactive adenopathy with no other specific diagnosis. However, in cases in which the child is acutely ill or the mass persists, diagnosis should be sought. Based on clinical presentation, blood and fungal cultures, polymerase chain reaction (PCR) for *Bartonella henselae,* and purified protein derivative (PPD) test should be considered. Imaging modalities of ultrasound and

CT scan may be helpful. If diagnosis is still uncertain and symptoms persist, FNA or open biopsy sent for microbiology and histopathology is the best way to provide definitive diagnosis.

INFECTIOUS CAUSES OF LATERAL NECK MASSES

Acute Lymphadenitis

Bilateral or diffuse acute lymphadenitis is usually caused by viral infection, but bacterial sources such as *Streptococcus pyogenes* or *Mycoplasma pneumoniae* can also be the pathogens. Clinical clues such as coexisting inflammation of the gingiva and oral cavity or rash suggest viral sources such as herpes simplex and cytomegalovirus. Occipital or posterior lymphadenitis is frequently associated with concurrent infection or inflammation of the scalp but may also be associated with rubella infection. Most viral causes are benign and resolve spontaneously.

Mononucleosis infection is a possibility and should be considered in the differential diagnosis. Imaging tests will often reveal multiple lymph nodes, which can be significant in size (6–12 cm). Diagnosis is suggested by elevated atypical lymphocytes on complete blood cell count and confirmed by heterophile antibody test (monospot, 87% sensitive, 91% specific). Antibody testing to viral-specific antibodies (97% sensitive, 94% specific) is preferred to the monospot in children younger than 5 years. If test results are negative but clinical suspicion remains, additional testing, such as PCR for Epstein-Barr virus DNA, can be useful. Confirming diagnosis is important so that other concerning processes, such as neoplasm, can be determined to be less likely on differential diagnosis. This may avoid surgical biopsy to rule out malignancy.

Unilateral or focal acute lymphadenitis is typically caused by bacterial infection. The 2 most common organisms are *Staphylococcus aureus* and *S pyogenes*. There appears to be a trend of increasing incidence of community-acquired methicillin-resistant *S aureus* in many populations. These bacterial infections can progress to form phlegmon or abscess. This causes increased tenderness, decreased neck range of motion, and palpable, tender neck mass. Sometimes there is overlying skin erythema and hyperemia. Ultrasound or CT scan with contrast is often indicated to assess extent of infection. Depending on the patient's clinical stability, surgical drainage may be indicated. Intravenous antibiotic therapy with appropriate coverage based on local antibiograms should be initiated. If a patient is clinically stable, a trial of antibiotic therapy prior to surgical drainage has the potential to avoid a surgical procedure. In these cases, the family and patient must be well informed and the patient should be monitored in the inpatient setting so that reimaging or surgical drainage can be performed quickly if needed. Additional information on deep neck space infections is in Chapter 13.

In neonates, acute unilateral lymphadenitis can be caused by group B streptococcal infection. This typically occurs in males who are febrile with erythematous skin changes and ipsilateral otitis media.

> **Pearl:** Palpable cervical lymphadenopathy is a common finding in children usually caused by reactions to viral infections in the head and neck. Most episodes will resolve spontaneously.

Chronic Lymphadenitis

Chronic lymphadenitis can be caused by various indolent pathogens. These can be challenging to diagnose, and suspicion for a neoplastic process must be maintained for cases refractory to medical management. Regular follow-up is necessary to track progress and order additional tests or place referrals as necessary. Following is a list of pathogens, their presentation, and treatment strategies.

Atypical Mycobacteria (Nontuberculous Mycobacteria)

These can be the cause of unilateral chronic lateral neck masses in children. Atypical mycobacteria include ubiquitous bacteria such as *Mycobacterium avium-intracellulare* and *Mycobacterium scrofulaceum* that are particularly present in midwestern and southwestern United States. These can breach mucosal and skin barriers through cuts or the teething process, which explains why cervical lymph nodes are most likely to be involved. Cases usually present with a single neck mass and characteristic overlying violaceous skin changes. Sometimes there can be spontaneous drainage resulting in a chronic fistula tract. Atypical mycobacteria lymphadenitis must be distinguished from active tuberculosis lymphadenitis. Atypical infections will generally have the following clinical characteristics compared with active tuberculosis:
1. No history of contact with active tuberculosis
2. Purified protein derivative result less than 15 mm
3. Normal chest radiography
4. Younger than 4 years

There have been reports of PPD cross-reactivity in the presence of atypical mycobacterial infections. Thus, definitive diagnosis must be made with histopathologic and microbiological analysis. This can be obtained with FNA or open biopsy. Treatment has traditionally been surgical excision or curettage with excellent results, but recent studies have demonstrated successful treatment with medical therapy or even observation alone in immunocompetent children.

Toxoplasma gondii

Toxoplasma gondii is widespread with prevalence as high as 90% depending on location. Humans can become infected by ingesting oocytes, often from cats or uncooked meats. Examination almost always reveals lymphadenopathy in the neck, with varying incidences of palpable lymphadenopathy in other lymph node regions. Most cases are asymptomatic and self-limiting. Serology testing is available but is rarely clinically indicated, and it can be difficult to prove that acute infection is responsible for current lymphadenopathy.

Bartonella henselae

A small gram-negative bacteria responsible for cat-scratch disease, *B henselae* infections typically occur in patients younger than 10 years, and predominant clinical feature is regional lymphadenopathy. A history of exposure to cats usually younger than 6 months or flea bites and evidence of a pustule at the inoculation site makes this diagnosis more likely. Diagnosis can be confirmed with PCR. Antibiotic therapy (macrolides or trimethoprim-sulfamethoxazole) is effective but often not necessary because many cases are self-limiting. Incision and drainage should be avoided because this can cause skin fistula tracts. If medical therapy is refractory, complete surgical excision should be performed.

HIV

HIV in children can present with chronic, generalized lymphadenopathy. This is often associated with splenomegaly. HIV serologies are part of the complete workup of chronic cervical lymphadenitis.

CONGENITAL CAUSES OF LATERAL NECK MASSES

Branchial Cleft Cysts

Relatively common, branchial cleft cysts account for nearly one-third of all congenital neck masses. The exact mechanism is not clear, but they are most likely caused by incomplete obliteration of branchial clefts in embryogenesis. They typically present in late childhood but can also

first become clinically apparent as an adult. Branchial cleft sinuses—
epithelialized tracts connecting to the pharynx or external auditory
canal—more commonly present in the first decade of life. Cysts of the
second branchial cleft account for 95% of the cysts. Second cleft cysts
present in the lateral neck anterior to the sternocleidomastoid muscle
(Figure 12-4). They may present as nontender cystic masses or as acute
infections with localized erythema and tenderness. A history of fluctuating size in the mass supports congenital etiology. Rare first branchial cleft cysts present as masses at the angle of the mandible and can
communicate with the external auditory canal. Third branchial cleft
cysts and sinuses are also rare and typically present as recurrent localized infections in the lower lateral neck adjacent to the ipsilateral lobe
of the thyroid gland. They can communicate with the pyriform sinus in
the pharynx (Figure 12-5). Recurrent infections of the low anterior neck
should prompt a laryngoscopy to look for a sinus tract at the time of
incision and drainage.

Ultrasound, CT, and magnetic resonance imaging (MRI) are useful to further evaluate the mass in relation to surrounding structures.
Ultrasound is a good initial test to confirm that the mass is cystic.

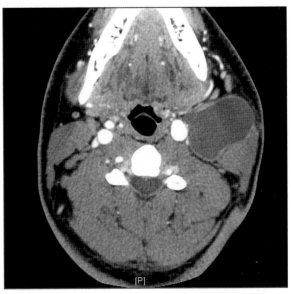

Figure 12-4. Axial computed tomography with contrast
of a 16-year-old boy with persistent fluctuating left
neck mass. Final pathology after complete excision
confirmed a second branchial cleft anomaly.

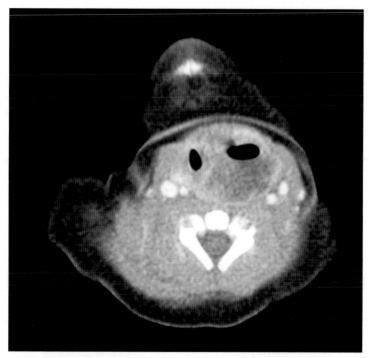

Figure 12-5. Axial computed tomography scan with contrast of a 3-year-old boy with acute onset of left neck mass. Note involvement of thyroid gland and air in mass consistent with infected pharyngeal piriform sinus tract anomaly (also referred to as a third branchial cleft anomaly).

Treatment is complete surgical resection. In the case of acute infection, it is preferred to treat medically with antibiotics because incision and drainage may cause scarring. In some cases, this cannot be avoided, and needle aspiration is often attempted to minimize scarring. Complete surgical resection can be performed with a high success rate if tissue is not actively inflamed.

Pseudotumor of Infancy and Congenital Muscular Torticollis

Pseudotumor of infancy (POI) (also referred to as sternocleidomastoid tumor of infancy or fibromatosis colli) and congenital muscular torticollis (CMT) are rare disorders involving unilateral contracture of the sternocleidomastoid muscle. Infants and children present with lateral neck mass, and prevalence is 0.4%. It is the third most common congenital musculoskeletal anomaly, after hip dislocation and clubfoot. Pseudotumor of infancy and CMT are similar entities, and distinction between the 2 has been vague. Recent literature has referred to POI in patients younger than 6 weeks and CMT if older at time of diagnosis. It can masquerade as neoplastic due to a palpable mass over the sternocleidomastoid muscle, which is present more commonly in infants younger than 6 weeks. Pathogenesis is unclear; theories point to mechanical factors of fetal positioning in utero or birth-related trauma. This is supported by associations with breech presentations and traumatic births.

History and physical examination are the key components to accurate diagnosis. Examination shows the head turned away from the affected side. This is because, for example, the right sternocleidomastoid muscle acts to rotate the head to the left. Examination will reveal a rock-hard mass within the sternocleidomastoid muscle. Ultrasound imaging can demonstrate fusiform enlargement of the sternocleidomastoid muscle if there is a question about diagnosis.

Initial treatment involves range-of-motion exercises for the infant younger than 2 months. Many cases resolve spontaneously. Physical therapy is likely to improve outcomes. For symptoms that persist despite therapy, further imaging can be obtained and surgical intervention is possible. Sternocleidomastoid tenotomy has been shown to be effective at releasing muscle heads. Surgical intervention should be performed when the patient is at least 12 to 18 months old. It is possible to develop facial and skull asymmetry as a result if symptoms persist past this time. The 12- to 18-month window allows ample time for spontaneous improvement to occur but also permits early surgical intervention to prevent facial asymmetry if necessary.

Thymic Cysts

These cysts result from thymic tissue implanting anywhere along the embryologic descent of the thymus from the third pharyngeal pouch. They are rare in the literature but may be more prevalent as they are often asymptomatic and noted incidentally. They are cystic and located to the left of midline. Occasionally they can be large and present with airway obstruction. Evaluation should begin with ultrasound in the stable patient. Surgical excision is the recommended treatment for symptomatic masses. Observation is an option if there are no symptoms in some cases.

Vascular and Lymphatic Malformations

These are discussed in Chapter 22.

MALIGNANT CAUSES OF LATERAL NECK MASSES

Malignancies occur at an incidence of 1 of every 7,000 children younger than 14 years; they represent the second leading cause of death in the 1- to 14-year age group following accidents. Within the head and neck, lymphomas are the most common malignancy encountered. There are many other types of rare malignant neoplasms that can present primarily or as metastatic lesions. Sarcomas and neuroblastomas make up a large portion of these uncommon malignancies.

Lymphoma

Lymphoma in the pediatric population accounts for 10% of all solid tumors in the United States. In regions where Epstein-Barr virus is endemic, Burkitt lymphoma is much more prevalent. Nearly half of pediatric lymphoma cases can present as a mass in the head and neck, according to a recent study in Korea. Other characteristics of lymphoma were found to be male predominance (2.5:1) and age older than 10 years. Hodgkin lymphoma usually presents with painless cervical lymphadenopathy. Follicular and small lymphocytic lymphomas are more likely to present with bilateral painless, soft, discrete, and small cervical nodes. Mucosa-associated lymphoid tissue lymphomas can present as isolated swelling of thyroid or salivary glands. These are sometimes associated with autoimmune disorders.

Imaging studies can show multiple, solid, enlarged lymph nodes (Figure 12-6). High clinical suspicion should be maintained in patients who first present with concerning signs. They should have close follow-up and be referred to a center where imaging studies to determine stage and best location for biopsy can be coordinated. Fine-needle aspiration and core biopsy are only useful if a positive result is obtained for lymphoma evaluation. Interpretation of cytology and samples must be done at an experienced laboratory, and the family must understand that the tissue sample may be inadequate for diagnosis. Open biopsy allows for the most accurate diagnosis when the specimen is sent fresh, in a saline solution.

Lymphoma can certainly present similar to benign cervical adenopathy, but careful attention to details of clinical presentation, examination findings, and worrisome imaging results permit appropriate workup and consideration for referral. More than half of patients with head and neck lymphoma also have involvement at extranodal sites, which include the posterior pharynx and Waldeyer ring, maxilla/mandible, paranasal sinuses, orbit, nasal cavity, and salivary glands. Radiologic findings suggestive of malignancy on ultrasound include

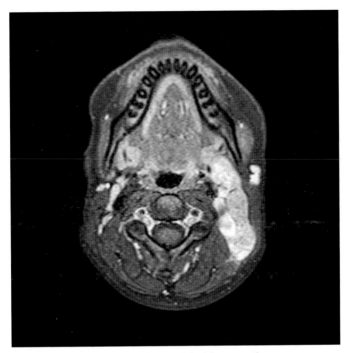

Figure 12-6. Axial image of T1-weighted magnetic resonance imaging with contrast of 13-year-old girl with lateral neck mass confirmed to be Hodgkin lymphoma on biopsy.

displacement of vessels, aberrant vessels, an avascular focus, and subcapsular vessels. These physical examination and radiologic findings coupled with a history of progressive cervical adenopathy or constitutional symptoms warrant a biopsy to obtain diagnosis. Retrospective studies of cervical adenopathy have based the decision to biopsy on concerning ultrasound findings and persistence of mass after 4 to 6 weeks despite antibiotic therapy. Fewer than 15% of patients met criteria for biopsy, and the majority of biopsy results show infectious or congenital etiologies. About 20% of the patients who met criteria and were biopsied resulted in a diagnosis of lymphoma, which correlated to approximately 2% of all patients who presented with cervical lymphadenopathy. Treatment is usually chemotherapy. Cure rates for Hodgkin lymphoma approach 90%.

Sarcoma

Sarcoma soft tissue tumors make up fewer than 20% of pediatric head and neck malignancies; rhabdomyosarcoma is the most common type encountered. It usually presents in patients younger than 6 years. Orbit is involved in one-third of cases and may cause proptosis. Treatment is usually multimodal with surgery, chemotherapy, or radiotherapy. Prognosis is a function of many factors including the ability to obtain negative margins on surgical resection. Non-rhabdomyosarcomas are very rare, with incidence of 2 to 3 cases per million. There are many types, including fibrosarcoma, chondrosarcoma, osteosarcoma, liposarcoma, leiomyosarcoma, and hemangiopericytoma.

Neuroblastomas

These neural tumors account for approximately 25% of malignant head and neck tumors in the pediatric population. The most common location is in the adrenal medulla. Depending on the stage at presentation, a combined treatment plan of surgery, chemotherapy, and radiotherapy can be developed. Despite advances in chemotherapy regimens, prognosis is poor overall because of the advanced stage at which many neuroblastomas become clinically apparent and are diagnosed.

Salivary Gland Tumors

These are discussed in Chapter 14.

INFLAMMATORY SYNDROMES

Chronic cervical lymphadenopathy may also be a manifestation of a number of inflammatory syndromes. Thorough history and physical examination can provide clues to systemic etiologies. Sarcoidosis, juvenile systemic lupus erythematous, Kawasaki disease, juvenile rheumatoid arthritis, Graves disease, and Rosai-Dorfman disease (histiocytosis) may present with cervical lymphadenopathy. Cervical adenitis has been reported after administration of phenytoin injection or after vaccinations. Periodic fever, aphthous stomatitis, pharyngitis, and cervical adenitis syndrome (periodic fever, aphthous stomatitis, pharyngitis, adenopathy [PFAPA]) should be included in the differential diagnosis in the setting of this constellation of symptoms. There are many other rare diseases, such as Kikuchi-Fujimoto disease and Kimura disease, which are possible causes of cervical adenitis with systemic symptoms.

■ Imaging

In cases in which diagnosis is uncertain and for possible surgical planning, imaging may be extremely helpful. For soft tissue masses, sonography is the initial imaging modality of choice due to its ability to delineate borders and relationship to vessels, as well as provide accurate descriptions of size, shape, and vascularity. There is no radiation exposure, and it is relatively inexpensive and can be done without sedation. If the mass is too large to capture on ultrasound or if more detail is required, CT or MRI may be indicated.

> **Pearl:** Ultrasound is the initial imaging modality of choice for evaluation of soft tissue neck masses in the pediatric population.

■ Treatment Options

Most persistent masses in the head and neck should be worked up with an imaging modality and evaluated by an otolaryngologist. Treatment options vary significantly. Observation may be the best initial management for many benign-appearing cervical adenopathies. Enteric and intravenous antimicrobial therapies play a large role in treatment of infectious etiologies. Surgical resection is the best option for problematic congenital neck masses. Open biopsy plays an important role in accurate tissue diagnosis of malignancies.

■ Natural History and Prognosis

Benign cervical adenopathy that resolves has no significant long-term negative sequelae associated with it. Surgical interventions for acute infections or congenital masses are associated with short hospital stays and minimal morbidity. Prognosis for malignancies of the head and neck varies greatly; they are best examined individually with a patient and family once staging and histopathology information is available.

■ Selected References

Albright JT, Pransky SM. Nontuberculous mycobacterial infections of the head and neck. *Pediatr Clin North Am.* 2003;50(2):503–514

Albright JT, Topham AK, Reilly JS. Pediatric head and neck malignancies: US incidence and trends over 2 decades. *Arch Otolaryngol Head Neck Surg.* 2002;128(6):655–659

Al-Dajani N, Wootton SH. Cervical lymphadenitis, suppurative parotitis, thyroiditis, and infected cysts. *Infect Dis Clin North Am.* 2007;21(2):523–541

Al-Khateeb TH, Al Zoubi F. Congenital neck masses: a descriptive retrospective study of 252 cases. *J Oral Maxillofac Surg.* 2007;65(11):2242–2247

Altıncık A, Demir K, Abacı A, Böber E, Büyükgebiz A. Fine-needle aspiration biopsy in the diagnosis and follow-up of thyroid nodules in childhood. *J Clin Res Pediatr Endocrinol.* 2010;2(2):78–80

Ayugi JW, Ogeng'o JA, Macharia IM. Pattern of congenital neck masses in a Kenyan paediatric population. *Int J Pediatr Otorhinolaryngol.* 2010;74(1):64–66

Bell AT, Fortune B, Sheeler R. Clinical inquiries. What test is the best for diagnosing infectious mononucleosis? *J Fam Pract.* 2006;55(9):799–802

Citak EC, Koku N, Demirci M, Tanyeri B, Deniz H. A retrospective chart review of evaluation of the cervical lymphadenopathies in children. *Auris Nasus Larynx.* 2011;38(5):618–621

Coppit GL 3rd, Perkins JA, Manning SC. Nasopharyngeal teratomas and dermoids: a review of the literature and case series. *Int J Pediatr Otorhinolaryngol.* 2000;52(3):219–227

Coventry MB, Harris LE. Congenital muscular torticollis in infancy; some observations regarding treatment. *J Bone Joint Surg Am.* 1959;41-A(5):815–822

Cushing SL, Boucek RJ, Manning SC, Sidbury R, Perkins JA. Initial experience with a multidisciplinary strategy for initiation of propranolol therapy for infantile hemangiomas. *Otolaryngol Head Neck Surg.* 2011;144(1):78–84

Emery C. The determinants of treatment duration for congenital muscular torticollis. *Phys Ther.* 1994;74(10):921–929

Fiedler AG, Rossi C, Gingalewski CA. Parathyroid carcinoma in a child: an unusual case of an ectopically located malignant parathyroid gland with tumor invading the thymus. *J Pediatr Surg.* 2009;44(8):1649–1652

Harris RL, Modayil P, Adam J, et al. Cervicofacial nontuberculous mycobacterium lymphadenitis in children: is surgery always necessary? *Int J Pediatr Otorhinolaryngol.* 2009;73(9):1297–1301

Herold BC, Immergluck LC, Maranan MC, et al. Community-acquired methicillin-resistant *Staphylococcus aureus* in children with no identified predisposing risk. *JAMA.* 1998;279(8):593–598

Hill DE, Chirukandoth S, Dubey JP. Biology and epidemiology of *Toxoplasma gondii* in man and animals. *Anim Health Res Rev.* 2005;6(1):41–61

Josefson J, Zimmerman D. Thyroid nodules and cancers in children. *Pediatr Endocrinol Rev.* 2008;6(1):14–23

Larsson LO, Bentzon MW, Berg Kelly K, et al. Palpable lymph nodes of the neck in Swedish schoolchildren. *Acta Paediatr.* 1994;83(10):1091–1094

Niedzielska G, Kotowski M, Niedzielski A, Dybiec E, Wieczorek P. Cervical lymphadenopathy in children—incidence and diagnostic management. *Int J Pediatr Otorhinolaryngol.* 2007;71(1):51–56

Nogová L, Reineke T, Eich HT, et al. Extended field radiotherapy, combined modality treatment or involved field radiotherapy for patients with stage IA lymphocyte-predominant Hodgkin's lymphoma: a retrospective analysis from the German Hodgkin Study Group (GHSG). *Ann Oncol.* 2005;16(10):1683–1687

Papadopouli E, Michailidi E, Papadopoulou E, Paspalaki P, Vlahakis I, Kalmanti M. Cervical lymphadenopathy in childhood epidemiology and management. *Pediatr Hematol Oncol.* 2009;26(6):454–460

Pryor SG, Lewis JE, Weaver AL, Orvidas LJ. Pediatric dermoid cysts of the head and neck. *Otolaryngol Head Neck Surg.* 2005;132(6):938–942

Ren W, Zhi K, Zhao L, Gao L. Presentations and management of thyroglossal duct cyst in children versus adults: a review of 106 cases. *Oral Surg Oral Med Oral Pathol Oral Radiol Endod.* 2011;111(2):e1–e6

Robson CD. Imaging of head and neck neoplasms in children. *Pediatr Radiol.* 2010;40(4):499–509

Roh JL, Huh J, Moon HN. Lymphomas of the head and neck in the pediatric population. *Int J Pediatr Otorhinolaryngol.* 2007;71(9):1471–1477

Rosenberg HK. Sonography of pediatric neck masses. *Ultrasound Q.* 2009;25(3):111–127

Scott KJ, Schroeder AA, Greinwald JH Jr. Ectopic cervical thymus: an uncommon diagnosis in the evaluation of pediatric neck masses. *Arch Otolaryngol Head Neck Surg.* 2002;128(6):714–717

Sridhara SK, Shah RK. Rosai-Dorfman in the submandibular salivary glands of a pediatric patient. *Laryngoscope.* 2010;120(Suppl 4):S228

Szinnai G, Meier C, Komminoth P, Zumsteg UW. Review of multiple endocrine neoplasia type 2A in children: therapeutic results of early thyroidectomy and prognostic value of codon analysis. *Pediatrics.* 2003;111(2):E132–E139

Tunkel DE, Domenech EE. Radioisotope scanning of the thyroid gland prior to thyroglossal duct cyst excision. *Arch Otolaryngol Head Neck Surg.* 1998;124(5):597–601

Wei JL, Schwartz KM, Weaver AL, Orvidas LJ. Pseudotumor of infancy and congenital muscular torticollis: 170 cases. *Laryngoscope.* 2001;111(4 Pt 1):688–695

Wexler LH, Helman LJ. Pediatric soft tissue sarcomas. *CA Cancer J Clin.* 1994;44(4):211–247

Wiersinga WM. Thyroid cancer in children and adolescents—consequences in later life. *J Pediatr Endocrinol Metab.* 2001;14(Suppl 5):1289–1298

Wolinsky E. Mycobacterial lymphadenitis in children: a prospective study of 105 nontuberculous cases with long-term follow-up. *Clin Infect Dis.* 1995;20(4):954–963

Zeharia A, Eidlitz-Markus T, Haimi-Cohen Y, Samra Z, Kaufman L, Amir J. Management of nontuberculous mycobacteria-induced cervical lymphadenitis with observation alone. *Pediatr Infect Dis J.* 2008;27(10):920–922

CHAPTER 13

Deep Neck Space Infections

Eric M. Jaryszak, MD, PhD, and Sukgi S. Choi, MD

■ Introduction

Deep neck infections are of primary interest in the pediatric population because of their frequency and potential for catastrophic complications. Proximity to major vascular structures, the mediastinum, and the central nervous system are reasons for concern in patients with deep neck infections. While the frequency of deep neck infection has decreased in recent years because of the advent and expansion of antimicrobial therapy, the problem still exists and requires a team approach using medical and surgical management.

As with many things in medicine, the diagnosis and management of deep neck infections is debated in the literature. Unfortunately, literature in the pediatric population is lacking. This can lead to a lack of consensus in the management of patients and a dogmatic approach to their care. Particularly, frequent questions arise about the selection of imaging modality, timing and duration of antibiotic therapy, and role of surgical therapy in the treatment of deep neck infections. The aim of this chapter is to summarize the literature and arrive at a comprehensive treatment algorithm for the management of patients with deep neck space infections.

■ Epidemiology

It is impossible to determine an incidence of deep neck infection because of the wide variety of etiologies and lack of criteria to establish the presence of an abscess. Deep neck infections tend to affect younger children, with a decreasing incidence as children get older. In a series of 169 pediatric patients undergoing surgical treatment of deep neck abscess, Coticchia et al noted an average age of 4.1 years at onset. There was a male predominance (56% vs 44%). White (54%) and black (43%) children were most commonly affected.

There are a multitude of factors that are considered predisposing, including premature birth, congenital cysts, immunosuppression, history of sepsis, and recent or current ear, nose, or throat infection. Twenty-eight percent of patients in the aforementioned series had one or more predisposing factors for deep neck infection, including two-thirds with a history of recent or current ear, nose, or throat infection. Low socioeconomic status and poor dental hygiene also may be predisposing factors for the development of deep neck infection.

◼ Anatomy

The neck is divided into compartments by the cervical fascia and anatomic structures (Figure 13-1). Knowledge of these compartments and their contents, as well as routes of spread to other compartments, is critical to triaging the care of patients with deep neck infections. Nomenclature of the fascial layers of the neck is confusing; a detailed explanation follows. The cervical fascia is separated into a superficial and deep layer. The superficial layer of the cervical fascia surrounds the platysma muscle and is continuous with the superficial muscular aponeurotic system, which invests the musculature of the face. This continues cranially as the temporoparietal fascia.

While the superficial layer of the cervical fascia is straightforward, the deep cervical fascia is more complex. The deep layer of cervical fascia is divided into 3 distinct layers (superficial, middle, and deep), which help to form the various spaces outlined as follows.

SUPERFICIAL LAYER

The superficial layer of the deep cervical fascia is also known as the investing layer. It encapsulates the neck, originating from the vertebral

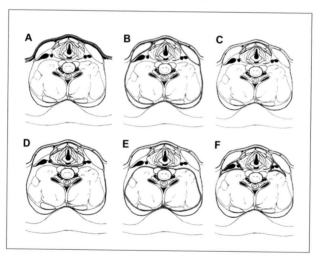

Figure 13-1. Cervical fascial planes highlighted in red. A, Superficial cervical fascia. B, Superficial layer of deep cervical fascia. C, Muscular division of the middle layer of deep cervical fascia. D, Visceral division of the middle layer of deep cervical fascia. E, Deep layer of deep cervical fascia. F, Carotid sheath. Modified from Vieira et al. *Otolaryngol Clin North Am.* 2008;41:459–483, with permission from Elsevier.

spinous processes and nuchal ligament, surrounding the trapezius muscles posteriorly and extending anteriorly to surround the sterno-cleidomastoid (SCM) muscles. Superiorly, this layer splits around the anterior belly of the digastric muscle. It also encapsulates the parotid and submandibular gland and forms the stylomandibular ligament.

MIDDLE LAYER

The middle layer of the deep cervical fascia, also known as the pretra-cheal fascia, is divided into a muscular layer, which invests the infrahy-oid strap muscles and travels inferiorly behind the sternum to fuse with the pericardium. The visceral layer surrounds the constrictor muscles and attaches to the skull base, forming the anterior border of the retro-pharyngeal space.

DEEP LAYER

The deep layer, or prevertebral fascia, originates from the spinous processes and surrounds the prevertebral muscles, brachial plexus, and subclavian artery. This deep layer splits starting at the skull base into a more anterior alar fascia, which forms the posterior border of the retropharyngeal space and the anterior border of the danger space, which extends from the skull base to the coccyx.

SPACES

Submandibular

The submandibular space actually comprises 2 spaces separated by the mylohyoid muscle: the sublingual space and the submaxillary space. These 2 spaces, however, communicate via the posterior margin of the mylohyoid muscle. Importantly, the tooth roots of the second and third molars lie below the mylohyoid line of the mandible, allowing infec-tions of these teeth to spread directly into the submaxillary compart-ment. The submaxillary space contains the submental space, which is the space confined by the anterior belly of the digastric muscle bilater-ally, mandible anterior, and hyoid bone posterior and inferior.

Parapharyngeal

The parapharyngeal space, or lateral pharyngeal space, is immediately adjacent to the lateral pharyngeal walls. It is the shape of an inverted pyramid that extends from the skull base down to its apex at the level of the hyoid bone. The medial border is the pharyngeal musculature. The lateral border is the mandible and pterygoid musculature.

Masticator

The masticator space lies between the masseter muscle laterally and the lateral pterygoid muscle medially. It is an extension of the temporal space and includes branches of the third division of the trigeminal nerve as well as the internal maxillary artery.

Buccal

The buccal space is contained between the buccopharyngeal fascia on the medial aspect of the buccinator muscle and the skin of the cheek laterally. It contains the parotid duct, facial artery, and buccal fat pad.

Parotid

This space is connected with the parapharyngeal or lateral pharyngeal space. The lateral border is the parotidomasseteric fascia, which is a component of the superficial layer of the deep cervical fascia. It contains not only the parotid gland but the facial nerve and external carotid artery branches.

Peritonsillar

The peritonsillar space is the space immediately lateral to the tonsil capsule between it and the muscular tonsillar fossa. The superior pharyngeal constrictor muscle and its surrounding pharyngobasilar fascia comprise the muscular tonsillar fossa.

Retropharyngeal

The retropharyngeal space is bordered posteriorly by the alar fascia, a component of the deep layer of the deep cervical fascia, and anteriorly by the visceral layer of the middle layer of the deep cervical fascia (Figure 13-2). The retropharyngeal space extends from the skull base to the mediastinum, obviating the concern for infections within this space and possible catastrophic intrathoracic complications. The retropharyngeal space is divided into a right and left side by a midline raphe. This is a key differentiating feature distinguishing between a process involving the retropharyngeal space compared

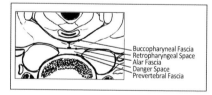

Figure 13-2. Divisions of the deep cervical fascia delineating the retropharyngeal and danger spaces. Note the midline raphe dividing the right and left retropharyngeal space which is absent in the danger space. Modified from Vieira et al. *Otolaryngol Clin North Am.* 2008;41:459–483, with permission from Elsevier.

with the danger or prevertebral spaces. As such, processes involving the retropharyngeal space generally respect the midline.

The retropharyngeal space contains lymph nodes that can be the origins of pathology within the space. Upper respiratory infections (URIs) can manifest with lymphadenopathy in the retropharyngeal nodes and ultimately suppurate. Expansion of infection out of the capsule of the lymph node can result in a rapid spread of infection down toward the mediastinum. Similarly, other pathology, including upper aerodigestive tract malignancies, can hide within these lymph nodes, so all that causes lymph node enlargement in this area is not necessarily infection.

Prevertebral

The prevertebral space is defined anteriorly by the prevertebral fascia. Its posterior border is the vertebral bodies of the spine and the anterior longitudinal ligament.

Vascular (Carotid)

The carotid space, also known as the visceral vascular space, is that which is contained by the carotid sheath. Beyond the major vascular structures, this space also contains cranial nerve X and the sympathetic trunk. The glossopharyngeal, spinal accessory, and hypoglossal nerves also exit the skull base in the carotid space until their exit at various points along its length.

Danger

The danger space is defined anteriorly by the alar fascia and posteriorly by the prevertebral fascia. This space extends down from the skull base to the coccyx.

■ Microbiology

The microbiology of deep neck infections can be divided into groups based on source of infection. Infections of odontogenic origin are distinctly different in terms of the inciting pathogen than are non-odontogenic infections. A review of 128 patients with bacteria isolated from their neck abscess revealed that 27 were of dental origin, while 22 had concurrent or recent infection of the upper airway including peritonsillar abscess (PTA), supraglottitis, and tonsillitis. The remaining 79 patients had another source of infection.

ODONTOGENIC INFECTIONS

Rega et al studied a series of deep neck infections secondary to an odon-togenic source. The review encompassed 103 patients who underwent surgical incision and drainage of deep neck infections. Interestingly, most patients presented with multiple-space abscesses, with the sub-mandibular being the most common space involved overall. In isolated single-space abscesses, the submandibular space (30%) was followed by the buccal space (27.5%) and lateral pharyngeal (parapharyngeal) space (12.5%). When multiple spaces were involved, the submandibular space (28%) was followed by the submental (14.8%), lateral pharyngeal (14.1%), buccal (12%), and sublingual (11.3%) spaces.

An average of 2.6 isolates were obtained per patient, including 5 fungal isolates *(Candida albicans* and *Aspergillus fumigatus)*. Most isolates were anaerobic (65.7%); however, the most commonly isolated organism was *Streptococcus viridans*. This was followed by *Prevotella, Staphylococcus,* and *Peptostreptococcus*. Sensitivity data presented in this study showed a high susceptibility of *S viridans* to penicillin and ampicillin, while the staphylococci were significantly less susceptible. Staphylococci were highly susceptible to ciprofloxacin (95%), clinda-mycin (90%), and vancomycin (100%). Sensitivity data were not avail-able for anaerobic isolates. In a smaller series of odontogenic infections, *S viridans* was shown to be the most common organism, followed by *Peptostreptococcus*.

NON-ODONTOGENIC INFECTIONS

Historically, the microbiology of deep neck infections has been reported by subsite of infection. Brook reported an average of 7.4 bacterial isolates per specimen in a group of 14 children. All 14 specimens contained anaerobic isolates, the most common of which were *Peptostreptococcus* and *Bacteroides* species. Interestingly, 12 of 14 speci-mens were mixed anaerobic/aerobic isolates. Most aerobic isolates were *Streptococcus* species and, again, there were nearly 2 aerobic isolates per specimen.

In a series of 117 children with head and neck space infections, Ungkanont et al presented a spectrum of head and neck space infec-tions. Sixty-seven percent of patients had cultures sent revealing *Streptococcus pyogenes, Staphylococcus aureus,* and *Bacteroides melanino-genicus* as the most common organisms isolated. Nine percent of cul-tures had no growth.

The literature on the microbiology of PTA is more robust. The largest series of 124 patients by Jousimies-Somer et al revealed an average of 4.4 isolates per specimen. Most cultures were mixed aerobic and anaerobic organisms. Of the aerobes, *S pyogenes* was isolated from 45% of patients, with *Streptococcus milleri* the second most common at 27%. *Fusobacterium* and *Prevotella* species were the most frequently isolated anaerobes.

Much attention recently has been paid to the role of resistant organisms, namely methicillin-resistant *S aureus* (MRSA) in deep neck space infections. There is a growing body of literature to suggest that there is a substantial rise in the proportion of *S aureus* isolates that are methicillin resistant. Thomason et al reported an increase in the incidence of MRSA in 245 patients undergoing incision and drainage of neck abscesses from 9% to 40% from 2001 to 2005. This is of great concern given this organism is not covered by first-line antibiotic therapy for refractory lymphadenitis or other URIs. Second, there is evidence to suggest that the organism may be more aggressive than its nonresistant counterparts. Wright et al reported that 32% of patients with retropharyngeal abscess (RPA) who had positive cultures grew MRSA. Furthermore, 6 of 8 patients developed mediastinitis.

In summary, the microbiology of deep neck infections varies in the location and suspected etiology of the infection. Anaerobic and aerobic organisms must be considered when selecting antimicrobial therapy. Finally, the incidence of community-acquired MRSA in deep neck infection is rising, and first-line therapy against this potentially more aggressive organism must be considered in the initial treatment of these infections.

■ Diagnosis

HISTORY AND PHYSICAL EXAMINATION FINDINGS

The presenting signs and symptoms of deep neck infection in children can vary widely. While adults may have specific localizing complaints, children are often difficult to interview and examine. Coticchia et al investigated the presenting signs and symptoms of 169 patients treated surgically for deep neck infection (Table 13-1). Neck mass (91%), fever (86%), and cervical adenopathy (83%) were common in all ages; however, there were some age-related shifts in presenting signs and symptoms. Children younger than 4 years were more likely to present with

(continued on page 284)

Table 13-1. Presenting Signs, Symptoms, and Investigations of Deep Neck Infection by Age Group (Average Age of Patients = 4 Years)

Presenting Sign, Symptom, and Investigation	Age Group, y				All Patients (n=169)
	<1 (n=33)	=1 to <4 (n=75)	=4 to <10 (n=44)	=10 to <19 (n=17)	
Agitation	17/31 (55)	36/75 (63)	6/34 (18)	1/16 (6)	60/138 (43)
Cough	10/30 (33)	24/68 (35)	5/42 (12)	3/17 (18)	42/157 (27)
Dehydration	2/32 (6)	3/72 (4)	3/44 (7)	1/17 (6)	9/165 (5)
Drooling	2/32 (6)	26/72 (36)	6/42 (14)	1/16 (6)	35/162 (22)
Dysphagia	1/6 (17)	20/39 (51)	16/28 (57)	12/16 (75)	49/89 (55)
Fever	28/33 (85)	63/75 (84)	37/42 (88)	14/16 (88)	142/166 (86)
Length of symptoms before admission, d	3.1	5.1	4.8	6.3	4.7
Lethargy	11/29 (38)	31/62 (50)	14/34 (41)	2/14 (14)	58/139 (42)
Leukocytes, mean, x 10^3 cells/µL	23.2	20.6	18.5	14.9	20.1
Lymphadenopathy	24/30 (80)	60/68 (88)	29/34 (85)	5/10 (50)	118/142 (83)
Nausea/vomiting	6/33 (18)	12/75 (16)	11/43 (26)	4/17 (24)	33/168 (20)
Neck mass	32/33 (97)	66/75 (88)	39/44 (89)	16/17 (94)	153/169 (91)

Table 13-1. Presenting Signs, Symptoms, and Investigations of Deep Neck Infection by Age Group (Average Age of Patients = 4 Years), continued

Presenting Sign, Symptom, and Investigation	Age Group, y				All Patients (n=169)
	<1 (n=33)	=1 to <4 (n=75)	=4 to <10 (n=44)	=10 to <19 (n=17)	
Neck stiffness	12/28 (43)	36/63 (57)	25/36 (69)	9/13 (69)	82/140 (59)
Oropharyngeal abnormalities	8/32 (25)	40/74 (54)	27/40 (68)	7/17 (41)	82/163 (50)
Poor oral intake	18/33 (55)	52/70 (74)	26/40 (65)	7/13 (54)	103/156 (66)
Positive CT scan of neck	21/23 (91)	57/60 (95)	29/34 (85)	11/14 (79)	118/131 (90)
Positive lateral neck radiograph	7/7 (100)	24/27 (89)	9/10 (90)	2/2 (100)	42/46 (91)
Respiratory distress	2/32 (6)	3/75 (4)	1/44 (2)	0/17 (0)	6/168 (4)
Retractions	2/32 (6)	3/75 (4)	1/44 (2)	0/17 (0)	6/168 (4)
Rhinorrhea	18/33 (55)	29/75 (52)	8/43 (19)	1/16 (6)	66/167 (40)
Sore throat	0/2 (0)	27/46 (59)	24/38 (63)	13/17 (76)	64/103 (62)
Stridor	2/32 (6)	2/75 (3)	1/44 (2)	0/17 (0)	5/168 (3)
Temperature, mean, °C	38.6	38.6	38.4	38.3	38.5

Abbreviation: CT, computed tomography.

Modified from Coticchia IM, Getnick GS, Yun RD, Arnold JE. Age-, site-, and time-specific differences in pediatric deep neck abscesses. *Arch Otolaryngol Head Neck Surg.* 2004;130(2):201–207. Copyright © American Medical Association. All rights reserved.

agitation, cough, drooling, lethargy, and rhinorrhea. Older children were more likely to have trismus and oropharyngeal abnormalities on examination.

The most common site of deep neck infection in infants and children is the peritonsillar space (49%). This is followed by infections of the retropharyngeal (22%), submandibular (14%), buccal (11%), and parapharyngeal (2%) spaces. Children younger than 1 year were more likely to have infections involving lymph nodes of the neck in the anterior or posterior triangles, whereas children older than 1 year were more likely to have infections of the retropharyngeal or parapharyngeal spaces. The anterior triangle is bordered medially by the midline and posteriorly and laterally by the SCM. The posterior triangle is bordered anteriorly by the SCM and posteriorly by the trapezius muscle.

In a series of patients 9 months or younger, Cmejrek et al also found that the most common location was anterior triangle. Furthermore, 13 of 17 scanned patients had some degree of airway compromise.

Immediate assessment of the airway by observation is paramount to the appropriate triage and care of these patients. There are several findings that are concerning for airway compromise: stridor, retractions, head in sniffing position (Figure 13-3), and excessive drooling. Care must be taken when considering airway management of these patients because a routine endotracheal intubation may result in a rupture of the abscess and catastrophic aspiration of pus. Coordination with anesthesiology and otolaryngology services is important when treating these complicated and critical patients.

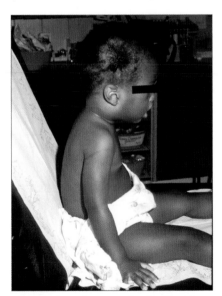

Figure 13-3. Photograph of patient in respiratory distress demonstrating the sniffing position. Courtesy Robert Allan Felter, MD, FAAP.

LABORATORY STUDIES

Laboratory evaluation can be useful not only in assisting in the diagnosis of patients with deep neck abscess but also for clinical monitoring of response to treatment. While intuitive, the use of laboratory studies in the diagnosis and monitoring of deep neck infections is not widely investigated in the pediatric population. Meyer et al reported a significantly higher white blood cell count (22.0 vs 18.4) in the abscess group, while there was no difference in C-reactive protein (CRP) levels (10.1 vs 10.6). A significant difference in white blood cell count between those with drainable fluid collections and those without was also reported by Miller et al. In summary, a white blood cell count can be useful in monitoring and decision-making processes in management of deep neck infections. There is not enough evidence at this time to consider routine monitoring with CRP levels in the care of these patients.

DIAGNOSTIC IMAGING

Imaging studies are extremely helpful in decision-making for the treatment of deep neck infections. There are multiple imaging modalities available, each with pros and cons.

Lateral Neck Radiography

Before the introduction of computed tomography (CT) imaging in 1972, lateral neck radiography was the cornerstone of diagnostic imaging for deep neck infections. Lateral neck radiography is simple, quick, and easily accessible, even in remote locations. The utility of lateral neck radiography in deep neck space infections has been debated. Surgically, it does not delineate anatomy the way a CT scan or an image from magnetic resonance imaging (MRI) would; however, one might argue that all that is needed from an imaging study is to determine if surgical intervention is required. Findings of prevertebral soft tissue thickening as well as air-fluid levels are indicative of deep neck space infection. Nagy and Backstrom reported that lateral neck radiographs had a sensitivity of 83% for determining the presence of a deep neck infection when compared with contrast-enhanced CT imaging. There is evidence to support the use of lateral neck radiography in the management of RPA. Boucher et al found that while CT was more sensitive, lateral neck radiography was more specific at determining an abscess. The study was limited because not all patients underwent incision and drainage, and those in the cellulitis group were those in whom no pus was seen at surgery and those who improved with antibiotic therapy alone. However, it does suggest that lateral neck radiography may have a role in the management of deep neck infections.

Pearl: Imaging findings concerning for deep neck infections are based on normative data. Wholey et al noted that the width of the prevertebral soft tissue at cervical vertebra 2 was 2 to 7 mm, and 5 to 14 mm at C6. Thicker soft tissues may indicate the presence of cellulitis or abscess in the retropharyngeal space.

Ultrasound

As otolaryngologists become increasingly familiar with ultrasound and as it is integrated into the residency curriculum, an increasing emphasis is being placed on it. There is evidence to suggest that ultrasound is better than CT or MRI at determining an abscess from a phlegmon. Glasier et al reviewed 11 cases in which ultrasound, in addition to another imaging modality (CT or MRI), was used for signs and symptoms of retropharyngeal infection. In the cases treated surgically, ultrasound was correct at determining the presence of pus 5 of 5 times, while contrasted CT or MRI was correct only 3 of 5 times. The inherent problems with ultrasonography include a significant dependence on the quality of the images and operator or technician, lack of anatomic detail optimal for surgical intervention, and difficulty interpreting images obtained independently by a technician rather than real-time observation.

Computed Tomography

Contrast-enhanced CT scan is the gold-standard imaging modality for the evaluation of deep neck space infections. It provides important information not only on the presence or absence of an abscess but also on the adjacent anatomy in anticipation of possible surgical treatment. Furthermore, CT scan demonstrates other potential complications, such as internal jugular vein thrombosis and mediastinitis.

The utility of CT imaging in delineating abscesses from cellulitis and phlegmon has been questioned. Stone et al reviewed 32 patients who underwent contrast-enhanced CT scan and surgical drainage. They showed that contrast-enhanced CT imaging had a sensitivity of 80.8% and a specificity of 62.5% in distinguishing between abscess and cellulitis. These numbers are consistent with those of Vural et al. At times it is difficult to ascertain whether something is an abscess or a contained pre-suppurative or suppurative lymph node. In the past, the determination of an abscess was made on the observation of a hypodense area with surrounding rim enhancement. This finding, however, has not been correlated to the finding of purulence at surgery. The presence of scalloping (Figure 13-4) of the enhancing rim, however, has been shown to increase the specificity of CT at predicting purulence but does not determine which patients will fail antibiotic therapy. Shefelbine et al determined that in the retropharyngeal space, when the volume of hypodensity within a necrotic lymph node measures less than 2 µL, treatment with medical management is usually successful. This confirmed an earlier study by Nagy et al.

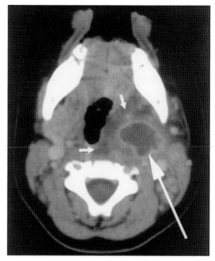

Figure 13-4. Axial contrast-enhanced computed tomography image showing scalloping of a left retropharyngeal fluid collection (large arrow) with associated edema (small arrows). Note that the edema bulges but does not cross the midline raphe of the retropharyngeal space. Modified from Kirse DJ, Roberson DW. *Laryngoscope.* 2001;111(8):1413–1422, with permission from John Wiley & Sons.

Magnetic Resonance Imaging

While the use of MRI in deep neck space infections is documented and potentially useful, the practicality of performing an MRI on all patients in whom a deep neck infection is suspected is limited. The expense and time required for imaging, particularly in the pediatric age group in which general anesthesia is frequently required for scanning, outweigh the enhanced soft-tissue definition. Furthermore, iodinated contrast agents and gadolinium are considered safe in the pediatric population, so preferences lie with obtaining CT imaging unless there is an absolute contraindication to receiving intravenous (IV) iodinated contrast.

■ Treatment

MEDICAL THERAPY

Antibiotic therapy is the cornerstone of treatment of all deep neck infections. While tailoring antimicrobial therapy to cases in which the origin of infection is known is ideal, frequently it is difficult to assess the exact source of the infection and, as a result, a comprehensive coverage of the most common organisms responsible for deep neck infections is an appropriate first step.

McClay et al reported a series of 11 patients with parapharyngeal, retropharyngeal, or combined abscesses defined by CT scan with a diameter greater than 1 cm in all dimensions. The maximum diameter abscess in this series was 3.9 cm. The patients were treated with clindamycin and, in most cases, cefuroxime. Ten of 11 patients (91%) had resolution of their symptoms with medical therapy alone by 8 days. The one patient who did not resolve underwent surgical drainage with successful drainage of purulence. Importantly, none of the patients in this series had evidence of airway compromise. In each case they reassessed patients' progress at 48 hours after the initiation of IV antibiotic therapy for signs of improvement. If none were noted, surgical intervention was considered.

In a larger series, Al-Sabah et al retrospectively reviewed 68 patients with a retropharyngeal infection based on CT scan. All patients received empiric clindamycin therapy. Only 25% of patients required surgical intervention. They concluded that all patients should receive a trial of conservative medical management for 72 hours, with surgery being reserved for those who do not respond. In total, on average, patients in the medical group received 5 days of IV antibiotic therapy and 10 days of oral therapy after discharge. The surgical patients received 6.5 days of IV therapy followed by 10 days of oral therapy after discharge. There were no recurrences.

Because of increasing incidence of MRSA, routine antibiotic therapy has evolved over the years. Now many institutions are recommending the empiric use of clindamycin with possible addition of a cephalosporin (cefuroxime or ceftriaxone) to account for this trend. Care must be taken to discern between community-acquired and hospital-acquired strains, which are frequently resistant to clindamycin and trimethoprim-sulfamethoxazole.

The literature suggests that patients with deep neck infections should receive an empiric trial of clindamycin for initial treatment of these infections. One may consider the addition of cefuroxime or ceftriaxone because these have been shown to be efficacious adjuvants. In many cases, these medications are able to mitigate the need for surgical intervention.

SURGICAL THERAPY

Peritonsillar Abscess

In addition to antibiotic therapy, frequently surgical options are required for the treatment of PTA. The surgical management of PTAs can be done on an outpatient basis, but attention must be paid to oral intake and pain control. There is a wide range of procedures that can be performed for PTA, from needle aspiration, to incision and drainage, to quinsy tonsillectomy, which is an immediate tonsillectomy in the setting of acute infection and abscess. The difficulty with children is the result of limited physical examinations in ill, noncooperative patients in whom performing procedures in the outpatient setting is troublesome. Additional problems arise in younger patients. The technique of needle aspiration, however, has been shown to be effective and safe in the pediatric population. Weinberg et al reported on 43 patients aged 7 to 18 years with PTA. Ninety-five percent of patients in this age group cooperated with the procedure. Pus was aspirated in 76% of patients, 87% of which resolved with this treatment and antibiotic therapy only. Only 2 patients (6%) required a quinsy tonsillectomy for persistent abscess in the needle aspiration group with a positive aspirate. Stringer et al noted a 92% cure rate with a single needle aspiration, compared with 93% for incision and drainage, with all failures requiring one additional treatment. No patients required tonsillectomy.

The role of needle aspiration is supported in the literature, but its utility in an uncooperative or younger child may be limited. Schraff et al suggest that needle aspiration in the operating room followed by incision and drainage to prevent inadequate drainage of the abscess is the better approach, with a 0% recurrence rate in 54 patients treated this way compared with 7% recurrence in the needle aspiration alone group.

Finally, the definitive management for PTA is tonsillectomy. In the setting of acute infection, this can be a difficult procedure when done as quinsy tonsillectomy. The literature advocating the use of quinsy tonsillectomy in the management of PTA is mixed. Schraff et al advocate the use of quinsy tonsillectomy (Figure 13-5). It is particularly useful in patients who have had previous tonsillitis/pharyngitis or symptoms of obstructive sleep apnea. Stringer et al reported, however, that if all PTAs were treated with immediate or interval tonsillectomy, up to 93% would be undergoing unnecessary surgery.

Whichever modality is chosen, surgical management of PTA is a successful therapeutic option in conjunction with antibiotic therapy. Needle aspiration, incision and drainage, and quinsy tonsillectomy are

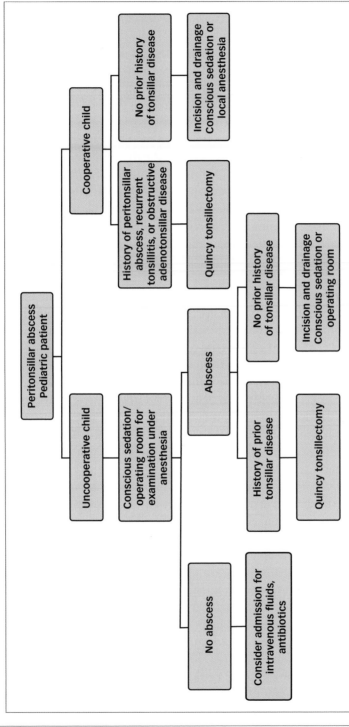

Figure 13-5. Algorithm for the management of the pediatric patient with a peritonsillar abscess. Modified from Schraff S, McGinn JD, Derkay CS. *Int J Pediatr Otorhinolaryngol.* 2001;57(3):213–218, with permission from Elsevier.

all efficacious options. Treatment of PTA may safely be performed as an outpatient with the understanding that oral intake and pain control are necessary to discharge a patient after treatment. Close follow-up is necessary to ensure complete resolution of symptoms.

Non-peritonsillar Abscess

Needle aspiration as a sole treatment modality for non-PTA head and neck infections was first reported by Herzon in 1985. Eight of 10 patients in this study were successfully managed with antibiotics and needle aspiration alone. Two patients required incision and drainage. Similar results were reported in a follow-up study including 25 patients.

This therapeutic option was assessed in children only by Brodsky et al. Nearly 56% of the 18 patients responded to needle aspiration alone, 80% of which had unilocular abscesses. Of the nonresponders, 71% were multiloculated. They proposed the treatment algorithm in Figure 13-6.

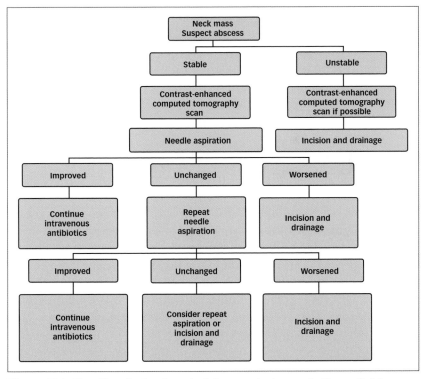

Figure 13-6. Algorithm for treatment of deep neck abscess in the pediatric patient. Stability based on the presence of respiratory compromise, severe systemic toxicity, or impending complications. Modified from Brodsky L, Belles W, Brody A, Squire R, Stanievich J, Volk M. *Clin Pediatr (Phila).* 1992;31(2):71–76. Reprinted by permission of SAGE Publications.

In a larger study of 35 patients, Serour et al successfully treated suppurative cervical lymphadenitis with a single-needle aspiration in 77% of cases. Eight patients required multiple aspirations, but all had complete regression of the nodes within 21 days with no relapse or scar formation. Ultrasound may be used for needle localization.

The main decision when proceeding to incise and drain a deep neck space abscess is the approach, ie, trans-oral versus transcervical versus both. This issue was investigated by Choi et al in 70 consecutive patients admitted and treated for lateral pharyngeal abscess (LPA), RPA, or both. Of the 58 patients with CT imaging findings consistent with LPA, RPA, or both, 36 underwent transoral drainage (12 RPA, 16 LPA, 8 both) with pus obtained in 28 (78%). No patient undergoing transoral drainage alone required revision surgery, and all patients were discharged from the hospital. The authors concluded that transcervical drainage for LPA or RPA should be reserved for disease that extends lateral to the great vessels or involves multiple deep neck spaces. The use of image guidance for abscesses in the medial parapharyngeal space has also been advocated as a useful adjunct.

Kirse and Roberson presented a series of 73 pediatric patients with RPA. Seventy were successfully treated with transoral surgical drainage. The authors concluded that 2 criteria should be met to proceed with safe transoral drainage. First, the abscess should be medial to the great vessels; second, it should be a confined process.

■ Complications and Special Considerations

MEDIASTINITIS

Mediastinitis is a potentially life-threatening complication of deep neck infection (Figure 13-7). While this is more of a problem for adults, it can be seen in children; if treated appropriately, children are more apt to recover fully without significant morbidity. *S aureus* appears to be the major pathogen in this process, and MRSA is a significant contributor. While most cases of mediastinitis are secondary to retropharyngeal space infections, direct extension of infection from an odontogenic source (Ludwig angina) may also occur.

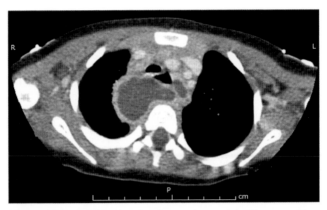

Figure 13-7. Axial contrast-enhanced computed tomography scan of the thorax demonstrating the extension of a retropharyngeal abscess into the mediastinum.

Pearl: The important factor in mediastinitis is the rapidity in which it can occur. If computed tomography imaging is concerning for mediastinal inflammation or suggests extension of the infectious process from the neck toward the chest, prompt surgical consultation of an otolaryngologist is paramount. When there is evidence of extension into the mediastinum, this should also involve cardiothoracic surgery colleagues for possible video-assisted thorascopic surgery with debridement and drainage.

CAROTID ARTERY RUPTURE AND PSEUDOANEURYSM

Carotid artery complications are rare but life-threatening sequelae of deep neck infection. There are very few reported cases of carotid artery rupture in the literature, particularly within the last decade. Pathogenesis is felt to be secondary to an arteritis, which ultimately results in a pseudoaneurysm formation (Figure 13-8) and subsequent rupture. While carotid artery pseudoaneurysm alone has been a more-reported complication in the literature, its incidence has also decreased with the advent of antibiotics. The mortality from these complications may be as high as 83%. While some signs of carotid

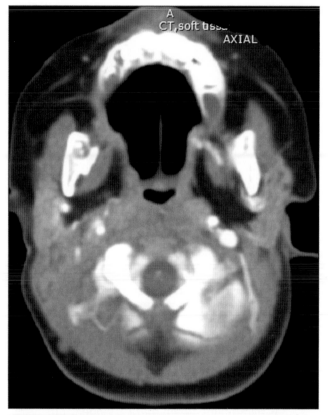

Figure 13-8. Axial contrast-enhanced computed tomography scan demonstrating an area of enhancement around the right carotid artery consistent with carotid pseudoaneurysm. This was confirmed by angiography.

artery pseudoaneurysm, such as an expanding pulsatile mass in the neck, worsening anemia, or a loud neck bruit, are obvious, other subtle findings include oropharyngeal ecchymoses, palsy of cranial nerves IX to XII, and an ipsilateral Horner syndrome. Assessment of the carotid artery on initial imaging and prompt surgical treatment of deep neck infections in the absence of improvement with conservative medical management are important.

LUDWIG ANGINA

First described by Wilhelm Frederick von Ludwig in 1836, Ludwig angina is a rapidly progressive cellulitis of the floor of mouth that, in Ludwig's time, was nearly universally fatal. Criteria for diagnosis were refined by Grodinsky in 1939. In 2000, Britt et al reviewed the literature, finding only 29 cases of Ludwig angina reported. Most cases were odontogenic in origin; however, 7 of 26 cases had no discernible etiology. This is in stark contrast with adults, in whom 90% of these infections are odontogenic in origin. The patients were treated surgically in 14 cases, most commonly via incision and drainage. Two patients received tracheostomy. There were 5 mortalities.

Airway management in Ludwig angina is controversial. In the past, it was advocated that all of these patients required tracheostomy. Britt et al noted, however, that 16 of 28 patients were managed with no artificial airway and only 2 required tracheostomy. Wound cultures from patients in this review were most commonly *Streptococcus* species, followed by gram-negative rods and anaerobes. Antimicrobial therapy, when initiated early, is the cornerstone of treatment, with surgical therapy, once the primary treatment, now an adjunctive treatment modality.

LEMIERRE SYNDROME

Lemierre syndrome is an unfortunate complication or progression of deep neck infection. Usually secondary to the bacteria *Fusobacterium necrophorum*, this syndrome, described initially in 1900 but characterized by Dr Lemierre in 1936, is characterized by anaerobic bacteremia, internal jugular vein thrombosis, and septic embolization secondary to infections in the head and neck. While uncommon, with an estimated incidence of between 0.6 and 2.3 per million population, it can have potentially devastating consequences. Treatment is surgical and medical. Surgery should be aimed at draining any pus that may be present in the surrounding deep neck spaces. Medical therapy is directed at treating the infection. While most cases are secondary to *Fusobacterium*, there are an increasing number of reports of *S aureus* being isolated, and thus coverage must address both organisms. Clindamycin is a good first-line choice for *Fusobacterium* and also covers sensitive and resistant strains of *S aureus*. Treatment with anticoagulation therapy is controversial.

DIABETES

Diabetes is the most common systemic disease associated with deep neck infection. Patients with diabetes have an altered distribution in the microbiology of deep neck infections. In a series of 128 patients (44 with diabetes), Huang et al reported that the most common organism isolated from cultures of deep neck infections in the diabetic patients was *Klebsiella pneumoniae,* even when the source was determined to be odontogenic. Care must be taken when treating patients with diabetes to cover *Klebsiella,* as clindamycin alone is not an effective therapy in these cases. The importance of adequate coverage in these patients stems from evidence that deep neck infections in diabetic patients may be more aggressive, have prolonged hospitalization, and have a higher complication rate.

■ Conclusion

Deep neck infections are potentially catastrophic problems that require a team approach for management. While there are certain cases, particularly those resulting in airway compromise, in which management is straightforward, for routine deep neck infections the approach has been more dogmatic. Contrast-enhanced CT imaging is preferred for deep neck infections because of anatomic definition and high sensitivity. Based on the literature, in general, patients with deep neck infections should have a trial of antibiotic therapy in the form of clindamycin with or without a cephalosporin. Failure to respond within 24 to 72 hours is an indication for otolaryngology consultation and possible surgical treatment. Peritonsillar abscess, on the other hand, is able to be managed safely as an outpatient in the cooperative child. Keep in mind special patient populations when treating these infections, and consider complications of deep neck infection if improvement is lacking or the clinical picture worsens significantly.

■ Selected References

Agarwal AK, Sethi A, Sethi D, Mrig S, Chopra S. Role of socioeconomic factors in deep neck abscess: a prospective study of 120 patients. *Br J Oral Maxillofac Surg.* 2007;45(7):553–555

Al-Sabah B, Bin Salleen H, Hagr A, Choi-Rosen J, Manoukian JJ, Tewfik TL. Retropharyngeal abscess in children: 10-year study. *J Otolaryngol.* 2004;33(6):352–355

Beningfield A, Nehus E, Chen AY, Yellin S. Pseudoaneurysm of the internal carotid artery after retropharyngeal abscess. *Otolaryngol Head Neck Surg.* 2006;134(2):338–339

Boucher C, Dorion D, Fisch C. Retropharyngeal abscesses: a clinical and radiologic correlation. *J Otolaryngol.* 1999;28(3):134–137

Britt JC, Josephson GD, Gross CW. Ludwig's angina in the pediatric population: report of a case and review of the literature. *Int J Pediatr Otorhinolaryngol.* 2000;52(1):79–87

Brodsky L, Belles W, Brody A, Squire R, Stanievich J, Volk M. Needle aspiration of neck abscesses in children. *Clin Pediatr (Phila).* 1992;31(2):71–76

Brook I. Microbiology of retropharyngeal abscesses in children. *Am J Dis Child.* 1987;141(2):202–204

Cable BB, Brenner P, Bauman NM, Mair EA. Image-guided surgical drainage of medial parapharyngeal abscesses in children: a novel adjuvant to a difficult approach. *Ann Otolaryngol Rhinol Laryngol.* 2004;113(2):115–120

Chen KC, Chen JS, Kuo SW, et al. Descending necrotizing mediastinitis: a 10-year surgical experience in a single institution. *J Thorac Cardiovasc Surg.* 2008;136(1):191–198

Chen MK, Wen YS, Chang CC, Lee HS, Huang MT, Hsiao HC. Deep neck infections in diabetic patients. *Am J Otolaryngol.* 2000;21(3):169–173

Choi SS, Vezina LG, Grundfast KM. Relative incidence and alternative approaches for surgical drainage of different types of deep neck abscesses in children. *Arch Otolaryngol Head Neck Surg.* 1997;123(12):1271–1275

Cmejrek RC, Coticchia JM, Arnold JE. Presentation, diagnosis, and management of deep-neck abscesses in infants. *Arch Otolaryngol Head Neck Surg.* 2002;128(12):1361–1364

Coticchia JM, Getnick GS, Yun RD, Arnold JE. Age-, site-, and time-specific differences in pediatric deep neck abscesses. *Arch Otolaryngol Head Neck Surg.* 2004;130(2):201–207

Davis GG. III. Acute septic infection of the throat and neck; Ludwig's angina. *Ann Surg.* 1906;44(2):175–192

Daya H, Lo S, Papsin BC, et al. Retropharyngeal and parapharyngeal infections in children: the Toronto experience. *Int J Pediatr Otorhinolaryngol.* 2005;69(1):81–86

Eykyn SJ. Necrobacillosis. *Scand J Infect Dis Suppl.* 1989;62:41–46

Felter RA, Waldrop RD. Emergent management of pediatric epiglottitis. Medscape Reference. http://emedicine.medscape.com/article/801369-media. Updated June 9, 2011. Accessed July 13, 2011

Glasier CM, Stark JE, Jacobs RF, et al. CT and ultrasound imaging of retropharyngeal abscesses in children. *AJNR Am J Neuroradiol.* 1992;13(4):1191–1195

Grodinsky M. Ludwig's angina: an anatomical and clinical study. *Surgery.* 1939;5:678–696

Har-El G, Aroesty JH, Shaha A, Lucente FE. Changing trends in deep neck abscess. A retrospective study of 110 patients. *Oral Surg Oral Med Oral Pathol.* 1994;77(5):446–450

Herzon FS. Management of nonperitonsillar abscesses of the head and neck with needle aspiration. *Laryngoscope.* 1985;95(7 Pt 1):780–781

Herzon FS. Needle aspiration of nonperitonsillar head and neck abscesses. A six-year experience. *Arch Otolaryngol Head Neck Surg.* 1988;114(11):1312–1314

Huang TT, Tseng FY, Yeh TH, Hsu CJ, Chen YS. Factors affecting the bacteriology of deep neck infection: a retrospective study of 128 patients. *Acta Otolarnyngol.* 2006;126(4):396–401

Hunt CH, Hartman RP, Hesley GK. Frequency and severity of adverse effects of iodinated and gadolinium contrast materials: retrospective review of 456,930 doses. *AJR Am J Roentgenol.* 2009;193(4):1124–1127

Inman JC, Rowe M, Ghostine M, Fleck T. Pediatric neck abscesses: changing organisms and empiric therapies. *Laryngoscope.* 2008;118(12):2111–2114

Jousimies-Somer H, Savolainen S, Mäkitie A, Ylikoski J. Bacteriologic findings in peritonsillar abscesses in young adults. *Clin Infect Dis.* 1993;16(Suppl 4):S292–S298

Kinzer S, Pfeiffer J, Becker S, Ridder GJ. Severe deep neck space infections and mediastinitis of odontogenic origin: clinical relevance and implications for diagnosis and treatment. *Acta Otolaryngol.* 2009;129(1):62–70

Kirse DJ, Roberson DW. Surgical management of retropharyngeal space infections in children. *Laryngoscope.* 2001;111(8):1413–1422

Lemierre A. On certain septicemias due to anaerobic organisms. *Lancet.* 1936;1:701–703

McClay JE, Murray AD, Booth T. Intravenous antibiotic therapy for deep neck abscesses defined by computed tomography. *Arch Otolaryngol Head Neck Surg.* 2003;129(11):1207–1212

Meyer AC, Kimbrough TG, Finkelstein M, Sidman JD. Symptom duration and CT findings in pediatric deep neck infection. *Otolaryngol Head Neck Surg.* 2009;140(2):183–186

Miller WD, Furst IM, Sàndor GK, Keller MA. A prospective, blinded comparison of clinical examination and computed tomography in deep neck infections. *Laryngoscope.* 1999;109(11):1873–1879

Nagy M, Backstrom J. Comparison of the sensitivity of lateral neck radiographs and computed tomography scanning in pediatric deep-neck infections. *Laryngoscope.* 1999;109(5):775–779

Nagy M, Pizzuto M, Backstrom J, Brodsky L. Deep neck infections in children: a new approach to diagnosis and treatment. *Laryngoscope.* 1997;107(12 Pt 1):1627–1634

Naidu SI, Donepudi SK, Stocks RM, Buckingham SC, Thompson JW. Methicillin-resistant *Staphylococcus aureus* as a pathogen in deep neck abscesses: a pediatric case series. *Int J Pediatr Otorhinolaryngol.* 2005;69(10):1367–1371

Ophir D, Bawnik J, Poria Y, Porat M, Marshak G. Peritonsillar abscess. A prospective evaluation of outpatient management by needle aspiration. *Arch Otolaryngol Head Neck Surg.* 1988;114(6):661–663

Rega AJ, Aziz SR, Ziccardi VB. Microbiology and antibiotic sensitivities of head and neck space infections of odontogenic origin. *J Oral Maxillofac Surg.* 2006;64(9):1377–1380

Schraff S, McGinn JD, Derkay CS. Peritonsillar abscess in children: a 10-year review of diagnosis and management. *Int J Pediatr Otorhinolaryngol.* 2001;57(3):213–218

Serour F, Gorenstein A, Somekh E. Needle aspiration for suppurative cervical lymphadenitis. *Clin Pediatr (Phila).* 2002;41(7):471–474

Shah RK, Chun R, Choi SS. Mediastinitis in infants from deep neck space infections. *Otolaryngol Head Neck Surg.* 2009;140(6):936–938

Shefelbine SE, Mancuso AA, Gajewski BJ, Ojiri H, Stringer S. Sedwick JD. Pediatric retropharyngeal lymphadenitis: differentiation from retropharyngeal abscess and treatment implications. *Otolaryngol Head Neck Surg.* 2007;136(2):182–188

Stone ME, Walner DL, Koch BL, Egelhoff JC, Myer CM. Correlation between computed tomography and surgical findings in retropharyngeal inflammatory processes in children. *Int J Pediatr Otorhinolaryngol.* 1999;49(2):121–125

Stringer SP, Schaefer SD, Close LG. A randomized trial for outpatient management of peritonsillar abscess. *Arch Otolaryngol Head Neck Surg.* 1988;114(3):296–298

Syed MI, Baring D, Addidle M, Murray C, Adams C. Lemierre syndrome: two cases and a review. *Laryngoscope.* 2007;117(9):1605–1610

Thomason TS, Brenski A, McClay J, Ehmer D. The rising incidence of methicillin-resistant *Staphylococcus aureus* in pediatric neck abscesses. *Otolaryngol Head Neck Surg.* 2007;137(3):459–464

Thompson JW, Cohen SR, Reddix P. Retropharyngeal abscess in children: a retrospective and historical analysis. *Laryngoscope.* 1988;98(6 Pt 1):589–592

Ungkanont K, Yellon RF, Weissman JL, Casselbrant ML, González-Valdepeña H, Bluestone CD. Head and neck space infections in infants and children. *Otolaryngol Head Neck Surg.* 1995;112(3):375–382

Vural C, Gungor A, Comerci S. Accuracy of computerized tomography in deep neck infections in the pediatric population. *Am J Otolaryngol.* 2003;24(3):143–148

Waggie Z, Hatherill M, Millar A, France H, Van Der Merwe A, Argent A. Retropharyngeal abscess complicated by carotid artery rupture. *Pediatr Crit Care Med.* 2002;3(3):303–304

Weber AL, Siciliano A. CT and MR imaging evaluation of neck infections with clinical correlations. *Radiol Clin North Am.* 2000;38(5):941–968

Weinberg E, Brodsky L, Stanievich J, Volk M. Needle aspiration of peritonsillar abscess in children. *Arch Otolaryngol Head Neck Surg.* 1993;119(2):169–172

Wholey MH, Bruwer AJ, Baker HL Jr. The lateral roentgenogram of the neck; with comments on the atlanto-odontoid-basion relationship. *Radiology.* 1958;71(3):350–356

Wright CT, Stocks RM, Armstrong DL, Arnold SR, Gould HJ. Pediatric mediastinitis as a complication of methicillin-resistant *Staphylococcus aureus* retropharyngeal abscess. *Arch Otolaryngol Head Neck Surg.* 2008;134(4):408–413

Yeow KM, Liao CT, Hao SP. US-guided needle aspiration and catheter drainage as an alternative to open surgical drainage for uniloculated neck abscesses. *J Vasc Interv Radiol.* 2001;12(5):589–594

CHAPTER 14

Salivary Gland Disorders in Children

Daniel L. Wohl, MD, and Eileen M. Raynor, MD

■ Introduction

Salivary glands are exocrine glands that produce and secrete saliva through their ducts into the oral cavity and oropharynx. Saliva provides lubrication and enzymes in support of food digestion along with having protective basic pH and anti-infectious properties. Salivary gland disorders in children are a relatively less common constellation of signs and symptoms encountered in a general pediatric practice. As one gains a clearer understanding of their basic cellular components and function and recognizes their role in head and neck physiology, identifying and managing benign and pathologic salivary gland disorders will become a more straightforward process.

■ Salivary Gland Developmental Anatomy

There are 3 major paired salivary glands—parotid, submandibular, and sublingual glands—plus hundreds of small, minor salivary glands, predominantly within hard and soft palate mucosa. Embryologically, all of these glandular structures are derived from ectoderm (stomodeum) or endoderm (foregut), which differentiate into the internal mucosal lining of the oral cavity and oropharynx. Major salivary glands secrete in response to autonomic nervous system stimulation during eating with intrinsic parasympathetic and sympathetic postganglionic innervation.

Parotid glands are the largest salivary glands. They occupy space lateral to the mandibular ramus and have deep lobes that extend (external) to the upper lateral pharynx—the parapharyngeal space. The parotid duct (Stensen duct) runs roughly horizontally and empties into the oral cavity opposite to where the maxillary second molar tooth is (or will be when it erupts). The facial nerve (cranial nerve VII) courses through the parotid gland and begins to separate into multiple branches within the body of the gland, creating a potential risk that must be accounted for when surgery is considered.

Submandibular glands are the second largest of the 3 major salivary glands. They develop lateral to the tongue and are located within the submandibular triangle. The submandibular duct (Wharton duct) courses horizontally through the floor of the mouth to exit near the midline with paired left and right puncta anterior to the lingual hilum. The submandibular gland resides immediately anterior to the hypoglossal nerve (tongue movement) and envelopes a portion of the facial artery, which ascends through the deeper aspect.

Sublingual glands are the smallest of the major salivary glands. They are relatively superficial, lying just deep to the mucosa of the anterior floor of the mouth. The sublingual glands empty their secretions via several ducts (ducts of Rivinus) into the floor of the mouth posterior to, but sometimes directly into, the submandibular gland ducts. Several hundred relatively small, minor salivary glands also are present throughout the oral cavity and oropharynx. These glands have short excretory ducts that empty saliva directly through the mucosa into their anatomic space.

■ Salivary Gland Physiologic Histology

Salivary gland physiology is a function of its cellular components. Each salivary gland is a variably sized aggregate of multiple salivary gland units that empty into collecting ducts that progressively coalesce into a common ductal structure. Each salivary gland unit is an organized multicellular complex with a proximal secretory acinus connected to a distal ductal element. Saliva is produced and stored by highly specialized serous and mucous glands in the acinus with surrounding myoepithelial cells able to help propel the fluid, when stimulated, through less complex but still metabolically active ductal apparatus.

Saliva is a complex solution of electrolytes, proteins, and enzymes, plus histocompatible antimicrobials and clotting factors. It has a high bicarbonate ion content, which creates alkaline pH. Saliva is mostly water; in general, the smaller the gland, the thicker the secretions. The parotid gland is composed of almost all serous glands, and its secretion has the highest water content with relatively lower mucin content, although still rich in enzymes. In contrast, the submandibular glands are a mixture of serous and mucous glands, and the sublingual glands are composed primarily of mucous glands with much greater viscosity to their secretions. Saliva has a baseline slow, steady production rate with production and flow stimulated first with the sight and smell of food, augmented by chewing and taste sensations, and continuing with esophageal- and gastric reflex–mediated responses. Depending on the size of the child, as much as between 250 and 1,500 mL of saliva may be secreted daily.

■ Salivary Gland Function

Components of saliva underscore their purpose. Saliva maintains moisture within the oral cavity and oropharynx, lubricating food, which helps with swallowing and solubilizing dry food to create taste. Its relative alkaline pH of 7.4 protects against acidic compounds, including regurgitated gastric secretions. Enzymes in saliva, such as starch amylases and lysozymes, help begin the food digestion process and inhibit bacterial growth. Additional antimicrobial activity, including IgA secretion, makes saliva a locally efficient component of the body's immune system. Overall, the multiple properties of saliva help protect against dental caries formation and provide insight into why minor mucosal injuries to the oral cavity and oropharyngeal mucosa generally heal on their own without infection.

Salivary gland dysfunction and disease, therefore, can manifest with altered salivary production, flow, or content with the potential for dry mouth (xerostomia), mucosal ulceration, and increased susceptibility to oral cavity or oropharyngeal infection. Dysfunction can result from primary or secondary ductal obstruction, such as from local inflammation, lithiasis (stones), or an intrinsic mass, with pain from ductal distension the primary presenting symptom, generally worse with eating. Although relatively uncommon in children, benign and malignant tumors may arise from any of the cellular components of salivary glands themselves or from any of the non-glandular components contained within the capsule, for example, within parotid glands that embryologically envelope lymph nodes and related vascular structures. In cases of salivary gland tumors, it is often presence of asymmetric swelling that brings the lesion to clinical attention. See Box 14-1 for a list of salivary gland disorders.

■ Physical Examination of Salivary Glands

Examination includes external and intraoral assessment of major salivary glands and visible oral cavity mucosa. Externally, first look for any asymmetric swelling and general appearance. Overlying skin should be observed for erythema, tenderness, dermal involvement, and edema. Bimanual palpation, with one hand externally and a gloved finger intraorally, can determine consistency, how much of the gland is involved, whether there is a fixed or mobile mass versus diffuse enlargement, as well as general texture of the gland.

Intraorally, inspection of the ducts should include buccal mucosa and floor of the mouth. Trauma related to cheek biting or dental appliances may cause ductal obstruction leading to fullness and erythema of the puncta as well as erythema and inflammation of surrounding mucosa. Salivary gland stones may be visible or palpable at the distal end of the duct and will look yellow or white. These are firm to palpation and often tender to touch. Evaluation of the ducts should also include visualization of salivary flow. By "milking" the suspicious gland

Box 14-1. Salivary Gland Disorders

Inflammatory
Acute
  Bacterial
    Suppurative sialadenitis
    Lymphadenitis/abscess
  Viral
    Mumps
    HIV
    Other
  Chronic
  Obstructive
    Sialectasis
    Sialolithiasis
    Mucocele
  Granulomatous
    Mycobacterial
    Actinomycosis
    Cat-scratch disease
    Sarcoidosis
    Toxoplasmosis
    Histoplasmosis
  Necrotizing sialometaplasia

Congenital
Dermoid
Branchial cleft cyst
Congenital ductal cyst
Agenesis of salivary gland

Autoimmune/systemic
Benign lymphoepithelial disease
Sjögren syndrome
Chronic sialorrhea
Cystic fibrosis
Allergy (shellfish, strawberry)

Neoplastic
Benign
  Pleomorphic adenoma
  Warthin tumor
  Lipoma
Malignant
  Mucoepidermoid carcinoma
  Acinic cell carcinoma
  Adenocarcinoma
  Adenoid cystic carcinoma
  Rhabdomyosarcoma
  Lymphoma
  Other
Vascular malformations
  Hemangioma
  Lymphatic malformations
  Arteriovenous malformations
  Other

from posterior to anterior in the parotid or pushing cranially for the submandibular gland, salivary flow can be noted from the puncta. An obstructed duct will not demonstrate adequate flow, and one may note an increase in edema around the ducts or puncta. Duct fluid with sialadenitis will appear milky or purulent, and systemic disorders that affect saliva, such as Sjögren syndrome or cystic fibrosis, may demonstrate thick mucoid saliva. Punctal erythema with clear saliva generally suggests viral etiology.

Cranial nerve function also needs to be assessed and documented. Facial nerve function in all divisions should be noted (cranial nerve VII). Tongue mobility and general somatic sensation should also be identified (12th and fifth cranial nerves). Facial or tongue weakness is a concerning sign and suggests a neoplastic process.

> **Pearl:** Facial nerve weakness and
> rapid enlargement of a salivary gland is
> highly suspicious of a malignant process.
> Solid lesions are more likely to be malignant
> in children than adults.

■ Diagnosis of Salivary Gland Disorders

DIAGNOSTIC IMAGING

Radiologic studies can provide useful information about diagnosis of a salivary gland disorder. Potential studies include plain radiography, sialography, ultrasonography, computed tomography (CT), and magnetic resonance imaging (MRI).

Plain radiographs have limited utility but can identify calcifications and sialoliths. Sialograms may be done using plain films or CT imaging. This study is used mainly to identify strictures or stones within the salivary ductal system. It is rarely indicated in the pediatric setting because of the need for general anesthesia and difficulty in cannulating the duct for infiltration of contrast material.

Computed tomography imaging is used to provide anatomic detail and assist in surgical planning. Early abscesses can be readily identified by CT imaging demonstrating a central hypodense area with ring enhancement. Intravenous (IV) contrast is needed to provide accurate information about vascularity or identifying abscess formation. Salivary gland masses may also be initially evaluated by CT imaging. Non-contrast CT is the study of choice to identify salivary gland stones. Sedation is rarely necessary except in uncooperative children. The procedure does expose the patient to ionizing radiation.

Magnetic resonance imaging gives excellent soft tissue detail and can directly identify the facial nerve within the confines of the parotid gland. Flow voids can be identified and help with determining the nature of vascular malformations. High-flow lesions, such as arteriovenous malformations and hemangiomas, are more readily delineated from low-flow lesions, such as lymphangiomas or hemangiopericytomas. Sedation and general anesthesia in infants and young children are usually necessary to achieve good-quality images free of motion artifact.

Ultrasonography is noninvasive and does not require radiation exposure or sedation but has limited utility in evaluating salivary gland conditions.

LABORATORY STUDIES

There are a variety of diagnostic laboratory tests that can assist in the diagnosis of salivary gland pathology. An elevated white blood cell count and C-reactive protein indicate infectious processes. Culture of saliva may identify pathogenic bacteria; however, these are often cross-contaminated with normal oral flora. In cases of bilateral parotid cystic lesions, HIV testing should be considered. Serology for sarcoidosis, cystic fibrosis, and Sjögren syndrome can also be useful if clinically suspicious.

BIOPSY

Fine-needle aspiration (FNA) biopsy, a useful outpatient procedure in evaluating salivary gland masses, has an overall diagnostic accuracy of 84%. Combined modality use of ultrasonography to guide biopsy has been demonstrated to improve specificity, which ranges from 95% to 100% for malignancies. This technique requires a cooperative older patient or a sedated younger child. When FNA is not feasible, surgical incisional biopsy to obtain a small sample is generally not recommended; rather, excisional biopsy is preferred in cases in which there is a risk of tumor spillage or the lesion is too small to access by needle biopsy. In cases of mycobacterial infection, FNA is useful for obtaining a DNA sample for cervicofacial abscesses in which the offending organism can be identified by polymerase chain reaction (PCR). For confirmation of Sjögren syndrome, excision of a minor salivary gland from the lip can demonstrate the same histopathologic features as larger salivary glands, thereby obviating the need for open biopsy with greater potential risk in major glands.

■ Treatment Options for Salivary Gland Disorders

INFLAMMATORY CONDITIONS

Viral Infections

Mumps

Prior to widespread vaccination, mumps was the most common salivary gland inflammatory disease in children around age 5 years. It is an acute, contagious illness causing painful bilateral parotid enlargement, fever, headache, and malaise. It is transmitted by contact with salivary droplets and has an 18- to 21-day incubation period. Saliva can shed virus up to 6 days before noticeable parotid swelling and 9 days afterward. Mumps can affect the central nervous system (CNS) and cause meningoencephalitis in 2% to 3%. Pancreatitis, sensorineural hearing loss, and orchitis are potentially severe sequelae. Treatment is usually supportive, consisting of adequate hydration, rest, respiratory isolation, and antipyretics. Immunity is lifelong.

HIV

Up to 30% of HIV-positive children have parotid involvement, consisting of lymphocytic infiltrates. Intraglandular lymphadenopathy and non-Hodgkin B-cell lymphoma are more common in these patients. Lymphoepithelial cysts can result in bilateral parotid enlargement. Aspiration of these cysts is indicated in enlargement, causing significant discomfort.

Other Viruses

Epstein-Barr virus may cause enlargement of intraparotid lymph nodes. Coxsackie A virus, echovirus, and cytomegalovirus can all cause viral parotitis. In cases of cytomegalovirus parotitis, the CNS, liver, and kidneys are also often affected.

Bacterial Infections

Acute Sialadenitis

Acute sialadenitis usually affects the parotid gland but can also be seen in the submandibular gland. It occurs in all ages of children and may be a solitary episode or recurrent. Patients present with an acutely swollen, firm and tender gland, associated with fever, difficulty eating due to pain, and dysgeusia. Dehydration and immunosuppression are common etiologies. Purulent saliva is expressed from the duct and culture is diagnostic. *Streptococcus viridans* and *Staphylococcus aureus* are the most common pathogens. Anaerobes are found in up to 50%. Treatment consists of systemic antimicrobial coverage, hydration, heat, massage, and sialogogues such as lemon drops or pickles, which stimulate salivary flow. In cases that do not resolve with these measures, progression to abscess formation needs to be considered. The gland will remain swollen and painful with overlying erythema. Computed tomography scan can be diagnostic. Imaging usually is not necessary, but CT scanning can be diagnostic. Surgical drainage of abscess is necessary to clear infection.

Acute Parotitis of Infancy

This usually affects premature newborns and the parotids preferentially because of the serous nature of saliva. Bacteriology is similar to that found in bacterial sialadenitis, and treatment is antimicrobial therapy and hydration. Resolution usually occurs within a week.

Juvenile Recurrent Parotitis

Children with juvenile recurrent parotitis often have intervening normal periods. There is a higher likelihood of congenital ductal abnormality, dental trauma, dehydration, or sialoliths. Children aged 3 to 6 years are most affected, and there is a higher male preponderance. *Streptococcus pneumoniae* and *Haemophilus influenzae* are the usual organisms isolated. Treatment is the same as that of suppurative parotitis. In recalcitrant cases, sialoendoscopy, lavage, dilation, or cortisone injection may be indicated. Endoscopy will demonstrate a white appearance of the ductal layers without a normal vascular cover. Ultrasonography can identify punctuate sialectasis found in recurrent parotitis. Computed tomography will demonstrate fibrosis of the gland and microcalcifications in the ductal system. In severe cases total gland resection may be indicated. Recurrent parotitis can be the initial manifestation of Sjögren syndrome.

Chronic Inflammatory Conditions

Sialectasis

Dilation of the small intercalated ducts can lead to salivary stasis and secondary bacterial infection. Symptoms are usually unilateral, although abnormal ducts are often found in both parotids. Clinical presentation is similar to that of acute parotitis. This can be an isolated finding or occur in association with juvenile recurrent parotitis.

Stricture

Generally related to trauma and occasionally from infection, intra-ductal calculi can also lead to stricture formation. Proximal dilation of the duct may be seen on radiographic imaging. Gland swelling is related to oral intake and slowly resolves over 1 to 2 hours after feeding. Endoscopic dilation often can resolve strictures of major ducts; gland excision is reserved for refractory cases.

Sialolithiasis

More common in adolescents than younger children, 80% occur in the submandibular gland. Boys are affected more than girls (3:1). Saliva from the submandibular gland is more viscous and contains more calcium and phosphorus. The duct has a longer, uphill course and takes a right-angle turn from the hilum of the gland. Stones usually contain a high concentration of calcium and are radiopaque. Children with cystic fibrosis do not have an increased preponderance to developing sialoliths. Symptoms include painful gland enlargement after eating, which subsides over several hours. The stone may be visualized at the duct puncta or palpated along the duct. Peripheral sialoliths may spontaneously extrude or may need surgical removal, usually consisting of dilation of the duct and stone extraction. Sialoendoscopy is a new technique that is useful for stone removal as well as stricture dilation. Hilar stones are generally larger and not palpable, causing diffuse gland enlargement. Treatment for these is usually gland excision. Plain radiography can identify 80% of submandibular calculi. Non-contrast CT is useful in equivocal cases.

With proper management, the majority of these conditions resolve without significant sequelae. Mumps can progress to cause CNS involvement and sensorineural hearing loss; therefore, vaccination is advocated for prevention. Recurrent sialadenitis can lead to fibrosis and discomfort, in some cases necessitating salivary gland resection. In these cases, surgical excision is usually curative. Sialoliths may extrude spontaneously and relieve obstruction, or they may be impacted within the salivary duct. Removal of the stone generally alleviates symptoms; however, they may occasionally recur.

Granulomatous Diseases

Granulomatous diseases of the salivary gland usually occur within intraparotid lymph nodes and can be localized or diffuse. Usually these are slowly progressive, and saliva appears normal.

Mycobacterial infections can cause overlying skin to become erythematous, often with a characteristic purple hue, with eventual skin breakdown and suppurative drainage with progressive growth. Nontuberculous mycobacteria cause 90% of such cases. Acid-fast bacillus staining may be positive but is not diagnostic of the strain of mycobacteria. Cultures are not always positive and can take up to 6 weeks to demonstrate growth, FNA and PCR amplification of DNA may be useful for early identification of species. Treatment consists of complete curettage or surgical excision of the granulomatous lesion to minimize facial nerve disruption. In diffuse infection or cases of *Mycobacterium tuberculosis*, long-term multidrug therapy is also usually indicated.

Actinomycosis involves salivary glands and results from intraoral trauma. Presentation is a painless mass, and cutaneous fistulae are common (61%). Yellow-white inclusions known as "sulfur granules" are diagnostic. Treatment consists of 6 courses of IV penicillin or erythromycin followed by multiple courses of oral antibiotics.

Cat-scratch disease, brucellosis, and histoplasmosis are other causes of granulomatous sialadenitis. Fine-needle aspirate biopsy can often confirm tissue diagnosis. In cases of sarcoidosis, parotid swelling may be initial presentation in up to 40% of patients. Swelling is persistent, and there is minimal discomfort. Facial paresis may be present in rare cases. Differentiation from a malignant process is necessary.

Prognosis is usually dependent on management of the underlying systemic condition. For atypical mycobacterial infections, gland removal or intralesional curettage and addition of antimycobacterial therapy in extensive disease is usually curative with no long-term sequelae. Management of salivary gland involvement due to sarcoidosis, Sjögren syndrome, or cystic fibrosis is aimed at supportive measures and systemic treatment of the specific disorder. Allergic reactions are usually managed by symptomatic medication intervention and avoidance of the offending food item.

CYSTIC LESIONS

Most cystic lesions of the salivary glands occur within the parotids, but they can occur in any glandular structure. They may be congenital or related to trauma, or result from inflammatory conditions.

Surgical excision or marsupialization usually results in cure. The exception may be a lymphoepithelial cystic lesion related to an HIV infection. These cysts may recur with variable frequency and are usually bilateral. Treatment in these cases is supportive and may involve needle aspiration for symptomatic lesions, and prognosis is related to overall condition of the patient.

Congenital, Non-acquired

Ranula

These mucous-retention cysts of the sublingual glands can present as a swelling in the floor of the mouth or in the submandibular triangle as they extend around the mylohyoid muscle ("plunging" ranula). Treatment consists of marsupialization or complete surgical excision of the cyst as well as excision of the offending sublingual gland.

First Branchial Arch Cysts

These uncommon lesions can present as parotid masses. Type 1 lesions are duplications of the external auditory canal and usually occur in the conchal bowl or postauricular sulcus, although they may present in the preauricular region as a draining sinus. Type 2 first branchial arch anomalies are even less commonly seen. They course from the infra-auricular region to the upper neck behind the mandible. The tract passes in close approximation to the facial nerve (cranial nerve VII), and abscess formation or chronically draining sinuses are common. Treatment consists of superficial parotidectomy with facial nerve preservation.

Acquired

Trauma

Blunt trauma may result in an intraglandular hematoma that can mimic a cyst. Penetrating trauma can result in disruption of the ductal structures, leading to salivary leakage or ductal cyst and stricture formation. Treatment is supportive for blunt trauma but may require evacuation of a sialocele or hematoma. In penetrating trauma, repair of the duct over a stent will often allow for good function of the salivary system. Direct nerve repair may be necessary in cases of parotid or cheek-penetrating traumatic injuries.

SYSTEMIC DISORDERS

Diffuse parotid swelling may be seen in a variety of conditions. Fatty infiltration of the gland may be found in diabetes. In up to 30% of patients with bulimia, bilateral symmetric parotid hypertrophy is demonstrated. Patients with cystic fibrosis have enlargement of the submandibular gland in 90% of cases. Multiple agents such as iodine and heavy metals can cause asymptomatic salivary gland enlargement.

Sjögren syndrome, an autoimmune disorder manifested by xerostomia, keratoconjunctivitis, and connective tissue disease, also produces diffuse nonpainful enlargement of the salivary glands. Biopsy shows lymphocytic infiltration and gland atrophy. There is an increased incidence of non-Hodgkin B-cell lymphoma and other lymphoproliferative disorders in these patients.

Food allergy, such as to shellfish and strawberries, can cause significant, sudden parotid gland edema along with urticaria, angioedema, or rash and an acute change in salivary viscosity. Patients usually have immediate type 1 hypersensitivity to the offending allergen, and parents and older children are often able to relate acute onset of swelling to the specific food.

> **Pearl:** Recurrent sialadenitis may indicate ductal stricture or a systemic disorder that requires further workup and evaluation. Subspecialty referral is indicated in these situations.

SOLID LESIONS

Less than 5% of salivary gland tumors occur in children younger than 16 years. Solid salivary gland tumors in children are more likely to be malignant, and the majority of these occur in parotid glands. These lesions can be subdivided into benign, low-grade malignancies, and high-grade malignancies.

Benign Tumors

Pleomorphic adenoma (benign mixed tumor) is the most common solid salivary gland tumor in children. It is composed of epithelial and myoepithelial cells. It generally occurs in the lateral aspect of the parotid gland and grows slowly with a firm, lobulated appearance. Diagnosis is usually made by FNA biopsy. Complete surgical excision with avoidance of tumor spillage and facial nerve presentation is the treatment. Recurrence can approach 20%.

Pleomorphic adenomas may also occur in minor salivary glands and can be confused for torus palatine when occurring in the palate. These lesions are smooth and not fixed to the overlying mucosa with a rubbery consistency. Imaging with CT or MRI can assist with surgical planning.

Other benign tumors include neurofibromas, Warthin tumors (papillary cystadenoma lymphomatosum), basal cell adenomas, and lipomas. These are all quite rarely found in salivary glands.

Embryomas are rare benign epithelial tumors that present within the first year of life. There is a fairly high potential for malignant transformation, and complete excision is the recommended treatment.

Most of these tumors exhibit slow growth and can initially be managed conservatively. Pleomorphic adenoma has a recurrence rate up to 20%, especially in cases of tumor spillage, and a 4% risk of malignant transformation if untreated over 20 to 30 years. Embryomas also have a high rate of malignant transformation within the first years of life, but complete excision is curative.

Malignant Tumors

Rapid growth and facial nerve weakness are signs specifically concerning for malignancy. Treatment of salivary gland malignancies usually consists of surgical excision, with cervical lymphadenectomy if regional metastases are present, and adjunctive external beam radiation.

Epithelial tumors occur more often in older children and adolescents, whereas sarcomas are more frequently identified in early childhood. Cranial nerve involvement and regional adenopathy are more indicative of high-grade malignancy. These are more likely in younger children.

Mucoepidermoid carcinoma and acinic cell carcinoma are the most common low-grade malignant salivary gland tumors in children. Both of these lesions are slowly growing and painless. They are more frequently found in the parotid.

High-grade mucoepidermoid carcinoma, adenocarcinoma, and adenoid cystic carcinoma are most likely to cause involvement of the facial nerve and fixation to surrounding structures. In the submandibular gland, hypoglossal or marginal mandibular nerve (lower facial nerve branch) weakness are signs suggestive of a malignant process.

Rhabdomyosarcoma is the most common sarcoma affecting salivary glands in the pediatric population. These can present in the area of the parotid gland and may initially be mistaken for primary parotid tumor. Diagnosis is confirmed by biopsy, and in this instance incisional biopsy may be more diagnostic than FNA. Resection followed by radiation and chemotherapy is generally the treatment of choice.

The parotid gland can also be a site for metastasis from facial or scalp primaries, including melanoma. Examination of these areas should be performed if malignancy is suspected.

Low-grade malignancies, such as acinic cell carcinoma, and low-grade mucoepidermoid carcinoma both have an excellent 5-year survival rate greater than 90%; however, 20-year survival rate drops to around 50% due to late recurrences.

High-grade lesions, including adenoid cystic carcinoma, high-grade mucoepidermoid carcinoma, and adenocarcinoma, have a high rate of spread to regional lymph nodes, neural involvement, and hematogenous spread. The 5-year survival for these lesions is around 80%, but long-term survival (>20 years) is significantly worse.

Rhabdomyosarcoma survival is directly related to tumor stage, with 8-year survival rates ranging from 80% for stage 1 to 72% for stage 2 and 25% to 40% for stage 3.

VASCULAR MALFORMATIONS

Hemangiomas

Hemangiomas account for up to 50% to 60% of pediatric salivary gland tumors. They generally present within the first year and have a rapid proliferative growth phase, followed by a stabilization period and finally an involution period, which is generally completed by age 7 years. These are composed of capillary spaces and solid cellular masses within glandular secretory segments. Up to 80% occur in the parotid and 18% to 20% in the submandibular. Up to 20% of these patients have multiple lesions. They present as erythematous, warm, compressible masses and do not cause facial nerve weakness. Saliva is normal on expression.

Ultrasound can suggest diagnosis of hemangioma; MRI is superior for assessing the nature and extent of the mass. Management varies with patient age as well as growth and extent of the mass.

Lymphatic Malformations

Lymphatic malformations may occur within the parotid gland or affect function of smaller salivary glands. They are soft, compressible, congenital lesions that present in the immediate perinatal period. They will increase in size in the setting of infection or trauma due to lymph accumulation within the lesion. Magnetic resonance imaging is the modality of choice to delineate the cystic nature of these lesions.

While small, asymptomatic lesions require no therapy, treatment should be considered for large lesions or those causing inflammation or functional compromise. Macrocystic lesions may be amenable to intralesional sclerotherapy; microcystic lesions generally require surgical intervention. Because lymphatic malformations in or near the salivary glands typically approximate the facial nerve, protection of the nerve during treatment is of utmost importance.

Arteriovenous malformations and low-flow venous malformations may occur in the area of the salivary glands but generally do not involve actual gland tissue. These lesions generally require a multidisciplinary approach involving interventional radiology.

Hemangiomas usually spontaneously regress and may completely resolve without any treatment. Systemic steroids, intralesional steroids, and propranolol have all been used effectively for large lesions with secondary symptomatic compromise. Long-term sequelae may include scarring of affected areas or persistent cosmetic deformity.

Lymphatic malformations may continue to grow with the child and can be severely debilitating. Use of sclerotherapy and surgical excision with preservation of local vital structures may prevent continued growth, and in limited lesions can be curative. Large lesions usually involve broad areas of anatomy and are not limited to salivary gland structures. In these cases, treatment is usually performed in multiple stages, and recurrence occurs in up to 15% of lesions that have been excised surgically, with persistent cosmetic and functional deformity not uncommon.

> **Pearl:** Malignant salivary gland tumors present with rapid growth and cranial nerve involvement and require immediate subspecialty referral. Solid tumors of the saliva glands are more likely to be malignant in the pediatric population.

> **Pearl:** Most salivary gland lesions in children have good prognosis with low likelihood of recurrence if treated appropriately. Exception is in high-grade malignancies; these should be managed aggressively with multimodality therapy.

■ Selected References

Al-Khafaji BM, Nestok BR, Katz RL. Fine-needle aspiration of 154 parotid masses with histologic correlation: ten-year experience at the University of Texas M.D. Anderson Cancer Center. *Cancer.* 1998;84(3):153–159

Bower CM, Dyleski RA. Diseases of the salivary glands. In: Bluestone CD, Stool SE, Alper CM, et al, eds. *Pediatric Otolaryngology.* 4th ed. New York, NY: Saunders; 2003:1251–1267

Buckmiller LM. Propranolol treatment for infantile hemangiomas. *Curr Opin Otolaryngol Head Neck Surg.* 2009;17(6):458–459

Casselman JW, Mancuso AA. Major salivary gland masses: comparison of MR imaging and CT. *Radiology.* 1987;165(1):183–189

Ericson S, Zetterlund B, Ohman J. Recurrent parotitis and sialectasis in childhood. Clinical, radiologic, immunologic, bacteriologic, and histologic study. *Ann Otol Rhinol Laryngol.* 1991;100(7):527–535

Garden AS, el-Naggar AK, Morrison WH, Callender DL, Ang KK, Peters LJ. Postoperative radiotherapy for malignant tumors of the parotid gland. *Int J Radiat Oncol Biol Phys.* 1997;37(1):79–85

Gayner SM, Kane WJ, McCaffrey TV. Infections of the salivary glands. In: Cummings CW, Fredrickson JM, Harker LA, et al, eds. *Otolaryngology-Head and Neck Surgery.* St. Louis, MO: Mosby-Yearbook; 1998:1234–1246

Ibrahim HZ, Handler SD. Diseases of the salivary glands. In: *Pediatric Otolaryngology.* New York, NY: Theime Medical Publishers; 2000:647–658

Lee KC, Cheung SW. Evaluation of the neck mass in human immunodeficiency virus-infected patients. *Otolaryngol Clin North Am.* 1992;25:1287–1305

Leverstein H, van der Wal JE, Tiwari RM, et al. Malignant epithelial parotid gland tumors: analysis and results in 65 previously untreated patients. *Br J Surg.* 1998;85(9):1267–1272

Megerian CA, Maniglia AJ. Parotidectomy: a ten year experience with fine needle aspiration and frozen section biopsy correlation. *Ear Nose Throat J.* 1994;73(6):377–380

Morgan DW, Pearman K, Raafat F, Oates J, Campbell J. Salivary disease in childhood. *Ear Nose Throat J.* 1989;68(2):155–159

Myer C, Cotton RT. Salivary gland disease in children: a review. Part 2: congenital lesions and neoplastic disease. *Clin Pediatr (Phila).* 1986;25(7):353–357

Nahlieli O, Shacham R, Shlesinger M, Eliav E. Juvenile recurrent parotitis: a new method of diagnosis and treatment. *Pediatrics.* 2004;114(1):9–12

Nozaki H, Harasawa A, Hara H, Kohno A, Shigeta A. Ultrasonic features of recurrent parotitis in childhood. *Pediatr Radiol.* 1994;24(2):98–100

Rice DH. Non-neoplastic diseases of the salivary glands. In: Paparella MM, ed. *Otolaryngology.* Philadelphia, PA: WB Saunders; 1991

Salomão DR, Sigman JD, Greenebaum E, Cohen MB. Rhabdomyosarcoma presenting as a parotid gland mass in pediatric patients: fine-needle aspiration biopsy findings. *Cancer.* 1998;84(4):245–251

Schuller DE, McCabe BF. Salivary gland neoplasms in children. *Otolaryngol Clin North Am.* 1977;10(2):399–412

Seibert RW, Seibert JJ. High resolution ultrasonography of the parotid gland in children. *Pediatr Radiol.* 1986;16(5):374–379

Shott SR. Salivary disease in children. In: Cotton RT, Meyer CM, eds. *Practical Pediatric Otolaryngology.* Philadelphia, PA: Lippincott-Raven Publishers; 1999:693–710

Smith RJH. Non-neoplastic salivary gland diseases. In: English GM, ed, *Otolaryngology.* Philadelphia, PA: JB Lippincott; 1994:1–29

Teresi LM, Kolin E, Lufkin RB, Hanafee WN. MR imaging of the intraparotid facial nerve: normal anatomy and pathology. *AJR Am J Roentgenol.* 1987;148(5):995–1000

Williams MA. Head and neck findings in pediatric acquired immune deficiency syndrome. *Laryngoscope.* 1987;97(6):713–716

Work WP. Cysts and congenital lesions of the parotid gland. *Otolaryngol Clin North Am.* 1977;10(2):339–343

Wotman S, Mercadante J, Mendel ID, Goldman RS, Denning C. The occurrence of calculus in normal children, children with cystic fibrosis, and children with asthma. *J Periodontol.* 1973;44(5):278–280

Wurster CF. Non-neoplastic salivary gland disorders. In: Gates GA, ed. *Current Therapy in Otolaryngology Head and Neck Surgery.* St. Louis, MO: Mosby-Yearbook; 1994:238–243

Yang WT, Ahuja A, Metreweli C. Sonographic features of head and neck hemangiomas and vascular malformations: review of 23 patients. *J Ultrasound Med.* 1997;16(1):39–44

Yeh S. The salivary glands. In: Ballenger JJ, ed. *Diseases of the Nose, Throat, Ear, Head & Neck.* Philadelphia, PA: Lea & Febiger; 1991:308–311

Airway and Swallowing

CHAPTER 15

Stridor in Infants and Children

Seth M. Pransky, MD, and Carrie L. Francis, MD

■ Introduction

Stridor is an abnormal sound produced by turbulent airflow through a partially obstructed supraglottis, glottis, or trachea. Stridor is a symptom, not a diagnosis or disease. The character of stridor and the respiratory phase in which it occurs will direct the workup and provide clues to the location and severity of anatomic or physiologic narrowing. Obstructing lesions or physiologic collapse in the supraglottis will result in high-pitched inspiratory stridor. The glottis and subglottis are fixed segments of the airway with little physiologic collapse. Noisy breathing generated by these lesions is appreciable in both phases of the respiratory cycle, resulting in biphasic stridor. The intrathoracic trachea and main stem bronchi undergo physiologic narrowing during expiration. Obstructing lesions at this level will also cause expiratory stridor.

The clinical history is key in directing the clinician to the cause of the stridor (Table 15-1). It is imperative to identify the precise underlying cause because appropriate management is dictated by an accurate diagnosis. The degree of respiratory distress and feeding difficulties on presentation will determine the extent of initial workup and urgency of intervention. Acute respiratory distress demands establishment of a secure airway regardless of the diagnosis, while stable patients can undergo a more thorough history and physical examination.

Stridor in infants and children is most commonly congenital (85%). Laryngeal lesions such as laryngomalacia (LM), vocal cord paralysis, and subglottic stenosis (SGS) make up most diagnoses. Tracheal abnormalities tend to be less frequent than laryngeal

Table 15-1. Differential Diagnosis of Pediatric Stridor	
Congenital	**Neoplastic**
Laryngomalacia	Subglottic hemangioma
Tracheomalacia	**Trauma/Toxin**
Laryngeal cleft	Foreign body—tracheal or esophageal
Vocal cord paralysis	Caustic ingestion
Glottic stenosis	Laryngotracheal trauma
Subglottic stenosis	**Infectious**
Subglottic cyst	Recurrent respiratory papillomatosis
Idiopathic	Croup (laryngotracheitis)
Vocal cord paralysis	Epiglottitis
Subglottic stenosis	Tracheitis
Intubation trauma	
Inflammatory	
Gastroesophageal reflux disease	
Eosinophilic esophagitis	

problems, with tracheomalacia (TM) and congenital vascular anomalies that result in external compression of the airway and subsequent stridor the anomalies most commonly seen.

■ History

A complete birth history is essential. This should include information about intubation, respiratory distress at time of birth, birth weight, prematurity, meconium aspiration, prolonged or difficult delivery, and birth injury (Table 15-2). History and length of neonatal intensive care stay or intubation in the neonatal period are critically important.

Table 15-2. History for Children With Stridor
Onset: acute, chronic, progressive
Fluctuation: positional changes that improve stridor
Age of onset
Prior respiratory problems ♦ Recurrent croup ♦ Aspiration ♦ Pneumonia ♦ Reactive airways disease
Birth history ♦ Ex-preemie ♦ NICU stay
Prior intubation
GERD symptoms
Sleep disordered breathing ♦ Snoring ♦ Nocturnal cough ♦ Witnessed apneas
Wheezing episodes
Feeding problems ♦ FTT, weight gain, choking episodes
Acute changes in clinical status ♦ Fever ♦ Respiratory distress ♦ Cough ♦ Drooling ♦ Change in voice or cry ♦ Decrease in oral intake ♦ Body position

Abbreviations: FTT, failure to thrive; GERD, gastroesophageal reflux disease; NICU, neonatal intensive care unit.

Even a transient intubation for meconium aspiration can be relevant to future development of stridor.

Age at symptom onset is important in guiding clinicians toward a diagnosis. Stridor that develops shortly after birth is likely to have a congenital etiology. Laryngomalacia, the most common laryngeal anomaly and source of congenital stridor, classically develops in the first 2 weeks of life. Bilateral vocal cord paralysis or congenital SGS are present and are usually symptomatic immediately after birth, while subglottic hemangioma (SGH) will result in symptoms after the first month of life. Acquired abnormalities usually develop later in infancy or childhood, most often associated with some form of airway trauma, manipulation, or intubation. Transient "acquired" causes of stridor, such as infectious croup, develop between ages 6 months to 6 years, with a peak incidence around age 2, and transient stridor that develops shortly after extubation may be secondary to edema. Symptoms related to acquired SGS can develop weeks to months after intubation injury.

Symptom progression or fluctuation is also an important factor that helps make diagnosis. Severity of stridor may progress in the case of SGH during its proliferative phase. In LM, the character of stridor will change with feeding, crying, and supine positioning and in intensity with growth of the infant. Acute decompensation and prolonged respiratory illness may be seen in cases of infectious problems and with developing SGS.

Quality of voice or volume of cry should always be documented. A change in voice (dysphonia) usually suggests pathology involving the vocal cords. In unilateral vocal cord paralysis, patients usually have a weak cry or "breathy" voice, while in bilateral vocal cord paralysis the cry is normally strong. Voice changes due to masses, such as granulomas or papillomas, are variable.

Parents should be questioned about feeding difficulties. For example, symptoms of choking, cough, regurgitation, or failure to thrive are present in severe LM. In unilateral vocal cord paralysis, cough, aspiration, and recurrent pneumonia can be present until the mobile, contralateral vocal cord compensates for the gap left by the nonmobile side. Similar symptoms may be present in children with tracheoesophageal fistula, in which TM is the cause of the stridor, and with laryngeal clefts in which redundant arytenoid mucosa may cause noisy breathing.

Symptoms related to sleep help distinguish pharyngeal obstruction from laryngeal, tracheal, or bronchial obstruction. Pharyngeal obstruction (stertor) generally worsens during sleep; laryngotracheal obstruction (stridor) is usually worse while awake and with activity.

Comorbidities, such as gastroesophageal reflux and neuromuscular or congenital heart disease, are also important because they may exacerbate patient symptoms.

■ Physical Examination

Physical examination begins with simple, direct observation of the patient. The clinician should always assess urgency based on signs of acute or progressive respiratory distress, such as tachypnea, nasal flaring, retractions, or cyanosis. Cyanosis is often a late sign of airway distress. These symptoms require immediate intervention to secure the airway independent of underlying diagnosis. Once a stable airway is established, the child will undergo a more thorough examination.

> **Pearl:** Have the parent or caregiver hold the child to calm him and help ensure an accurate evaluation. This is especially helpful if the child is in respiratory distress.

Auscultation is the next step in evaluation. It provides information about symmetry and efficiency of breath sounds. In addition to the lungs, it is important to sequentially listen over the nares, mouth, and neck. The latter is facilitated using the rubber tubing from a "headless" stethoscope, from which the diaphragm and head are removed. Attention to the character of stridor and its respiratory phase is paramount. This allows the clinician to more accurately determine the site of anatomic abnormality by identifying the location of maximal noise. This, in turn, may direct the clinician to the underlying cause of stridor. The patient may also be placed in various positions to assess the effect on stridor. For example, stridor associated with LM improves in the prone position. In unilateral vocal cord paralysis, lying down on the side of normal vocal cord mobility may reduce severity of the stridor.

■ Additional Evaluation

While history and physical examination may suggest the most likely diagnosis, further evaluation may be necessary. The primary care practitioner must determine his or her comfort level in directing this evaluation based on the characteristics and severity of the child's stridor. For example, children whose symptoms are classic for LM or croup and whose symptoms are minimal may reasonably be managed medically with close follow-up. In such cases, the primary care practitioner may choose to order studies that help confirm the diagnosis. However, when the stridor or associated symptoms do not suggest a particular pathology or symptoms are severe, otolaryngologic consultation, including endoscopic assessment, should be the next step.

Radiographs, in certain cases, can contribute to the evaluation of a child with stridor. In children whose history and physical examination are highly suggestive of LM and whose stridor is of mild severity, radiographs of the airway and chest may be useful in assessing the likelihood of more distal causes of stridor. Posteroanterior and lateral neck x-rays may also be useful in evaluation of laryngeal infection. In supraglottitis, the radiograph will show an enlarged epiglottis protruding from the anterior wall of the hypopharynx, a finding known as the thumb sign (Figure 15-1). In children with croup, imaging usually demonstrates a steeple sign reflecting inflammation of the subglottis (Figure 15-2). However, such films must be performed using high kilo-voltage and may be very technique sensitive. When feeding difficulties are present, barium esophagogram may reveal a vascular ring; radiographs and pH probe studies may also aid in diagnosing gastroesophageal reflux that may contribute to stridor.

The primary care practitioner may also choose to assess the severity of pathology based on objective data. Pulmonary function, pulse oximetry, and apnea monitoring may help determine those children whose stridor requires more immediate attention.

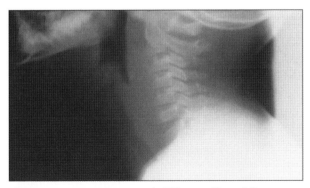

Figure 15-1. In acute supraglottitis, swelling of the epiglottis results in the thumb sign observed on lateral radiographs of the neck.

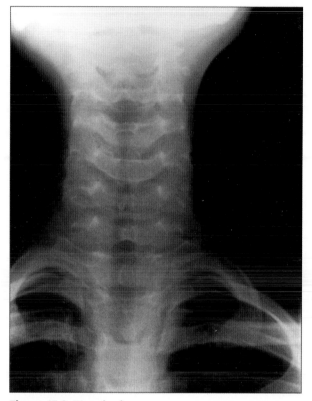

Figure 15-2. Steeple sign.

■ Endoscopy

In most cases, otolaryngologic consultants will perform flexible fiber-optic endoscopy (Figure 15-3) during their initial clinic evaluation. Flexible fiber-optic endoscopy allows excellent assessment of the supraglottic and glottic larynx and is easy to perform. In neonates and very young infants, endoscopy can often be performed transorally. Older infants and children typically require topical nasal decongestion and local analgesia for transnasal laryngoscopy.

Flexible fiber-optic endoscopy facilitates assessment of the tongue base, vallecula, pyriform sinus, and supraglottic and glottic larynx, with attention to presence of secretions and vocal cord mobility. However, visualization of the glottis may occasionally be compromised by pathology, excess secretions, or overhanging epiglottis, and the subglottis and trachea are rarely well seen. Vocal cord mobility can also be difficult to assess in the neonate.

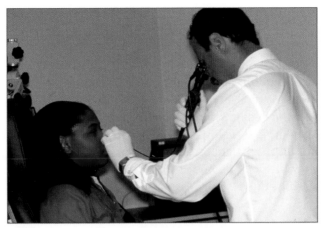

Figure 15-3. Flexible fiber-optic laryngoscopy is performed in most children without difficulty.

Operative direct laryngoscopy and bronchoscopy (DLB), the most definitive assessment, is routinely performed but may not be necessary for every child with stridor. There are multiple indications for DLB (Table 15-3). The role of surgery is to establish diagnosis when stridor is not otherwise explained and to direct appropriate surgical intervention. Additionally, DLB is used to evaluate for synchronous lesions. In patients with chronic stridor, synchronous lesions have been reported to occur in anywhere from 7.5% to 60% of patients. Synchronous lesions are usually suspected when the clinical picture is not fully explained by the diagnosis provided by other means. Risks of endoscopy are fortunately rare and are mostly related to the underlying pathology necessitating an evaluation. These include postoperative

Table 15-3. Direct Laryngoscopy and Bronchoscopy Indications
To establish a diagnosis (when other measures fail)
To evaluate for synchronous lesions (usually suspected when the clinical picture is not fully explained by the diagnosis provided by other measures)
Concern for subglottic lesion
Severe or progressive stridor
Cyanosis or apnea concerns
Radiologic abnormalities
Concern for foreign body
Parental or physician anxiety

edema, respiratory infection, possible need for extended treatment with steroids, lengthened hospitalization, airway injury causing SGS or glottic web, and voice abnormalities.

The key limitation of operative endoscopy is that it may not assess the airway in its normal physiologic state. This can make evaluation of dynamic changes, such as vocal fold movement or TM, difficult. To completely assess the dynamic component of laryngeal mobility, the patient may need flexible endoscopy at the beginning or end of the operative endoscopy with the patient breathing spontaneously. Similarly, TM can be assessed with spontaneous ventilation using a flexible bronchoscope or rigid telescope only.

■ Common Causes of Stridor

LARYNGOMALACIA

Laryngomalacia is the most common congenital laryngeal anomaly and cause of stridor in infants. It is generally a self-limited process, but when severe it may cause life-threatening airway obstruction or failure to thrive. Laryngomalacia is classically characterized by an omega-shaped epiglottis, short aryepiglottic folds, and cuneiform cartilage prolapse (Figure 15-4). Laryngomalacia is a clinical entity distinct from TM, which is far less common; *the term* laryngotracheomalacia *has no clinical significance and should not be used in medical parlance.*

Most cases of LM are mild and treated expectantly with positioning and medical therapy for comorbidities such as gastroesophageal reflux. Authors have reported that the range of infants with LM requiring surgical intervention varies between 11% and 22%. Endoscopic techniques,

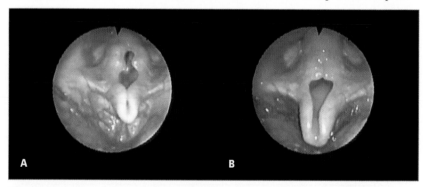

Figure 15-4. Two phases of obstruction in a patient with laryngomalacia. (A) The epiglottis is curled tightly on itself while the vocal folds and posterior laryngeal cartilages are open. (B) The epiglottis has unfurled somewhat, while the posterior laryngeal cartilages have prolapsed over the vocal folds.

most commonly supra-glottoplasty, have now largely displaced the tracheostomy as the gold-standard operative treatment. These procedures have successful outcomes in the range of 38% to 100%. Multiple etiologic theories of LM exist, though it is still unclear whether neurologic or anatomic pathology or both play a role in the symptomatic child.

The classic presentation of LM is intermittent inspiratory staccato type of stridor that worsens with feeding, agitation, excitement, or supine positioning. Stridor usually develops during the first 2 weeks of life, and most will present by 4 months of age. The natural course of LM is for stridor to peak over 6 to 8 months then spontaneously resolve by 12 to 24 months of age. Associated sequelae include respiratory symptoms, such as desaturations, tachypnea, retractions, and recurrent respiratory infection, and feeding difficulties. In the most severe cases of LM, apnea, cyanosis, or cor pulmonale can occur; fortunately, such cases are rare.

Feeding difficulties have been reported as the second most common symptom in LM. The most common signs of feeding difficulties include cough, choking, gastroesophageal regurgitation, nasal obstruction, nasopharyngeal reflux, and poor weight gain. Other signs include recurrent emesis, aspiration, oxygen desaturations with feeding, and slow and laborious feeding associated with failure to thrive. Though no causal effect has been established, gastroesophageal reflux disease (GERD) and laryngopharyngeal reflux (LPR) are the most common comorbidities in LM.

Laryngomalacia can usually be diagnosed from the clinical history and presentation. The key anatomic findings of LM—an omega-shaped epiglottis, cuneiform prolapse, and foreshortened aryepiglottic folds—are confirmed on flexible fiber-optic laryngoscopy (FFL). It is important to note that the diagnosis of LM requires the anatomic findings and the pattern of inspiratory collapse producing stridor.

Most infants have mild LM with intermittent stridor and occasional feeding symptoms like cough, occasional choking, or regurgitation. Fewer than 8% have an associated comorbidity (eg, GERD, cardiac, neurologic disease, craniofacial syndrome). If indicated, following GERD precautions with or without acid suppression has been effective in controlling symptoms. Disease progression occurs in up to 30% within 2 months after diagnosis. Therefore, these patients should be followed for the development of respiratory sequelae or persistent feeding difficulties.

Moderate LM patients typically present with stridor and have the highest rate of feeding symptoms. The most common feeding symptom is postprandial regurgitation. Acid suppression successfully resolves most feeding symptoms, but these patients should be monitored closely for refractory symptoms. Most symptoms will resolve within 12 months, but up to 28% require surgical intervention for disease progression within 2 months. Half of these patients will have an associated comorbidity. Common indications for intervention include aspiration, cyanosis with feeding, and failure to thrive unresponsive to acid suppression.

Severe LM presents with stridor, cyanosis, or apnea during feeding. Because of airway obstruction and a discoordinate suck-swallow-breathe mechanism, these patients may develop failure to thrive, aspiration, and frequent respiratory illnesses or pneumonia. Other respiratory sequelae include apparent life-threatening events, retractions, or rarely chronic hypoxia and cor pulmonale. Half will have a comorbidity, and up to 80% of these patients may have a secondary airway lesion. Gastroesophageal reflux disease management should be optimized because these patients may develop postoperative feeding issues related to scarring and surgical alteration to the complex neural pathways that provide tonicity to laryngeal cartilages. All of these patients undergo surgical intervention.

Treatment of LM is tailored to the patient and pattern of collapse. The primary surgical therapy for LM is supra-glottoplasty, an endoscopic procedure designed to open the larynx by dividing shortened aryepiglottic folds or reducing redundant arytenoid mucosa. These procedures are routinely performed endoscopically with a micro-debrider, CO_2 laser, or cold-knife instrumentation.

DISCOORDINATE PHARYNGOLARYNGOMALACIA

This entity was first described in the late 1990s. It is defined as severe LM with complete supraglottic collapse during inspiration, without shortened aryepiglottic folds or redundant mucosa, and with associated pharyngomalacia. Normal pharyngeal patency is maintained by pharyngeal muscle activity influenced by the cerebral cortex in response to neural and chemical inputs. An immature central nervous system (CNS) leads to depressed pharyngeal dilator muscle activity, resulting in pharyngolaryngomalacia. Children with neurologic abnormalities, like cerebral palsy, may carry this diagnosis. In short, discoordinate pharyngolaryngomalacia is symptomatically similar to LM and physiologically neurologic in nature. Treatment options include continuous positive airway pressure (CPAP)/bilevel positive airway pressure

(BiPAP) or tracheostomy. Surgical techniques traditionally used for LM (ie, aryepiglottic fold division) are not useful and may make airway obstruction worse.

TRACHEOMALACIA

The pathophysiology and natural history associated with TM is quite different from that of LM. While LM typically produces inspiratory stridor that resolves spontaneously with growth, stridor associated with TM is expiratory. It is often accompanied by a characteristic harsh, "brassy" cough caused by intrathoracic location of collapse. Other important respiratory features of TM include tracheal wheeze that does not respond to and may even worsen with bronchodilator therapy, neck hyperextension, dyspnea, and recurrent respiratory tract infections. Reflex apnea, or "dying spells," are vagally mediated neural reflexes occurring in the area of compression that cause total occlusion of the trachea and apnea that may progress to cardiac arrest. It can be associated with feeding. Recurrent respiratory infections result from respiratory obstruction and impaired clearance of secretions. Not infrequently, these children will present in the neonatal intensive care unit (NICU) as children who are difficult to ventilate because of tracheal collapse occurring distal to the end of the endotracheal tube. In addition, many children with TM have feeding difficulty, poor weight gain, and failure to thrive.

Primary TM results from a congenital deformity of the tracheal rings. The lack of mature cartilaginous support results in dynamic collapse. Increased intrathoracic pressure and flaccid cartilaginous rings decrease anteroposterior diameter of the airway, causing a flattening of the normal trachea. This may be segmental in nature and can extend into the main bronchi. The cartilage-membranous ratio shifts from the normal 4:1 to 2:1 (Figure 15-5). Secondary TM usually has an appearance of asymmetric flattening on endoscopy and occurs as a result of extrinsic compression from congenital vascular anomalies. The most common etiology of secondary TM is innominate artery compression (Figure 15-6). Diagnosis and type of TM is confirmed by tracheoscopy in a spontaneously breathing patient so that the dynamic collapse is readily visible. Primary TM will have more of a "fish-mouth" shape, while extrinsic compression will cause asymmetric flattening of tracheal rings (figures 15-6 and 15-7). The latter patients should undergo a thorough cardiac workup, including computed tomography (CT) angiogram of the thorax to rule out any anatomic causes of external compression such as congenital vascular anomalies or mediastinal masses.

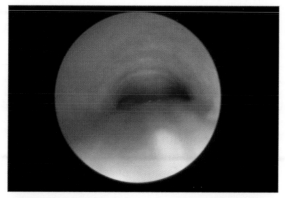

Figure 15-5. Tracheomalacia. Note abnormally low ratio of cartilaginous to membranous trachea.

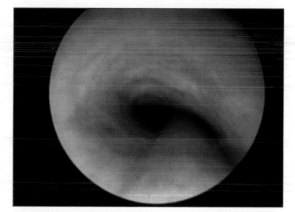

Figure 15-6. Asymmetric flattening of trachea due to innominate artery compression.

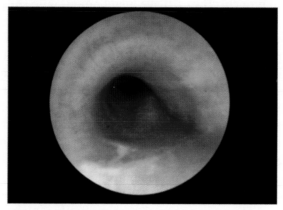

Figure 15-7. Compression of trachea by vascular ring including right-sided aortic arch.

In most cases of primary TM, symptoms will improve as the tracheobronchial tree grows. However, patients may be symptomatic for years. Treatment involves observation, control of associated comorbidities (eg, GERD), and positive-pressure ventilation to stent airways open (CPAP/BiPAP). Severe cases associated with reflex apnea, airway obstruction, or frequent respiratory illnesses may require tracheostomy with custom-length tubes to bypass the distal collapse. Stents are primarily palliative due to considerable morbidity secondary to granulation formation, or stent displacement. Secondary TM is treated with correction of the vascular anomaly, followed by conservative management similar to primary TM. In spite of surgical correction, stridor may be present for years because of residual TM. Gormley et al followed patients for 9 years postoperatively and found that 75% had complete resolution of symptoms.

VOCAL CORD PARALYSIS

True vocal cord paralysis (TVP) is the second most common cause of stridor in infants and children, occurring in 3% to 10% of cases. True vocal cord paralysis in children is classified as congenital or acquired, complete or partial, and unilateral or bilateral. Congenital bilateral vocal cord paralysis should be suspected in cases of immediate respiratory distress after delivery. Acquired paralysis can be seen most often after prolonged intubation and cardiac or thoracic surgery. Unilateral and bilateral paralysis can be related to neurologic abnormalities. Spontaneous recovery is possible and may occur 6 weeks to as long as 5 years after the insult.

Bilateral vocal cord paralysis usually results in airway obstruction rather than aspiration problems. Respiratory distress is more severe in these cases because vocal cords are frequently fixed in the adducted position. In severe cases, securing the airway immediately is required. Voice, cry, and feeding may be normal in bilateral vocal cord paralysis because of the anatomic position of the vocal cords. Causes may be idiopathic or iatrogenic (surgical or intubation), or a result of CNS anomalies (eg, Arnold-Chiari malformation, posterior fossa lesions), and peripheral nervous system insults (eg, myasthenia gravis, muscular dystrophy).

Children with unilateral vocal cord paralysis frequently have breathiness, dysphonia, or an abnormal cry. Unilateral paralysis rarely causes airway obstruction because the non-paralyzed vocal cord is able to abduct. Concerns center around feeding and airway protection; patients are at high risk for aspiration and must be followed closely while awaiting compensation of the other vocal cord. If no compensation occurs or the respiratory status begins to decline, the role of surgery becomes important. Additionally, an inadequate cough may result in aspiration, pooling of secretions, poor pulmonary clearance, and recurrent pneumonia. Paralysis may be idiopathic, iatrogenic (surgical or intubation), or related to a neoplasm, cardiovascular anomaly, or mediastinal lesions.

An evaluation of TVP should assess the entire course of the recurrent laryngeal nerve. This should begin with a complete history and physical and neurologic examination. Flexible fiber-optic laryngoscopy is the gold standard in vocal cord mobility evaluation. Repeat FFL, if limited during the initial assessment, may be required to obtain the correct diagnosis. Imaging is useful in identifying cardiovascular or CNS anomalies. Assessment for Arnold-Chiari malformation is critical because vocal cord paralysis, usually bilateral, will resolve with management of the CNS abnormality. A video fluoroscopic swallow study or endoscopic evaluation of swallowing may show evidence of laryngeal penetration or aspiration. Barium examinations may provide evidence of vascular ring.

Bilateral paralysis can sometimes be managed expectantly if the patient is stable with minimal symptoms or sequelae. Weight gain and feeding issues along with the status of the respiratory tract must be closely monitored in these instances. Surgical management is usually needed for more overt airway obstruction. Tracheostomy is the standard intervention for bilateral vocal cord paralysis; however, newer endoscopic treatments have had some success over the years. Cordotomy and arytenoidectomy are performed endoscopically. Open procedures include posterior laryngeal expansion or recurrent laryngeal reinnervation procedures.

Unilateral paralysis can be observed while awaiting spontaneous recovery. In asymptomatic patients, speech production and quality become more important from a psychological and functional standpoint as they age. Voice therapy may be helpful. Feeding difficulties and aspiration related to uncompensated glottic gap may dictate intervention if feeding therapy and thickener have been unsuccessful. Vocal cord injections with a temporary or semipermanent material have been used in unilateral TVP. Thyroplasty is a surgical procedure in which an implant is used to medialize the vocal fold in unilateral TVP. Both are used to improve voice quality and prevent feeding difficulties and aspiration.

SUBGLOTTIC HEMANGIOMA

Subglottic hemangiomas comprise most airway vascular anomalies. They appear as a stain at birth in the subglottis, then enter a proliferative phase with rapid grow over the first 6 to 12 months of life, followed by involution. The involution phase may take years. In the subglottis these lesions will produce biphasic stridor. Unfortunately, there is often a delay in diagnosis because of frequent misdiagnoses of asthma or croup.

The classic presentation is the onset of croup symptoms beginning at 6 to 8 weeks of age. Additionally confusing, respiratory distress and stridor often respond to typical croup therapy—humidified air, nebulizers, and steroids. Unlike croup, however, children with SGH usually have no fever or associated upper respiratory illness. The clinician should suspect SGH when classic croup symptoms are prolonged or not responding to standard treatment, when croup occurs prior to 6 months of age, or when croup recurs before 12 months of age. If a patient younger than 6 months is hospitalized for croup, an ear, nose, and throat referral should be made to investigate alternate explanations, including SGH. An accurate diagnosis is important because the airway can be threatened during the proliferative phase.

Once the history and physical examination are complete, comprehensive airway endoscopy is indicated for diagnosis and treatment. Classic endoscopic appearance of SGH is a smooth submucosal subglottic mass (Figure 15-8). Lesions causing bilateral involvement may be mistaken for a "soft" SGS. Biopsy is not essential; however, CT angiography or magnetic resonance imaging may be considered to evaluate uncertain cases or assess the degree of extraluminal extent.

Initial management is establishment of a secure airway and initiation of medical or surgical therapy. In mild cases, medical therapy may be sufficient. In more obstructed airways or those in which intralesional injection is performed, a brief period of endotracheal intubation may be necessary. The choice of initial therapy depends on the patient's clinical situation and experience of the managing clinician.

Management using oral propranolol has largely supplanted systemic steroids as the mainstay of medical therapy. Since the serendipitous discovery of its inhibitory effect on hemangioma growth in 2008, several authors have demonstrated the efficacy of propranolol in the control of airway hemangioma. The ideal initiation protocol and dosing regimen have yet to be established; however, maintenance doses are generally 2 to 3 mg/kg/day divided 2 to 3 times a day. Primary care practitioners

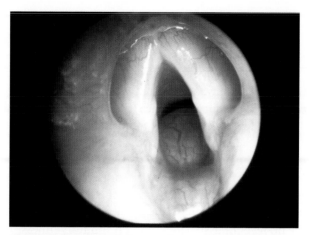

Figure 15-8. Subglottic hemangioma emanating from posterior tracheal wall.

should monitor such patients for bradycardia or hypoglycemia that may accompany increases in dose. Steroids also have been shown to control the growth of hemangiomas and cause regression; however, used systemically at doses of 2 to 4 mg/kg/day, side effects are common. Short bursts may be useful in the setting of an upper respiratory tract infection when mucosal edema exacerbates already compromised airway, or in patients who do not respond well to propranolol. In rare cases of severe, life-threatening hemangioma, interferon and vincristine are available. Both are used infrequently because of risk of toxicity or irreversible complications.

Surgical therapy most commonly involves endoscopic partial resection with a laser or micro-debrider or open surgical excision, often in combination with intralesional steroid injection. Intralesional steroid injections are frequently helpful but may need to be repeated every few months. Laser therapy and intralesional steroids have success rates in the 80% range. Open surgical excision with or without cartilage grafting requires considerable expertise to prevent complications. Tracheostomy is an option when other modalities fail, or to establish an airway urgently when clinicians experienced in hemangioma management are not readily available.

POST-INTUBATION INJURIES

Given the number of intubations in neonates, post-intubation injuries are seen frequently. Premature neonates with respiratory difficulties often have this problem. Risk factors for injury include NICU history, frequent and prolonged intubation, emergent intubations by less experienced personnel, and recurrent self-extubation. Stridor, respiratory distress, history of recurrent or prolonged croup, and multiple comorbidities (eg, genetic syndrome, GERD) are factors that may lead to intubation and result in an injury. Symptoms may present months to years from the time of injury.

Subglottic Cysts

Subglottic cysts (Figure 15-9) are common post-intubation injuries. Cyst development begins with mucus gland hypertrophy and duct blockage. Cysts typically occur along the posterior lateral subglottic wall and can be multiple. They present with stridor and airway obstruction, which may increase with an upper respiratory infection. They can be removed using a variety of endoscopic techniques, including micro-debrider, cup forceps, and various lasers.

Anterior Commissure Web

Anterior commissure webs (Figure 15-10) can be acquired after intubation and may also extend into the subglottis. Children present with a weak, hoarse cry or perhaps stridor. Acute respiratory distress rarely occurs because the posterior glottis is widely patent. Surgical treatment is endoscopic division of the web and can be performed with sharp instruments or a laser.

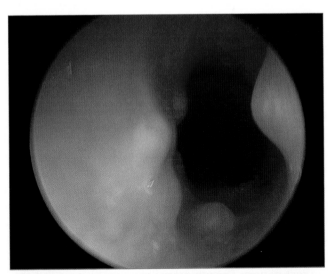

Figure 15-9. Subglottic cysts are most common in neonates with a history of prematurity and endotracheal intubation.

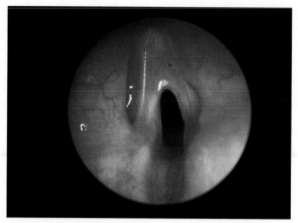

Figure 15-10. Glottic webs may be congenital or acquired. Anterior webs often cause dysphonia alone; with greater posterior involvement of the larynx, stridor becomes increasingly apparent.

Posterior Glottic Injury/Interarytenoid Web

Intubation resulting in arytenoid injury may cause granulation that progresses to adhesion, or ulceration that progresses to posterior glottic scar (Figure 15-11). While the former requires only simple division, the latter is more serious and difficult to manage. Posterior glottic stenosis may be mistaken for bilateral vocal cord paralysis because it results in bilateral true vocal fold immobility, which in turn can lead to acute respiratory distress and airway obstruction. To distinguish this entity from vocal cord paralysis, operative endoscopy and palpation of the arytenoid are required. Posterior glottic expansion, cordectomy, arytenoidectomy, or tracheostomy can be used to manage this injury.

Subglottic Stenosis

Acquired SGS has a reported incidence as high as 17% after intubation in an intensive care setting and is a problem with tremendous variation in its presentation and severity. The clinical picture may range from mild biphasic stridor and endoscopic findings of subglottic inflammation that respond to steroids and expectant management, to severe stenosis that requires surgical intervention. The classic history is failed extubation in a premature neonate after prolonged ventilation. Fortunately, incidence of this disease is decreasing with improved NICU ventilation techniques. The typical progression to stenosis begins with edema, granulation, ulceration, perichondritis/chondritis, and scarring leading to stenosis. The subglottis is most commonly involved because

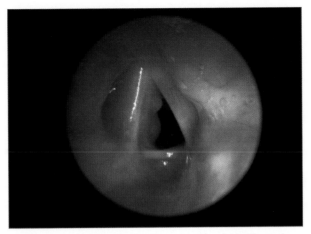

Figure 15-11. Posterior glottic scar and subglottic cysts in a patient with a history of perinatal intubation.

this is the only portion of the airway that is cartilaginous circumferentially (cricoid ring).

When SGS is suspected, complete airway endoscopy from the nasopharynx to carina is indicated. When stenosis is found, the endoscopist makes note of the length of the stenosis, location of the stenosis (ie, glottic, subglottic, or tracheal), character of the stenosis (soft and early versus firm and mature), and grade of stenosis based on involved cross-sectional area.

Grade I (0%–50% obstruction) and asymptomatic grade II (50%–70% obstruction) stenoses can frequently be managed expectantly with medical therapy, including antibiotics, anti-reflux medications, and intermittent steroid bursts to manage acute inflammation. Symptomatic grade II and select mild grade III (70%–99% obstruction) stenoses are amenable to multiple endoscopic modalities, including dilation with or without laser excision. Steroids and antibiotics are used in conjunction with endoscopic procedures to decrease inflammation and control granulation, and mitomycin C is occasionally applied topically to minimize scarring by inhibiting fibroblast proliferation.

More severe grade III and grade IV (no discernible lumen) stenoses, and those that fail to respond to endoscopic treatments, are candidates for open surgical procedures. The most common open surgical procedures are laryngotracheal reconstruction with rib cartilage augmentation and cricotracheal reconstruction. General medical status, comorbid conditions, and parental expectations will dictate timing of surgery; tracheotomy may be necessary to maintain airway until these issues are addressed. Children with congenital or acquired SGS frequently have cardiac or pulmonary comorbidities as well as other sequelae of prematurity. It is imperative that a multidisciplinary approach be taken. These patients should have complete pulmonary, cardiac, pediatric surgery, or gastroenterology consultations as deemed necessary.

CONGENITAL AIRWAY ANOMALIES

There are several common congenital airway anomalies that should be mentioned.

Congenital Subglottic Stenosis

In addition to acquired lesions of the subglottis that result from endotracheal injuries, SGS can be congenital. Endoscopically, the subglottis appears abnormally narrow and has an elliptical-shaped cricoid ring in the absence of scar (Figure 15-12). Incidence of congenital SGS has been reported as occurring in up to 2% of neonates. Presentation of neonates with congenital SGS is very similar to those presenting with acquired SGS. Neonates with severe congenital SGS may require intubation secondary to respiratory distress, making the diagnosis of congenital SGS difficult. However, patients with mild congenital SGS have symptoms without history of intubation. Mild cases of congenital SGS are often outgrown without any surgical intervention.

Laryngeal Cleft

Laryngeal clefts (also called laryngotracheoesophageal clefts) are a midline defect representing failure of formation of the posterior laryngeal wall and the common wall separating the trachea and esophagus. These children may have stridor but are primarily symptomatic because of aspiration and inability to handle their secretions. A cleft should be suspected whenever a child develops chronic cough with feeding, failure to thrive, recurrent aspiration pneumonia, and stridor early in life. Diagnosis is made by lateral distraction of the arytenoid cartilages during airway endoscopy. Clefts are classified as types I to IV based on the extent of laryngeal involvement. Type I clefts extend to the vocal cords; type II clefts extend into the subglottis but do not involve the entire cricoid; type III clefts involve the entire cricoid cartilage and extend into the cervical trachea; and type IV clefts extend deep into the thoracic trachea and are often fatal.

Treatment varies with the extent of the cleft. Type I clefts can often be observed but are occasionally treated by endoscopic repair or injection of filler. Type II clefts may be also be amenable to endoscopic

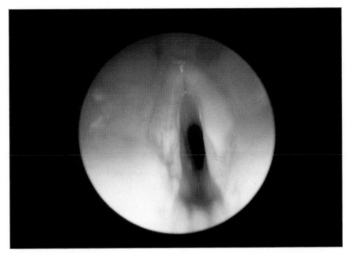

Figure 15-12. Elliptical cricoid causing subglottic narrowing and stridor in an infant.

repair but more commonly require open repair (laryngofissure) with posterior buttressing. Type III and IV clefts present immediately after birth and are life threatening, requiring immediate open surgical intervention. Type IV clefts must be approached via thoracotomy.

Patients with laryngeal clefts should be screened for cardiovascular defects. Such patients also require acid suppression. Dysphagia studies should be performed to determine the safety of swallowing and risk of aspiration. If oral feeding is unsafe, a feeding tube can be placed.

Vascular Rings/Slings

Children with cardiovascular anomalies often manifest stridor and some degree of airway obstruction related to their abnormal mediastinal vasculature. The 3 most common anomalies are aberrant innominate artery (most common), double aortic arch, and aberrant right subclavian artery that may course posterior to the esophagus, otherwise called dysphagia lusoria. These children present similarly to those with TM. They have harsh expiratory stridor and characteristic cough and may experience dying spells. Evaluation should include esophagram and imaging of the thoracic vasculature by CT angiography. When identified on tracheobronchoscopy, a fish-mouth appearance of the trachea is seen with pulsatile compression. If there is an aberrant innominate artery, compression will be anterior; if a double aortic arch or aberrant right subclavian, compression (Figure 15-7) will be from the posterior aspect of the trachea. Symptomatic children require open vascular decompression.

Congenital Tracheal Stenosis

Congenital tracheal stenosis (CTS) develops as a structural abnormality inherent to the trachea itself resulting in a narrowing of the trachea that produces airway obstruction. In most cases, the narrowed segment of the trachea is characterized by complete cartilaginous rings that involve a segment of the trachea of variable length (Figure 15-13).

The spectrum of respiratory symptoms in CTS ranges from isolated intermittent stridor to acute life-threatening events requiring cardio-pulmonary resuscitation. Rarely, air exchange may be so compromised that extracorporeal membrane oxygenation may be necessary. Symptoms generally appear within the first few weeks of life. Patients are often misdiagnosed as having croup; however, croup is exceedingly rare among neonates. Failure to thrive results from the caloric demand of increased work of breathing combined with poor feeding. Congenital tracheal stenosis is frequently associated with other congenital malformations of the pulmonary, cardiovascular, and gastrointestinal systems. A pulmonary artery sling is present in 30% to 50% of patients and should be ruled out before a definitive management plan is established.

The diagnosis of CTS is usually established by bronchoscopy performed to evaluate the etiology of the stridor. The trachea will appear funnel shaped and passage of a telescope or bronchoscope will be restricted. Once identified, it is important not to cause inflammation in the narrowed segment from trauma from the scope or an endotracheal tube used to secure the airway. The airway is best secured with an endotracheal tube place with the tip proximal to the narrowed

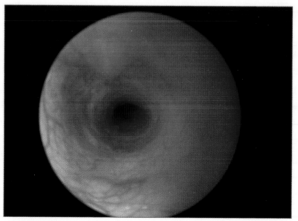

Figure 15-13. Congenital tracheal stenosis. Note funnel shape of trachea and absence of membranous trachea at narrowing.

segment; generally, neither intubation nor tracheotomy is useful because of the severity of the stenosis or the distal location of the obstruction. Following endoscopy, CT scanning with 3-D reconstruction may be used to establish the length and diameter of the stenotic segment.

Management strategies include conservative measures and surgery. In milder cases, stridor may be tolerated and acute exacerbations treated with systemic and inhaled steroids. However, more severe cases require surgical intervention. In short-segment stenosis, it is often possible to resect the narrowed portion of the trachea and suture together the portions of normal caliber. Long-segment stenosis usually requires a slide tracheoplasty in which the stenosis is divided horizontally and the cut ends are slid over one another and sutured, widening and shortening the trachea.

RECURRENT RESPIRATORY PAPILLOMATOSIS

Recurrent respiratory papillomatosis (RRP) is the most common benign neoplasm of the larynx in children and the second most frequent cause of childhood hoarseness (after vocal cord nodules). It is caused by the human papillomavirus (HPV), most commonly serotypes 6 and 11. The incidence of RRP is 4.3 per 100,000 children in the United States.

The earliest and most common presenting symptom is dysphonia or hoarseness. Progression of the disease to involve the posterior glottis results in stridor. Less common symptoms include dyspnea and acute respiratory distress, which are more likely to occur in young children with an upper respiratory tract infection. Diagnosis is most often made around 3 years of age, but correct diagnosis may be delayed for years, with affected children often treated initially for asthma or recurrent croup. Although RRP most commonly involves the larynx (Figure 15-14), it can occur anywhere within the aerodigestive tract. Spread of the disease beyond the larynx to the tracheobronchial airway occurs in up to 30% of cases. Malignant transformation is extremely rare.

When a patient with stridor also presents with prolonged hoarseness, diagnosis of RRP should be considered. Such patients should be referred for flexible laryngoscopy, where the classic findings of exophytic cauliflower-like warty growths are identified.

Children with RRP are challenging to manage because the disease is characterized by frequent recurrence and need for repetitive surgical intervention. The psychological and emotional effects on the child and family are often significant. Beyond multiple procedures, the dysphonia

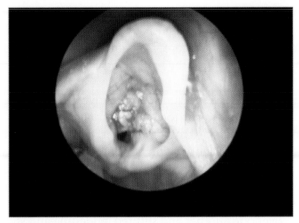

Figure 15-14. Respiratory papillomatosis most commonly involves the larynx.

generated affects education and social interaction, and bulky disease can cause life-threatening airway obstruction.

Multiple surgical modalities exist for removal of the papilloma with the basic principles always to create a safe and patent airway, decrease spread of disease and avoid tracheostomy, reduce tumor burden, preserve voice quality, and increase the interval between surgical procedures. For the most severe cases of RRP, medical adjuvant therapy is available. These therapies should be considered when a patient requires more than 4 surgeries in a 12-month period or is experiencing airway obstruction despite full surgical therapy. Intralesional cidofovir is currently the most widely used adjuvant and has found to be successful in many cases. Interferon therapy has also been used with some degree of success. As with any disease, prevention is the best cure. Gardasil, a quadrivalent vaccine against HPV serotypes 6, 11, 16, and 18, is currently Food and Drug Administration approved and available to males and females to help prevent HPV infection and reduce the incidence of cervical cancer. As vaccine use increases, the by-product should be a reduction in the number of children developing RRP.

VOCAL CORD DYSFUNCTION

Vocal cord dysfunction (VCD) is a functional disorder of the larynx characterized by paradoxical adduction of the vocal cords during inspiration. Affected patients experience frequent, episodic attacks of dyspnea, hoarseness, cough, wheezing, chest tightness, inspiratory stridor, and anxiety. The symptoms are usually preceded by physical activity or intense emotion and may be mistaken for asthma, and in fact, 30% of patients with asthma have symptoms of VCD. However, the stridor associated with VCD does not respond to therapies for asthma. Rather, these patients tend to improve with anxiolytics, relaxation, and breathing techniques.

Patients with VCD typically demonstrate no laryngoscopic abnormalities unless they are symptomatic at the time of the procedure. During symptomatic intervals, flexible laryngoscopy demonstrates pathognomonic inspiratory anterior vocal cord closure with posterior chink, or opening. This obstruction decreases laminar airflow through the glottis and produces an inspiratory wheeze or stridor similar to that heard in those with asthma, making the 2 entities difficult to differentiate symptomatically. In asthma alone, however, a posterior glottic chink is not seen. Flow-volume loops obtained during symptomatic periods of wheezing show a limitation of inspiratory flow suggestive of variable extrathoracic obstruction (inspiratory loop flattening).

Several different causes of VCD have been described including brain or brain stem injury, conversion disorder, malingering, and irritant induced. If a brain abnormality is suspected, a more thorough evaluation and imaging should be obtained. Vocal cord dysfunction may be a low-grade form of laryngospasm in response to the irritation from gastroesophageal reflux.

Vocal cord dysfunction often is a diagnosis of exclusion. Flexible laryngoscopy is performed in the absence of symptoms to assess the larynx for other possible causes of stridor. Asthma should also be definitively ruled out in these patients. Occasionally, performing the laryngoscopy and pulmonary functions tests under exercise conditions (treadmill or stationary bike) will elicit the classic findings.

Medical therapy for acute exacerbations of VCD includes heliox, a gaseous mixture of oxygen and helium that is less dense than air and reduces turbulence in the airway, as well as topical lidocaine and anxiolytics to break the cycle of hyperactive laryngeal adduction and muscle contractions. Long-term management of VCD requires a multidisciplinary approach involving speech therapy, psychiatric support, and physician education about the syndrome. Speech therapy techniques are aimed at focusing attention on expiration and abdominal breathing rather than on inspiration and laryngeal breathing. Therapy with early recognition of symptoms allows relaxation of neck, shoulder, and chest muscles and promotes normal laryngeal breathing.

■ Conclusion

Stridor in infants and children may have varied presentation and clinical course. Acute respiratory distress should be addressed immediately by securing the airway. More stable presentations can be evaluated more thoroughly. Several historic facts should be considered in initial assessment including birth history, age of onset, intubations, progression, and feeding difficulties. Physical examination should begin with initial observation of the patient and proceed systematically. Differential diagnosis is extensive, but careful history and physical examination can lead the astute clinician toward the correct diagnosis. Flexible fiber-optic laryngoscopy and operative endoscopy are useful procedures to make diagnosis. Treatment is directed toward specific diagnosis and must take into account the general health status of the patient and associated comorbidities. A multidisciplinary approach including pediatric otolaryngology, pediatric surgery, speech pathology, occupational therapy, intensivist, pulmonology, anesthesiology, cardiology, and gastroenterology is often used to optimize care and promote good results.

■ Selected References

Buckmiller LM. Update on hemangiomas and vascular malformations. *Curr Opin Otolaryngol Head Neck Surg.* 2004;12(6):476–487

Buckmiller LM, Munson PD, Dyamenahalli U, Dai Y, Richter GT. Propranolol for infantile hemangiomas: early experience at a tertiary vascular anomalies center. *Laryngoscope.* 2010;120(4):676–681

Choi SS, Zalzal GH. Changing trends in neonatal subglottic stenosis. *Otolaryngol Head Neck Surg.* 2000;122(1):61–63

Cotton RT. Management of subglottic stenosis. *Otolaryngology Clin North Am.* 2000;33(1):111–130

Cotton RT, Myer CM. *Practical Pediatric Otolaryngology.* Philadelphia, PA: Lippincott-Raven; 1999:637–660

de Jong AL, Kuppersmith RB, Sulek M, Friedman EM. Vocal cord paralysis in infants and children. *Otolaryngology Clin North Am.* 2000;33(1):131–149

Derkay CS, Wiatrak B. Recurrent respiratory papillomavirus: a review. *Laryngoscope.* 2008;118(7):1236–1247

Dickson JM, Richter GT, Meinzen-Derr J, Rutter MJ, Thompson DM. Secondary airway lesions in infants with laryngomalacia. *Ann Otol Rhinol Laryngol.* 2009;118(1):37–43

Friedman EM, Vastola AP, McGill TJ, Healy GB. Chronic pediatric stridor: etiology and outcome. *Laryngoscope.* 1990;100(3):277–280

Froehlich P, Seid AB, Denoyelle F, et al Discoordinate pharyngolaryngomalacia. *Int J Pediatr Otorhinolaryngol.* 1997;39(1):9–18

FUTURE I/II Study Group, Dillner J, Kjaer SK, et al. Four year efficacy of prophylactic human papillomavirus quadrivalent vaccine against low grade cervical, vulvar, and vaginal intraepithelial neoplasia and anogenital warts: randomised controlled trial. *BMJ.* 2010;341:c3493

Goldman J, Muers M. Vocal cord dysfunction and wheezing. *Thorax.* 1991;46(6):401–404

Gormley PK, Colreavy MP, Patil N, Woods AE. Congenital vascular anomalies and persistent respiratory symptoms in children. *Int J Ped Otorhinolaryngol.* 1999;51(1):23–31

Hartley BE, Cotton RT. Paediatric airway stenosis: laryngotracheal reconstruction or cricotracheal reconstruction? *Clin Otolaryngol Allied Sci.* 2000;25(5):342–349

Hartzell LD, Richter GT, Glade RS, Bower CM. Accuracy and safety of tracheoscopy for infants in a tertiary care clinic. *Arch Otolaryngol Head Neck Surg.* 2010;136(1):66–69

Ho AS, Koltai PJ. Pediatric tracheal stenosis. *Otolaryngol Clin North Am.* 2008;41(5):999–1021

Hoff SR, Schroeder JW Jr, Rastatter JC, Holinger LD. Supraglottoplasty outcomes in relation to age and comorbid conditions. *Int J Pediatr Otorhinolaryngol.* 2010;74(3):245–249

Jephson CG, Manunza F, Syed S, Mills NA, Harper J, Hartley BE. Successful treatment of isolated subglottic hemangioma with propranolol alone. *Int J Ped Otorhinolaryngol.* 2009;73(12):1821–1823

Léauté-Labrèze C, Dumas de la Roque E, Hubiche T, Boralevi F, Thambo JB, Taïeb A. Propranolol for severe hemangiomas of infancy. *N Engl J Med.* 2008;358(24):2649–2651

Lindstrom DR 3rd, Book DT, Conley SF, Flanary VA, Kerschner JE. Office-based lower airway endoscopy in pediatric patients. *Arch Otolaryngol Head Neck Surg.* 2003;129(8):847–853

Maschka DA, Bauman NM, McCray PB Jr, Hoffman HT, Karnell MP, Smith RJ. A classification scheme for paradoxical vocal cord motion. *Laryngoscope.* 1997;107 (11 Pt 1):1429–1435

Moungthong G, Holinger LD. Laryngotracheoesophageal clefts. *Ann Otol Rhinol Laryngol.* 1997;106(12):1002–1011

Myer CM 3rd, O'Connor DM, Cotton RT. Proposed grading system for subglottic stenosis based on endotracheal tube sizes. *Ann Otol Rhinol Laryngol.* 1994;103(4 Pt 1):319–323

Newman KB, Mason UG 3rd, Schmaling KB. Clinical features of vocal cord dysfunction. *Am J Respir Crit Care Med.* 1995;152(4 Pt 1):1382–1386

Pezzettigotta SM, Leboulanger N, Roger G, Denoyelle F, Garabédian EN. Laryngeal cleft. *Otolaryngol Clin North Am.* 2008;41(5):913–933

Rameau A, Foltz RS, Wagner K, Zur KB. Multidisciplinary approach to vocal cord dysfunction diagnosis and treatment in one session: a single institutional outcome study. *Int J Pediatr Otorhinolaryngol.* 2012;76(1):31–35

Richter GT, Thompson DM. The surgical management of laryngomalacia. *Otolaryngol Clin North Am.* 2008;41(5):837–864

Richter GT, Wootten CT, Rutter MJ, Thompson DM. Impact of supraglottoplasty on aspiration in severe laryngomalacia. *Ann Otol Rhinol Laryngol.* 2009;118(4):259–266

Rutter MJ, Cohen AP, de Alarcon A. Endoscopic airway management in children. *Curr Opin Otolaryngol Head Neck Surg.* 2008;16(6):525–529

Sakakura K, Chikamatsu K, Toyoda M, Kaai M, Yasuoka Y, Furuya N. Congenital laryngeal anomalies presenting as chronic stridor: a retrospective study of 55 patients. *Auris Nasus Larynx.* 2008;35(4):527–533

Schroeder JW Jr, Bhandarkar ND, Holinger LD. Synchronous airway lesions and outcomes in infants with severe laryngomalacia requiring supraglottoplasty. *Arch Otolaryngol Head Neck Surg.* 2009;135(7):647–651

Stern Y, Cotton RT. Evaluation of the noisy infant. In: Cotton RT, Myer CM, eds. *Practical Pediatric Otolaryngology.* Philadelphia, PA: Lippincott-Raven Publishers; 1999:471–476

Tadié JM, Behm E, Lecuyer L, et al. Post-intubation laryngeal injuries and extubation failure: a fiberoptic endoscopic study. *Intensive Care Med.* 2010;36(6):991–998

Thompson DM. Abnormal sensorimotor integrative function of the larynx in congenital laryngomalacia: a new theory of etiology. *Laryngoscope.* 2007;117(6 Pt 2 Suppl 114):1–33

Thompson DM. Laryngomalacia: factors that influence disease severity and outcomes of management. *Curr Opin Otolaryngol Head Neck Surg.* 2010;18(6):564–570

Zoumalan R, Maddalozzo J, Holinger LD. Etiology of stridor in infants. *Ann Otol Rhinol Laryngol.* 2007;116(5):329–334

CHAPTER 16

Speech and Voice Disorders

Steve Maturo, MD, and Christopher Hartnick, MD

■ Introduction

The development of speech and voice in children has a significant effect on social and educational development. The inability to communicate clearly affects the psychological and emotional well-being of the growing child. Children with speech and language disorders are more likely to have psychiatric disorders and become incarcerated. The effect on society also stretches to adulthood, when 70% of those adults who have speech disorders or difficulty being understood are unemployed, and adults with speech problems were found to be in a lower income group at a rate 1.5 times greater than controls. In a highly verbally communicative society it is unacceptable to adapt an attitude of benign neglect of childhood speech and voice disorders given the potential lifelong effect on future personal interactions and vocation choices.

Speech and voice disorders encompass a broad category of diagnoses and are often confused as being a single disorder. Prior to diagnosing a voice or speech disorder, basic definitions of each should be provided. *Voice* is the sound produced from the larynx, whereas *speech* is the sound created by modification of the voice as it travels through the oropharynx, nasopharynx, and oral cavity (Figure 16-1). Articulation and resonance issues are considered speech disorders. Voice and speech are complicated processes that begin with a column of air generated from within the lungs and expressed through the vocal cords, on to the pharynx, oral cavity, and nasopharynx. Alterations at the level of the larynx leads to a *voice problem*, while changes after the air column has passed through the larynx is a *speech problem*. Voice and speech are highly complicated processes that also require voluntary and involuntary neural inputs.

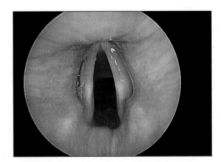

Figure 16-1. Normal-appearing vocal cords. The vocal cords make up a portion of the larynx or voice box.

The purpose of this chapter is to give an overview of speech and voice disorders in children. Most children with speech and voice disorders can be helped with a multidisciplinary team approach that include pediatricians, otolaryngologists, pulmonologists, gastroenterologists, speech-language pathologists, teachers, and psychologists. Although most speech and voice disorders are benign processes, they can have a lasting effect on the overall development of the growing child if left untreated.

> **Pearl:** In modern society an individual's voice is the primary means of communication. Voice not only provides a sense of health but also is related to one's self-identity.

■ Epidemiology

The prevalence of voice disorders in the pediatric population ranges between 3% and 10%. Studies have shown a slightly higher incidence in boys (7.5%) than girls (4.6%). One-third of all patients (including adults) suffering speech or voice problems are of kindergarten age. The incidence of specific diagnosis is age dependent.

In the newborn, the most common "voice" concern is a weak or hoarse cry. Most evaluations of newborns are done out of concern for airway or breathing abnormalities, but a hoarse cry is suggestive of an anatomic disorder that warrants further evaluation. One of the more common causes of hoarseness in a neonate is vocal cord paresis. Unilateral vocal cord paresis is most likely iatrogenic due to cardiothoracic surgeries or idiopathic, but in the absence of surgery an evaluation of the brain stem anatomy should be performed to rule out anatomic anomalies, such as Arnold-Chiari malformation. Other, less common causes of a hoarse cry in newborns include laryngeal webs (figures 16-2 and 16-3), transglottic hemangiomas (figures 16-4 and 16-5), and laryngeal clefts. Cleft lip and palate, one of the more common birth disorders, is not a diagnosis that usually requires urgent evaluation, but appropriate referral to a craniofacial team is necessary to ensure that the child has optimal treatment to obtain the best possible speech as he grows older (see Chapter 11, Cleft Lip and Palate, for an in-depth discussion) (figures 16-6 and 16-7). Children who have had their cleft palate repaired at a younger age will usually have some form of velopharyngeal insufficiency (VPI) characterized by a hypernasal voice in which air escapes through the nose. This becomes apparent as the child begins to develop speech and as her vocabulary expands.

The most common voice condition in children of preschool and elementary school age is vocal nodules (Figure 16-8). Approximately 50% of children with chronic hoarseness have vocal nodules; they are more

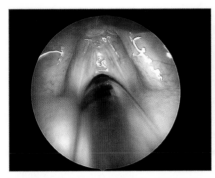

Figure 16-2. Two-week-old with weak cry and stridor due to laryngeal web giving an appearance that the vocal cords are fused. Endotracheal tube is in place.

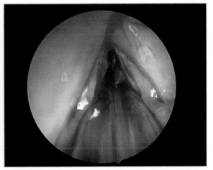

Figure 16-3. Laryngeal web divide with the anterior commissure of the glottis now open.

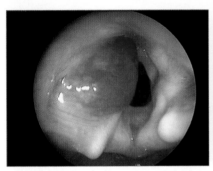

Figure 16-4. A left-sided supraglottic hemangioma. Notice the normal right vocal cord.

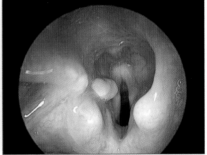

Figure 16-5. Six weeks after oral propranolol therapy and laser excision of supraglottic hemangioma.

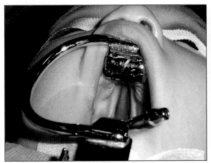

Figure 16-6. Ten-month-old with a complete secondary cleft palate. The structure in the middle of the cleft is the vomer.

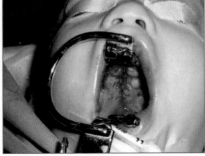

Figure 16-7. Completion of cleft palate repair. Child will be followed closely for the next 5 to 10 years to ensure proper speech development.

commonly seen in boys by a 2:1 ratio until the teenage years, when girls are more affected. Vocal cord nodules are usually caused by vocal abuse. The most common benign tumor of the larynx in children is juvenile-onset recurrent respiratory papilloma (JORRP) (Figure 16-9). Although recurrent respiratory papilloma (RRP) is a benign tumor, if left untreated it can lead to airway obstruction, thus pointing to the importance of a thorough evaluation of children with voice concerns lasting more than a few weeks or any concerns associated with breathing problems. In fact, the average child diagnosed with RRP has symptoms for at least 1 year prior to definitive diagnosis. Other, more common laryngeal abnormalities causing altered voice or speech in preadolescent children include vocal cord cysts and polyps.

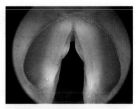

Figure 16-8. Bilateral vocal cord nodules in the classic area of the anterior third of the vocal cords. These will improve with voice therapy; surgery is rarely, if ever, necessary.

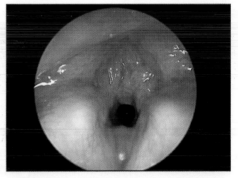

Figure 16-9. Papilloma obstructing majority of airway. Vocal cords are not visible.

The focus of this chapter is speech and voice disorders. However, a common concern of parents with young children is fluency disorders, the most common being stuttering. The most frequent age that children begin to stutter is around 3 years, with boys affected more than girls. Mild dysfluency is common in many children, but further evaluation is warranted when children are struggling to talk and episodes are frequent. Children who stutter have speech characterized by repetition of words, prolongation of words, and inability to start words. Secondary signs of stuttering may be the development of facial or body tics as a response to the tension of stuttering. The child may become withdrawn and less socially outgoing out of fear or embarrassment. The underlying cause of stuttering is likely a combination of genetic and environmental factors. There have been case reports of children developing stuttering after beginning stimulant and asthma medications, but this is the rare case, and stuttering resolved after the medication was discontinued. The optimal treatment of stuttering is debated, but involvement of a speech pathologist with behavioral therapists can provide relief to children who stutter.

In adolescents and teenagers, functional voice disorders, rather than organic pathology, are most common. Functional dysphonia and puberphonia are the most common. Puberphonia is the continued presence of the preadolescent voice in the child who has completed puberty. Most often this condition has a significant psychological component that is responsive to voice therapy. Functional dysphonia or muscle tension dysphonia presents with an altered voice or, in some cases, aphonia with a normal laryngeal and neurologic evaluation. Most often there is a significant emotional component to this disorder, but it may also be brought on by an organic disorder such as vocal nodules or a recent upper respiratory tract infection that causes laryngeal and extralaryngeal muscle hyperfunctioning. Again, this disorder is best treated with speech and behavioral therapy. One of the more unrecognized functional disorders in adolescents is paradoxic vocal fold motion (PVFM). This entity involves the adduction of the vocal cords during inspiration, resulting in dyspnea and shortness of breath. Paradoxic vocal fold motion is most commonly seen in highly achieving young females with otherwise normal physical examinations, although the rare case of brain stem or neuronal injuries has been reported. Habit cough is another diagnosis most commonly made in adolescence and sometimes presents as speech and voice concerns. Habit cough is typically a diagnosis of exclusion in which the cough is usually only present during awake hours and does not respond to typical asthma medications, and the patient has normal imaging and pulmonary function studies.

> **Pearl:** Most speech and voice disorders in children are due to benign disease, but they should not be ignored by the treating physician.

■ Presenting Symptoms

A voice problem exists when the quality of the voice is not appropriate for the age or sex of the child. There are limited data in the pediatric literature about what constitutes a normal voice, but concerns about pitch, loudness, or quality may be the presenting complaint. The most common presenting voice or speech symptom is a complaint of persistent hoarseness, but other complaints include hypernasality or hyponasality, cough, throat clearing, and snoring.

Although it is not usually difficult to determine a voice or speech disorder, the challenge becomes what symptoms are concerning enough to warrant further investigation (Box 16-1). As with any medical evaluation, the key factors of the history include time of onset, duration, aggravating factors, and progression. Furthermore, caregivers may not realize what a normal voice sounds like or understand the effect that an abnormal voice has on a child's development. Finally, troublesome symptoms include voice changes that accompany breathing difficulties, stridor, cyanotic episodes, hemoptysis, dysphagia, odynophagia, and persistent hoarseness lasting longer than a few weeks. History of trauma to the neck with voice changes is a concerning presentation, as the first thought should be potential airway embarrassment.

The typical history of a young child with vocal cord nodules causing hoarseness is a voice that worsens with increased use and improves with rest. The hoarseness may become more frequent, yet it is unlikely that airway or swallowing difficulties are ever associated. Another common finding may include a child who is competing to be heard in a household with older siblings. Parents of children with VPI will most often complain that the child cannot be understood and has difficulty with articulating certain letters, commonly s and p. Of specific mention is the child who has PVFM. Most often this child presents with refractory asthma that does not respond to frequently prescribed inhalers and has minimal changes on pulmonary function tests. This child, usually an academically or athletically talented adolescent female, has breathing or voice changes during periods of stress, such as athletic competitions.

Box 16-1. Indications for More Urgent Referral to an Otolaryngologist

♦ Shortness of breath
♦ Stridor
♦ Hemoptysis
♦ Aspiration
♦ Odynophagia
♦ Dysphagia
♦ Failure to thrive
♦ Cyanotic episodes
♦ Apparent life-threatening events

Finally, one must get a sense of the voice and speech concerns of the child and caregiver. In the infant who has not yet developed voice or speech, a weak cry may be the only symptom. Young children may be shy and avoid speaking, but with some help from the parents and some patience, the basic voice and speech of the child can be ascertained. Older children and teenagers may be embarrassed by the sound of their voice. A useful tool employed by pediatric otolaryngologists who treat children with voice disorders is a validated survey to determine the effect of the vocal disorder on the child's quality of life (Figure 16-10). Although the specifics of this survey may not be as important to the general pediatrician, it may be a useful screening document prior to the first visit for the family to determine the concern of the voice complaints.

> **Pearl:** Airway or breathing concerns in a child who presents with speech or voice disorders should prompt a more urgent evaluation by an otolaryngologist.

■ Physical Examination

To accurately identify a speech or voice disorder, a thorough head and neck examination is of utmost importance. Initially, a general assessment of the overall health of the child must be made. Rapid or difficult breathing may be perceived as a voice problem, but this presentation may require a more urgent evaluation and securing of the airway. Urgent evaluations may also need to be made in the setting of recent trauma in which an injury to the head or neck may result in voice or speech alterations and point to more life-threatening injuries to the airway or neurovascular system.

Most pediatricians are adept at recognizing children with craniofacial abnormalities. Many syndromic children have laryngeal manifestations that may not be readily apparent, but vocal quality may be a concern of the parents that is not addressed because of multiple other medical issues of these children. Children with gross sensory or motor delay, whether it is readily apparent or picked up on a general examination, may be associated with speech and voice disorders.

One of the areas often overlooked in evaluating the child with speech or voice disorders is hearing. A common complaint among families is that their child speaks too loud or is hard to understand. A thorough evaluation of the ears along with formal audiologic testing

Please answer these questions based on what your child's voice (your own voice, if you are the teenage respondent) has been like over the past 2 weeks. Considering how severe the problem is and how frequently it happens, please rate each item below on how "bad" it is (that is, the amount of each problem that you have). Use the following rating scale:

1 = None, not a problem (10)

2 = A small amount (7.5)

3 = A moderate amount (5)

4 = A lot (2.5)

5 = Problem is "as bad as it can be" (0)

6 = Not applicable

Because of my voice…	How much of a problem is this?
Q11) My child has trouble speaking loudly or being heard in noisy situations.	1 2 3 4 5
Q12) My child runs out of air and needs to take frequent breaths when talking.	1 2 3 4 5
Q13) My child sometimes does not know what will come out when he or she begins speaking.	1 2 3 4 5
Q14) My child is sometimes anxious or frustrated (because of his or her voice).	1 2 3 4 5
Q15) My child sometimes gets depressed (because of his or her voice).	1 2 3 4 5
Q16) My child has trouble using the telephone or speaking with friends in person (because of his or her voice).	1 2 3 4 5
Q17) My child has trouble doing his or her job or schoolwork (because of his or her voice).	1 2 3 4 5
Q18) My child avoids going out socially (because of his or her voice).	1 2 3 4 5
Q19) My child has to repeat himself or herself to be understood.	1 2 3 4 5
Q20) My child has become less outgoing (because of his or her voice).	1 2 3 4 5

Figure 16-10. Pediatric voice-related quality-of-life survey.

is recommended to rule out a hearing problem. More common middle ear conditions in children younger than 7 years are chronic otitis media with effusion and recurrent ear infections, both conditions that general pediatricians are very familiar treating and referring to otolaryngologists for possible surgical management.

An evaluation of the nose and oral cavity can identify anatomic lesions that usually result in resonance or articulation disorders. Examination of the anterior nares could reveal enlarged turbinates or obstructive masses causing a change in airflow. Within the oral cavity, the palate should be examined to ensure there is no cleft and that the soft palate does not appear foreshortened. Mobility of the tongue and size of the tonsils should also be noted. Examination of the neck and palpation for masses that could be compressing the laryngeal structures are also important. Particular attention should be focused on the thyroid gland, especially in teenage girls, in whom the incidence of thyroid disease and cancer becomes more common. A general neurologic examination focusing on the cranial nerves should also be stressed. Although sometimes difficult to examine in the young child, a general assessment of most of the cranial nerves can be made by observing the child. Any abnormalities should be further investigated with appropriate imaging, such as a computed tomography scan or magnetic resonance imaging.

A complete evaluation of the nasal cavity, nasopharynx, oropharynx, and larynx is only available through the use of flexible nasopharyngoscopy. The nasopharyngoscope is not a common tool in a general primary care office, but it is an essential component of the physical examination once a child is referred to an otolaryngologist. This examination is relatively painless and is tolerated by most children when a gentle approach is used. The techniques and possible findings are beyond the scope of this chapter, but nasopharyngoscopy can be carried out in the majority of children in the office setting, avoiding the need for an evaluation in the operating room or endoscopy suite. The need for further investigation, such as audiometry, pulmonary function tests, and pH probe studies, will be brought about through answers elucidated from a thorough history. More pediatric centers have established airway and swallowing clinics where collaboration is carried out among pediatric otolaryngology, pulmonology, and gastroenterology, along with pediatric audiology and speech-language pathologists. This multidisciplinary collaboration provides not only a convenience benefit for families but a truly comprehensive approach to speech and voice disorders.

> **Pearl:** The goal of the general physical examination in the pediatric patient with a speech or voice disorder is to identify a condition that may require a more urgent evaluation.

■ Differential Diagnosis

The differential diagnosis of children with voice or speech disorders is vast, and most anatomic abnormalities are impossible to diagnosis without direct visualization with a nasopharyngoscope or evaluation in the operating room. As has been stressed throughout this chapter, the key is to always consider any possible airway pathology that is affecting the voice. As with many diagnoses in children, age plays an important factor in determining an appropriate differential diagnosis. It must be noted, though, that not all voice and speech disorders are primarily caused by the structures of the larynx and upper airway. A thorough history to identify more common afflictions that can affect the voice and speech should be covered. Some of the more common diagnoses not directly related to airway structures include frequent upper respiratory tract infection, gastroesophageal reflux, and allergies. Most pediatricians are comfortable diagnosing these more common entities, but close follow-up is warranted and further evaluation is needed if the child's voice or speech is not improving after treatment.

Box 16-2 lists the most common diagnoses separated into newborn/infant, child, and adolescent categories. As has been stressed throughout this chapter, troubling symptoms include airway and swallowing findings. Newborns have not developed a speech or voice, but any report of hoarseness should prompt an otolaryngologic evaluation. Also, many of the conditions present in the newborn are not diagnosed until the baby begins developing vocalization.

> **Pearl:** Age is the most important consideration when formulating a differential diagnosis in the pediatric patient presenting with a voice or speech disorder.

Box 16-2. Common Diagnoses That Cause Speech and Voice Disorders

Newborn/Infant
- Vocal fold immobility (caused by paresis/paralysis)
- Gastroesophageal reflux disease
- Laryngomalacia
- Laryngeal hemangioma
- Laryngeal web
- Laryngeal cysts
- Laryngeal cleft
- Juvenile-onset recurrent respiratory papilloma
- Cleft lip/palate
- Velopharyngeal insufficiency
- Ankyloglossia (tongue-tie)

Child
- Voice abuse/misuse
- Vocal cord nodules
- Upper respiratory infections
- Juvenile-onset recurrent respiratory papilloma
- Vocal cord cysts/polyps
- Stuttering
- Velopharyngeal insufficiency
- Tonsil/adenoid hypertrophy
- Laryngeal web
- Vocal cord granuloma
- Vocal fold immobility (caused by paresis/paralysis)
- Ankyloglossia
- Muscle tension dysphonia

Adolescent
- Voice abuse/misuse
- Vocal cord nodules
- Muscle tension dysphonia
- Puberphonia
- Paradoxic vocal fold motion
- Laryngitides due to smoking
- Gastroesophageal reflux disease
- Thyroid disease

■ Treatment Options

Treatment options for voice and speech disorders depend on the specific diagnosis and include behavioral, medical, and surgical therapy. Most childhood speech and voice disorders are treated with speech therapy. The decision to proceed with surgery is not one to be taken lightly because interventions on the growing vocal cord can have life-long effects that may be worse than the initial presenting symptom. One underlying theme in the evaluation and treatment of children with speech or voice disorders is the importance of a team approach in which various behavioral, medical, and surgical skill sets are combined and applied in an individualized manner.

Voice therapy is the most common management approach in children with voice disorders because of voice abuse or misuse and hyperfunctional states. Although there is debate about the efficacy of voice therapy in children, it is the most common treatment modality used. Even in the rare child in whom surgery is carried out, voice therapy plays a major role in the perioperative period and in secondary prevention strategies. Voice therapy programs vary according to training and experience of the speech-language pathologist, but certain underlying facets are demonstrated in most programs. The approach to a child with a speech or voice disorder is not the same as the approach taken with an adult. Family and school involvement is necessary, and age-appropriate activities with emphasis on behavioral changes lead to successful results.

Medical therapy most commonly includes treatment of gastroesophageal reflux disease and allergies if symptoms are present. Most pediatricians are familiar with the signs and symptoms of allergies, and it would be the unique child who presented with the sole manifestation of allergies as a complaint of hoarseness. Treatment with common antihistamine and intranasal steroid medications usually results in success, but further evaluation by an allergist for persistent symptoms may be necessary. Empiric treatment with proton pump inhibitors for benign laryngeal disease, such a vocal cord nodules or mild to moderate laryngopharyngeal reflux, is controversial, as no prospective studies have demonstrated efficacy, but the relative safety profile of this medication makes it a common choice among otolaryngologists for children. The role of medical management for most other laryngeal disorders in children is limited, but adjuvant therapies in JORRP should be noted. Juvenile-onset recurrent respiratory papilloma is considered a surgical disease with the goals of providing a safe airway while balancing minimal effect on the child's developing voice. A certain subset of children, though, require multiple, frequent surgeries to maintain a safe airway. In these children, multiple adjuvant medical therapies have been tried to prevent frequent surgical trips, but success has been limited. The difficulty lies in the fact that this a rare disease encountered in numbers insufficient for individual centers to carry out large-scale studies. Success has been reported with intralesional injection of certain medications, but the search still continues for a medication that provides relief with limited side effects.

The role of surgery depends on the specific diagnosis. As mentioned previously, the most common diagnosis, vocal cord nodules, is not a surgical disease because voice therapy and medical management are usually successful. Microscopic laryngoscopy in the operating room may necessary to diagnosis a child with presumed nodules who is refractory to speech therapy, but manipulation of the growing vocal cord likely will result in more harm than good. Specific phonosurgical procedures for such conditions as unilateral vocal cord paresis, laryngeal webs, respiratory papillomas, and vocal cord granulomas are beyond the scope of this chapter. For children with speech disorders, surgeries involving the tonsils, adenoid, and soft palate are frequently employed. A child with hyponasal speech (ie, decreased nasal airflow) or with recurrent postnasal drip affecting voicing may be a candidate for adenoidectomy. A tonsillectomy is rarely carried out for speech disorders but may be done in instances of children with VPI who are candidates for palate procedures. Finally, palate lengthening and augmenting procedures have been shown to have improved voicing outcomes on patients with VPI.

Behavioral therapy most often is used in conjunction with speech therapy. Children with PVFM will most likely be treated successfully by an experienced speech-language pathologist. In those children with a psychological component such as anxiety, treatment may also be supplemented by child psychologists or psychiatrists. We have found that first acknowledging the voice or speech component of this disorder makes the child and caregivers more responsive to seeking psychological counseling along with speech therapy.

> **Pearl:** Most children with speech or voice disorders are treated successfully with speech therapy. Adjuvant medical and surgical therapy may be required depending on the underlying cause of the disorder.

■ Natural History and Prognosis

Natural history and prognosis of speech and voice disorders in children is best described in general terms based on specific diagnoses. Overall, most children with dysphonia caused by vocal cord nodules will improve by the time they reach puberty, but at least 10% will not. It is this subset of children who may require surgery or, at the very least, a thorough multidisciplinary approach to their voice pathology. Similarly, newborns with idiopathic unilateral vocal fold paresis usually improve with time and without any intervention. Children with a vocal fold paralysis caused by iatrogenic injury tend to compensate well and have minimal voice and speech deficits. Temporary and permanent procedures are available for the child with vocal fold paralysis. These procedures have been demonstrated to have good results when applied to the appropriate patient. Juvenile-onset recurrent respiratory papilloma is a challenging disease, especially in children with severe disease who require multiple visits to the operating room and consideration for adjuvant medical therapy. In most children, the disease burden runs its course by their teenage years, but in a small minority of children JORRP progresses to the lungs, ultimately resulting in death. Adolescents with functional voice disorders are usually successfully treated with speech and behavioral therapy. In the adolescent with a recalcitrant voice disorder, consultation with a child psychiatrist may be worthwhile to investigate any ongoing issues.

Hopefully, we have stressed the importance that although most speech and voice disorders in children are benign processes, the negative effect on educational, social, and psychological development can last into adulthood. Understanding the potential effects and applying appropriate treatment, such as behavioral or psychological counseling, can improve the child's and caregiver's quality of life. Certainly, there is debate concerning optimal approaches in certain childhood voice and speech disorders. More basic science and clinical research devoted to the relatively nascent field of pediatric voice and speech disorders will hopefully result in better outcomes in the future for children.

> **Pearl:** Most children with speech or voice disorders can be successfully treated. The most important element of speech and voice disorders is identifying that there is a problem.

■ Selected References

Baker BM, Blackwell PB. Identification and remediation of pediatric fluency and voice disorders. *J Pediatr Health Care.* 2004;18(2):87–94

Blumin JH, Keppel KL, Braun NM, Kerschner JE, Merati AL. The impact of gender and age on voice related quality of life in children: normative data. *Int J Pediatr Otorhinolaryngol.* 2008;72(2):229–234

Boseley ME, Cunningham MJ, Volk MS, Hartnick CJ. Validation of the pediatric voice-related quality-of-life survey. *Arch Otolaryngol Head Neck Surg.* 2006;132(7):717–720

Cardin PN, Roulstone S, Northstone K, ALSPAC Study Team. The prevalence of child-hood dysphonia: a cross-sectional study. *J Voice.* 2006;20(4):623–630

Daya H, Hosni A, Bejar-Solar I, Evans JN, Bailey CM. Pediatric vocal fold paralysis: a long-term retrospective study. *Arch Otolaryngol Head Neck Surg.* 2000;126(1):21–25

Gray SD, Smith ME, Schneider H. Voice disorders in children. *Pediatr Clin North Am.* 1996;43(6):1357–1384

Hirschber J, Dejonckere PH, Hirano M, Mori K, Schultz-Coulon HJ, Vrticka K. Voice disorders in children. *Int J Pediatr Otorhinolaryngol.* 1995;32(Suppl):S109–S125

Hooper CR. Treatment of voice disorders in children. *Lang Speech Hear Serv Sch.* 2004;35(4):320–326

Mori K. Vocal fold nodule in children: preferable therapy. *Int J Pediatr Otorhinolaryngol.* 1999;49(Suppl 1):S303–S306

Newman KB, Mason UG 3rd, Schmaling KB. Clinical features of vocal cord dysfunction. *Am J Respir Crit Care Med.* 1995;152(4 Pt 1):1382–1386

Ruben RJ. Valedictory—why pediatric otorhinolaryngology is important. *Int J Pediatr Otorhinolaryngol.* 2003;67(Suppl 1):S53–S61

St. Louis KO, Hansen GR, Buch JL, Oliver TL. Voice deviations in coexisting communication disorders. *Lang Speech Hear Serv Sch.* 1992;23:82–87

CHAPTER 17

Drooling and Salivary Aspiration

Corrie E. Roehm, MD, and Scott R. Schoem, MD

■ Introduction

Sialorrhea, or drooling, is defined as an inability to control oral secretions and is a common difficulty in pediatric patients with neuromuscular disorders. Pathologic sialorrhea is defined as saliva beyond the margin of the lip in patients older than 4 to 5 years who are in an alert state. This is not necessarily caused by an increased volume of saliva (hypersalivation) but by a lack of coordinated control of saliva by the oropharyngeal and tongue musculature that control the voluntary oral phase of swallowing. An inability to direct saliva into the posterior oropharynx for swallowing leads to anterior pooling of secretions with eventual spilling. Similarly, pooling in the posterior oropharynx with decreased swallowing may lead to laryngeal spilling and aspiration of secretions. Major causes of sialorrhea in pediatric patients include cerebral palsy, mental retardation, and other causes of neurologic or neuromuscular dysfunction. Drooling has a broad effect on the patient and her family and caregivers, increasing daily care needs of cleaning and clothing and bib changes. This requires a higher level of care at more time and cost, and often restricts the activities of patients and their caregivers. Many patients have lip and facial chapping that can lead to skin maceration, bleeding, and secondary infections. Visible drool detracts from the patient's physical appearance and can impair speech and social interactions, often reducing normal physical contact. Most importantly, sialorrhea involves an increased risk for aspiration and secondary pneumonia or pneumonitis with potentially devastating morbidity.

■ Salivation

Normal salivation involves production of 1 to 1.5 L daily, requiring approximately 600 swallows a day, with the potential for up to 10 times more volume with salivary stimulation. Ninety percent of saliva is made by the submandibular, parotid, and sublingual glands, with 10% contribution from minor salivary glands. Saliva consists of mucous and serous fluid in varying proportions based on the producing gland. The serous component has a lower calcium content and contains amylase for carbohydrate digestion of starch into maltose, while the more viscous mucous component provides lubrication and contains higher calcium levels. Saliva functions include enzymatic digestion of carbohydrates, lubrication of mucosal membranes, cleansing food debris, immune function with secretory IgA, and protecting dentition with calcium and phosphate mineralization and breaking down bacterial cell walls with lysozyme. The parotid gland produces thinner, more serous saliva, while the submandibular and sublingual glands secrete a thicker mixture of mucous and serous saliva. Salivation is stimulated by a reflex arch in the autonomic nervous system ultimately signaling through acetylcholine-driven muscarinic M_3 receptors of the cholinergic system. Cranial nerves V, VII, IX, and X bring afferent stimulation from chemoreceptors and mechanoreceptors in the oropharynx and upper gastrointestinal tract to the inferior and superior salivary nuclei in the medulla oblongata. The parotid gland is innervated by the ninth cranial nerve traveling from the inferior salivatory nucleus through the tympanic cavity on the tympanic segment of the glossopharyngeal nerve (Jacobson nerve), then through the lesser petrosal nerve, the otic ganglion, and along the auriculotemporal nerve to the gland. The submandibular, sublingual, and minor salivary glands are innervated by the seventh cranial nerve from the superior salivatory nucleus with fibers traveling with chorda tympani along lingual nerves to the submandibular ganglion, finally terminating in the gland. Parasympathetic signaling stimulates saliva production within all of the glands, while the sympathetic system prompts contraction of the smooth muscle in salivary ducts for expulsion of saliva from the glands and specific production of the submandibular gland's thicker saliva.

■ Etiology

Sialorrhea is affected by a number of physical and anatomic factors, including oral motor dysfunction or oral sphincter deficiency, inadequate swallowing capacity, poor posture, hypoglossia, dental malocclusion, impaired nasal airway, and general hypotonicity. Altered concentration and diminished oral sensation can decrease a patient's awareness of the need to swallow and also lead to sialorrhea. Potential etiologies can be categorized as causes of decreased swallowing or increased saliva production (Table 17-1). Cerebral palsy is one of the main diagnoses associated with decreased swallowing, with 10% to 37% of pediatric cerebral palsy patients affected. Other common causes of decreased swallowing include mental retardation and orthognathic abnormalities such as anterior open bite and macroglossia. Increased saliva production (hypersalivation) can be triggered by oral irritation, mouth breathing from nasal airway obstruction, gastroesophageal reflux disease (GERD), or cholinergic stimulation from medication side effects (eg, anticonvulsants; antipsychotics, particularly clozapine and

| Table 17-1. Causes of Sialorrhea ||
Decreased Swallowing	Increased Saliva Production
Neurologic disorders ♦ Cerebral palsy ♦ Causes of mental retardation—Down syndrome ♦ Facial paralysis (Bell palsy) ♦ Encephalopathy ♦ Heavy metal neurotoxicity—mercury, thallium, copper, arsenic, antimony ♦ Wilson disease ♦ Angelman syndrome ♦ Pseudobulbar palsy ♦ Bulbar palsy	♦ Oral irritation—ulcerations, infection, trauma, dental appliances ♦ Medication side effects—cholinergic effects from anticonvulsants, clozapine, risperidone, nitrazepam, bethanecol ♦ Gastroesophageal reflux disease ♦ Organophosphate toxicity
Anatomic abnormalities ♦ Macroglossia **Orthodontic problems—anterior open bite, lip seal incompetence** **TMJ ankylosis** **Surgical defects following major head and neck resections**	

Abbreviation: TMJ, temporomandibular joint.

risperidone; nitrazepam; bethanecol) or organophosphate and heavy metal (eg, mercury, thallium) toxicity.

■ Assessment

Assessing a patient with sialorrhea and deciding on appropriate management involves an evaluation of the severity of drooling and the chronicity and progression of any underlying etiology. The amount of drooling can be quantified with direct measurement of saliva volume, with several different techniques or with multiple grading methods to assess its frequency, severity, and any complications (Table 17-2). Examples of these scales include the Teacher's Drooling Scale, Blasco's Scale, and Drooling Impact Scale (Figure 17-1). Immediate visual evaluation can show active drooling, perioral skin irritation, or maceration, with a complete examination including a nasal examination for potential nasal airway obstruction, evaluation of dentition for caries and malocclusion, tongue size and any active thrusting, and assessment of head posture and position. Answering a number of questions in the patient's

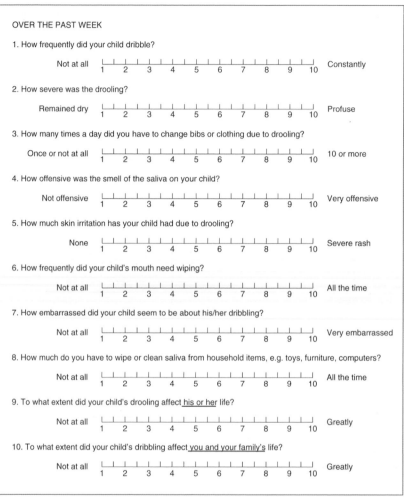

Figure 17-1. Drooling impact scale. From Reid SM, Johnson HM, Reddihough DS. The Drooling Impact Scale: a measure of the impact of drooling in children with developmental disabilities. *Dev Med Child Neurol.* 2010;52(2):e23–e28, with permission from John Wiley & Sons.

history is useful in identifying treatable causes of sialorrhea and helping direct treatment decisions (Box 17-1).

The first step of treatment is to address immediately treatable underlying conditions (ie, GERD, nasal obstruction from adenoid hypertrophy, allergic rhinitis) and eliminate medications with known hypersalivation side effects when possible, with follow-up of a patient's sialorrhea through serial evaluations and scaling of its

Table 17-2. Drooling Scales

Teacher's Drooling Scale[a]		Drooling Frequency and Severity Scale[b]	
Grade	Symptom	Severity	Frequency
1	No drooling	1—Dry, never drools	1—Dry, never drools
2	Infrequent drooling, small amount	2—Mild (only wet lips)	2—Occasional drool (not every day)
3	Occasional drooling, intermittent all day	3— Moderate (lips and chin)	3—Frequent drool, every day
4	Frequent drooling but not profuse	4—Severe (clothing)	4—Constant drool (all day)
5	Constant drooling, always wet	5—Profuse (clothing, tray)	5—Constant drool, wet pillow in morning

[a]Reprinted with permission from Camp-Bruno JA, Winsberg BG, Green-Parsons AR, Abrams JP. Efficacy of benztropine therapy for drooling. *Dev Med Child Neurol.* 1989;31(3):309–319.
[b]Reprinted with permission from Thomas-Stonell N, Greenberg J. Three treatment approaches and clinical factors in the reduction of drooling. *Dysphagia.* 1988;3:73–78

Box 17-1. Questions to Ask to Direct Treatment Decisions

◆ How frequent/severe is the drooling?
◆ Is the underlying cause of sialorrhea temporary?
◆ Will the patient outgrow the problem, or will it likely remain the same or worsen?
◆ Does the patient eat orally or through non-oral means (eg, gastric feeding tube)?
◆ Does the patient have functional oral communication?
◆ Is there any history of possible aspirations (eg, choking or coughing on saliva, particularly at night; prior pneumonia)?
◆ Does the patient have any evidence of gastroesophageal reflux disease that could stimulate salivation?
◆ Could any current medications cause hypersalivation or have cholinergic effects?
◆ Is the patient's nasal airway obstructed, leading to mouth breathing and open mouth?

severity. If drooling is persisting or is moderate or severe on initial evaluation, it will be managed more effectively with multidisciplinary input from speech therapists, pediatricians, pediatric dentists, and otolaryngologists.

■ Management

Treatment of sialorrhea depends on the severity of the problem and temporary versus permanent underlying etiologies and age, with the goal of eliminating excessive saliva and spilling while maintaining a moistened, healthy oral cavity. In patients younger than 5 years who are otherwise healthy, reassurance is appropriate because drooling will tend to resolve with time. The remainder of patients can be treated in a progressive manner to maximize conservative measures before considering more aggressive options in unresponsive cases (Box 17-2). This includes oral stimulation programs with speech therapy to improve oro-motor coordination and proprioception, decrease tongue thrusting, and prompt jaw and lip closure. Behavior modification can be useful in patients who are aware and cooperative enough to participate in posture training and positioning to improve oral closure and posterior salivary flow. Swallowing prompts with auditory signals or other cues, teaching oral motor skills and oral awareness, or palatal training appliances can guide the patient to better control lip and jaw closure and tongue movements and decrease drooling.

MEDICATION

Medications to reduce saliva production are the next therapeutic option in patients who do not improve with behavior modification and speech therapy. One key pharmacologic target to control drooling is the postganglionic muscarinic M_3 receptor, where parasympathetic action of acetylcholine normally stimulates salivary glands to increase saliva production. Several antimuscarinics that block this action have been shown to effectively inhibit salivation. They include benztropine, benzhexol hydrochloride (trihexyphenidyl), glycopyrrolate, and scopolamine (Table 17-3). However, the action of antimuscarinic pharmacologics is not selective. Their effects on extra-salivary muscarinic receptors and on smooth muscles that are responsive to acetylcholine may cause systemic effects including dilation of pupils, increased heart rate, decreased gut motility, urinary retention, and reduced sweating. Headache, irritability, confusion, nausea, tachycardia, blurred vision, xerostomia, and decreased taste are several of the most common side effects, and these anticholinergics are contraindicated in patients with glaucoma, obstructive uropathy, gastrointestinal obstruction, myasthenia gravis, or asthma to prevent exacerbations. Studies available in the literature showing the effectiveness of scopolamine, benztropine, and

Box 17-2. Progressive Management of Drooling

♦ Oral stimulation programs
♦ Behavior modifications
♦ Medication
♦ Botulinum toxin injections or surgical treatment

Table 17-3. Medications

Medications	Doses Available	Dosage	Side Effects
Glycopyrrolate	1- or 2-mg tablets	Adults: start 0.5 mg orally 1 to 3 times daily; titrate as needed (maximum dose, 8 mg/d) Children: 0.04 mg/kg per dose 2 to 3 times a day; titrate as needed	Xerostomia, blurred vision, hyperactivity, irritability, constipation, urinary retention
Scopolamine	1.5-mg transdermal patch	One patch every 3 days	Xerostomia, blurred vision, irritability, dizziness, constipation, urinary retention
Benztropine	0.5-, 1-, or 2-mg tablets, 1 mg/mL injection	Average 3.8 mg daily[a]	Xerostomia, blurred vision, constipation, tachycardia, urinary retention, disorientation, rash
Benzhexol hydrochloride	2-, 5-mg tablets, 2/5-mL elixir	2 to 3 mg twice daily[b]	Blurred vision, dizziness, urinary retention

[a]Camp-Bruno JA, Winsberg BG, Green-Parsons AR, Abrams JP. Efficacy of benztropine therapy for drooling. *Dev Med Child Neurol.* 1989;31(3):309–319
[b]Reddihough D, Johnson H, Staples M, Hudson I, Exarchos H. Use of benzhexol hydrochloride to control drooling of children with cerebral palsy. *Dev Med Child Neurol.* 1990;32(11):985–989

glycopyrrolate as pharmacologic options for sialorrhea often have limitations of small study numbers and non-standardized outcome measurements, but glycopyrrolate may have an advantage over the others because it has fewer side effects. Benztropine is a synthetic compound structurally similar to atropine that was effective in approximately 65% of 20 patients in a study by Camp-Bruno et al, with 15% (3 patients) discontinuing the medication for significant systemic side effects; long-term data on effect length and adverse effects were not measured. Scopolamine has been shown to reduce drooling in patients with developmental delays and with cerebral palsy, specifically, with more than 50% reduction of drooling volume in 53% of patients. Scopolamine has not been studied for long-term use and also causes systemic effects, with unique side effects, including temporary toxic psychosis, in addition to classic antimuscarinic effects. Using a separate mechanism, clonidine patches have also been shown to be effective at reducing hypersalivation from antipsychotic medications by increasing adrenergic activity. Glycopyrrolate is a quaternary ammonium antimuscarinic structurally related to atropine that does not easily cross the blood-brain barrier, decreasing central side effects but maintaining the ability to decrease drooling scores by approximately 50% in one study by Bachrach et al. Blasco et al found a 90% rate of reduction in drooling, with 28% rate of side effects leading to discontinuation of treatment and a wide effective dose range from 0.01 to 0.82 mg/kg in a pediatric study population. Dosing of antimuscarinic medications must be balanced to control drooling while avoiding adverse side effects, if possible, and may be variable over time as drooling volumes change. Decreasing saliva production to the degree of xerostomia is often uncomfortable for patients, can make speech and eating more difficult, and can lead to long-term complications, including dental caries.

OTHER TYPES OF TREATMENT

For patients with severe sialorrhea or poor responses to more conservative measures, therapies aimed at more prolonged reduction or elimination of salivary gland function should be considered, including botulinum toxin injections and surgery. Radiation therapy has been used historically in treating sialorrhea in geriatric patients aiming to render the salivary glands nonfunctional with damage to serous acinic cells. However, this modality is not practically applicable in pediatric sialorrhea because of potential alteration of midface growth and increased malignancy risk 10 to 15 years following exposure. Botulinum toxin injections are a more recent addition to the treatment options for pediatric sialorrhea and use the action of a neurotoxin produced by *Clostridium botulinum* bacterium to decrease salivation. This toxin causes proteolytic cleavage of SNAP-25, an enzyme involved in vesicle fusion and acetylcholine release at the presynaptic membrane. Inhibition of acetylcholine action at the synapse establishes a temporary functional denervation of the salivary glands and prevents salivary stimulation for several weeks to months following injection. Placement of injections can be completed with or without ultrasound guidance but usually requires general anesthesia for pediatric patients. Various injection methods and dosing have been reported, including single 5 U botulinum toxin A doses into the superficial parotid glands bilaterally, with 55% of patients showing perceived benefit. Wilken et al used 2 approximately 15 U botulinum toxin A or B injections into the anterior and posterior parotid and approximately 15 U into the submandibular gland and demonstrated an 83% reduction in Teacher's Drooling Scores at 4 weeks and sustained reduction in drooling with 2- to 6-month injection intervals. One controlled trial evaluating botulinum toxin efficacy and scopolamine efficacy in pediatric sialorrhea patients used weight categories for dosing of submandibular gland injections (15 U/gland for patients weighing less than 15 kg; 20 U/gland for 15 to 25 kg; 25 U/gland for heavier than 25 kg), with 61% response rate 2 weeks after botulinum toxin injections and causing fewer side effects than scopolamine treatment in the same study group. Comparisons of botulinum toxin A to toxin B show no significant difference in efficacy; however, more research is needed to determine optimal pediatric dosing for maximal efficacy and minimal risk of complications. These studies further defined the side effect profile of botulinum toxin injections with rare, mild complications including mild xerostomia, thickened saliva, transient flu-like symptoms, and short-lived injection site tenderness. Thickened saliva is likely from preferential injection of the parotid gland, eliminating its thin serous saliva production, instead of the submandibular gland, which produces thicker, mucous saliva. More serious side effects reported were facial nerve weakness, oral closure, and chewing difficulty from masseter muscle weakness, likely from diffusion of toxin from parotid injection sites, and dysphagia from systemic botulinum toxin effects on pharyngeal musculature. Patients responding to botulinum toxin injections can avoid more invasive surgical procedures, but injections still require general anesthesia in most pediatric patients and recurring injections for prolonged effect.

Surgery

Surgery is often considered when less invasive or non-permanent treatment options fail to decrease drooling after 6 months of treatment in patients older than 5 to 6 years, to allow for full maturity of oropharyngeal motor coordination. It is also more useful in patients unable to engage in behavioral or postural therapies or when aspiration, pneumonia, and other serious sequelae of drooling occur. One important factor to consider when choosing a surgical procedure for a drooling patient is the presence of aspiration, in which posterior ductal rerouting may be less useful with its potential for posterior salivary pooling, theoretically increasing the risk of aspiration. For patients who have undergone maximal nonsurgical and surgical sialorrhea therapies with continuing severe aspiration problems and significant morbidity, laryngotracheal separation and tracheotomy provide definitive protection for the pulmonary tree from the upper aerodigestive tract and its secretions.

However, with advances in the treatment of drooling over the past several decades, this procedure is rarely necessary.

Historically, a variety of surgical procedures have been used in the treatment of sialorrhea to interrupt innervation or gland ductal drainage, redirect ductal drainage, or remove glands entirely. Techniques have evolved over time attempting to improve postoperative results and avoid the risk of additional complications. These procedures can be categorized as salivary reduction or salivary diversion procedures (Table 17-4). One procedure for sialorrhea that is no longer used is transtympanic nerve sectioning to interrupt fibers carrying salivary stimuli, including bilateral tympanic neurectomy transecting Jacobson nerve of the glossopharyngeal nerve (cranial nerve [CN] IX) and the chorda tympani nerve section of the facial nerve (CN VII). This procedure was performed under local anesthesia, was quick to complete, and resulted in no external scars. Improvement rates of 74% in one study by Mullins et al in 1979 showed more significant resolution of

Table 17-4. Surgical Options for Sialorrhea		
	Advantages	**Disadvantages**
Salivary reduction		
Nerve sectioning	Fast procedure, under local anesthesia	Nerve regrowth can result in need for repeated sectioning; poor results, procedure abandoned.
Ductal ligation	Simple procedure, decreases flow predictably	Temporary gland swelling, potential for sialocele or sialoliths
Gland excisions	Excellent reduction in salivary volume	Increased procedure complexity and risk to surrounding structures (eg, facial nerve branches, hypoglossal and lingual nerves), external scar, higher risk of xerostomia, dental caries
Salivary diversion		
Submandibular duct rerouting	No external scar, reduces anterior pooling/spillage	Risk of anterior caries, ranula if sublingual gland not excised, duct obstruction, potential aspiration risk
Parotid duct rerouting	No external scar, reduces anterior pooling/spillage of thin saliva	Risk of sialocele, potential aspiration risk, duct obstruction, parotid and facial swelling, parotitis

drooling in patients who underwent careful transection of the complete tympanic plexus of Jacobson nerve. Grewal et al concluded in 1984 that combining both nerve sections was more effective at preventing nerve regrowth and recurring sialorrhea, but overall published success rates of nerve section studies fell between 50% and 80%. Risks of the nerve transection procedures included an unavoidable loss of taste in the anterior two-thirds of the tongue innervated by facial nerve fibers within chorda tympani, potential xerostomia, dental caries, tympanic membrane perforations, otitis media, or recurrence of drooling from nerve regeneration.

Salivary duct surgery for sialorrhea was introduced in 1967 by Theodore Wilkie with parotid duct relocation to the tonsillar fossa to redirect salivary flow to the posterior oropharynx. This method was modified by Wilkie and Brody several years later to include submandibulectomy (removal of both submandibular glands), resulting in an 85% reduction in drooling but an associated 35% rate of adverse effects. Bilateral submandibulectomy became a logical surgical target because the submandibular glands produce approximately 70% of saliva volume, and excision of the glands reliably and dramatically reduced salivary volume. However, gland removal procedures—submandibulectomy, parotidectomy, and sublingual gland excisions—involve risk of external scarring, irreversible xerostomia, and facial nerve injury. Subsequently, salivary ductal ligation became popular because of easy access to the gland ducts trans-orally with minimal dissection and reliable reduction in saliva volume. Ligation works by inducing gland atrophy from functional obstruction to reduce saliva production and block salivary flow immediately, with 4-duct ligation studies reporting rates of 64.1% improvement in drooling. Complications include mild temporary swelling and discomfort. Submandibular ductal ligations result in higher rates of sialoliths (salivary stones) because of more mucous saliva with the higher calcium content and viscosity of submandibular gland saliva, and the upward slanting course of Wharton duct causing retention of particulates. Four-duct ligation procedures with suture ties are advantageous for ease of access to the ducts for ligation and predictable decreases in saliva production. Duct clipping and laser photocoagulation have been investigated as potential procedural variations of ductal ligation aiming to decrease surgical time and extent of dissection even further.

■ Conclusion

Drooling in the pediatric patient is a complex problem with many potential etiologies, and treatment requires an understanding of the underlying causes and a multidisciplinary approach to the treatment and possible complications of drooling. Treatment options range from behavioral changes, to medications, to botulinum toxin injections, and surgery, but many of the treatment options have side effects that must be considered along with the potential for an improvement in drooling. Patients derive the most benefit from an individualized approach to their drooling to remove correctible causes, avoid irreversible procedures and known side effects where possible, and address potential aspiration risk.

■ Selected References

Bachrach SJ, Walter RS, Trzcinski K. Use of glycopyrrolate and other anticholinergic medications for sialorrhea in children with cerebral palsy. *Clin Pediatr (Phila).* 1998;37(8):485–490

Benson J, Daugherty KK. Botulinum toxin A in the treatment of sialorrhea. *Ann Pharmacother.* 2007;41(1):79–85

Blasco PA, Stansbury JC. Glycopyrrolate treatment of chronic drooling. *Arch Pediatr Adolesc Med.* 1996;150(9)932–935

Borg M, Hirst F. The role of radiation therapy in the management of sialorrhea. *Int J Radiat Oncol Biol Phys.* 1998;41(5)1113–1119

Bothwell JE, Clarke K, Dooley JM, et al. Botulinum toxin A as a treatment for excessive drooling in children. *Pediatr Neurol.* 2002;27(1):18–22

Camp-Bruno JA, Winsberg BG, Green-Parsons AR, Abrams JP. Efficacy of benztropine therapy for drooling. *Dev Med Child Neurol.* 1989;31(3):309–319

Chang CJ, May-Kuen Wong AA. Intraductal laser photocoagulation of the bilateral parotid ducts for reduction of drooling in patients with cerebral palsy. *Plast Reconstr Surg.* 2001;107(4):907–913

Crysdale WS. Management options for the drooling patient. *Ear Nose Throat J.* 1989;68(11):820–830

El-Hakim H, Richards S, Thevasagayam MS. Major salivary duct clipping for control problems in developmentally challenged children. *Arch Otolaryngol Head Neck Surg.* 2008;134(5):470–474

Freudenreich O. Drug-induced sialorrhea. *Drugs Today (Barc).* 2005;41(6):411–418

Garrett JR, Proctor GB. Control of salivation. In: Linden RWA. *The Scientific Basis of Eating.* 1998:135–155

Grewal DS, Hiranandani NL, Rangwalla ZA, Sheode JH. Transtympanic neurectomies for control of drooling. *Auris Nasus Larynx.* 1984;11(2):109–114

Hockstein NG, Samadi DS, Gendron K, Handler SD. Sialorrhea: a management challenge. *Am Fam Physician.* 2004;69(11):2628–2634

Jongerius PH, Joosten F, Hoogen FJ, Gabreels FJ, Rotteveel JJ. The treatment of drooling by ultrasound-guided intraglandular injections of botulinum toxin type A into the salivary glands. *Laryngoscope.* 2003;113(1):107–111

Jongerius PH, van den Hoogen FJ, van Limbeek J, Gabreels FJ, van Hulst K, Rotteveel JJ. Effect of botulinum toxin in the treatment of drooling: a controlled clinical trial. *Pediatrics.* 2004;114(3):620–627

Jongerius PH, van Tiel P, van Limbeek J, Gabreels FJ, Rotteveel JJ. A systematic review for evidence of efficacy of anticholinergic drugs to treat drooling. *Arch Dis Child.* 2003;88(10):911–914

Klem C, Mair EA. Four-duct ligation: a simple and effective treatment for chronic aspiration from sialorrhea. *Arch Otolaryngol Head Neck Surg.* 1999;125(7):796–800

Lewis DW, Fontana C, Mehallick LK, Everett Y. Transdermal scopolamine for reduction of drooling in developmentally delayed children. *Dev Med Child Neurol.* 1994;36(6):484–486

Mier RJ, Bachrach SJ, Lakin RC, Barker T, Childs J, Moran M. Treatment of sialorrhea with glycopyrrolate: a double-blind, dose-ranging study. *Arch Pediatr Adolesc Med.* 2000;154(12):1214–1218

Mullins WM, Gross CW, Moore JM. Long-term follow-up of tympanic neurectomy for sialorrhea. *Laryngoscope.* 1979;89(8):1219–1223

Pena AH, Cahill AM, Gonzalez L, Baskin KM, Kim H, Towbin RB. Botulinum toxin A injection of salivary glands in children with drooling and chronic aspiration. *J Vasc Interv Radiol.* 2009;20(3):368–373

Reddihough D, Johnson H, Staples M, Hudson I, Exarchos H. Use of benzhexol hydrochloride to control drooling of children with cerebral palsy. *Dev Med Child Neurol.* 1990;32(11):985–989

Reed J, Mans CK, Brietzke SE. Surgical management of drooling: a meta-analysis. *Arch Otolaryngol Head Neck Surg.* 2009;135(9):924–931

Scully C, Limeres J, Gleeson M, Tomás I, Diz P. Drooling. *J Oral Pathol Med.* 2009;38(4):321–327

Talmi YP, Finkelstein Y, Zohar Y. Reduction of salivary flow with transdermal scopolamine: a four-year experience. *Otolaryngol Head Neck Surg.* 1990;103(4):615–618

Tscheng DZ. Sialorrhea—therapeutic drug options. *Ann Pharmacother,* 2002;36(11):1785–1790

Wilken B, Aslami B, Backes H. Successful treatment of drooling in children with neurological disorders with botulinum toxin A or B. *Neuropediatrics.* 2008;39(4):200–204

Wilkie TF. The problem of drooling and cerebral palsy: a surgical approach. *Can J Surg.* 1967;10(1):60–67

Wilkie TF, Brody GS. The surgical treatment of drooling. A ten-year review. *Plast Reconstr Surg.* 1977;59(6):791–797

CHAPTER 18

Chronic Cough in Children

Ian N. Jacobs, MD

■ Introduction

Cough is one of the most common reasons for which patients seek medical attention. It accounts for 8.5% of all visits to a primary care practitioner, resulting in an enormous financial burden due to time missed from work and medical expenditures. Most cases are caused by self-limited illnesses resulting from viral infections of the upper respiratory tract that resolve within 2 to 3 weeks. However, prolonged cough is a potential cause of discomfort for the child, anxiety for the parent, and sleep disturbance for both. Fear of a significant underlying pathology and the potential for injury are frequent parental concerns, and indeed chronic cough may portend a more serious disorder.

■ Mechanism

Cough is the sudden and violent expulsion of air in late inspiration after the complete closure of the laryngeal sphincter. This results in the rapid expulsion of deep lung gaseous contents and facilitates clearance of abnormal secretions and infections, as well as expulsion of foreign bodies. Cough also prevents foreign material from entering the trachea in the first place.

Cough requires a neurologically competent larynx and pharynx as well as diaphragm and chest wall. Patients with vocal cord paralysis or loss of afferent sensation of the larynx may not have a competent cough and may be susceptible to aspiration and lower airway problems. Patients with diaphragmatic paralysis also may not be able to generate an effective cough.

Cough is mediated by the cough reflex arc (Figure 18-1). Cough receptors are found in varying concentrations in the mucosa of the entire respiratory tract, including the larynx, trachea, bronchi, pharynx, and nasal passages. Sensory fibers of the afferent limb, when stimulated by incidental contact or pressure with a foreign body or noxious agent, transmit impulses to the cough center in the medulla. Efferent impulses, in turn, travel from the medulla to the end organs, including the diaphragm, intercostals muscles, laryngeal adductors, and external chest wall muscles, via the vagus and phrenic nerves. This results in a violent Valsalva maneuver, which acts to expel debris or the noxious offending agent. The cough reflex is weak in premature neonates and develops by about age 5 years; this fact correlates with 5 years as the age at which accidental nut aspiration becomes less common.

Pearl: Children younger than 5 years should not be fed nuts because their gag reflex is not yet mature enough to protect the airway against aspiration.

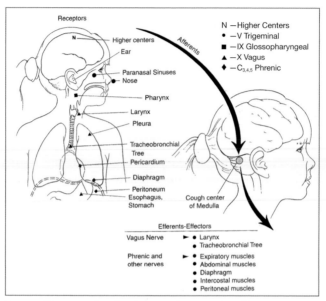

Receptors

N —Higher Centers
• —V Trigeminal
■ —IX Glossopharyngeal
▲ —X Vagus
♦ —C₃,₄,₅ Phrenic

Higher centers
Afferents
Ear
Paranasal Sinuses
Nose
Pharynx
Larynx
Pleura
Tracheobronchial Tree
Pericardium
Diaphragm
Peritoneum
Esophagus, Stomach
Cough center of Medulla

Efferents-Effectors

Vagus Nerve ► • Larynx
• Tracheobronchial Tree

Phrenic and other nerves ► • Expiratory muscles
• Abdominal muscles
• Diaphragm
• Intercostal muscles
• Peritoneal muscles

Figure 18-1. Cough reflex mechanism. From Holinger LD, Sanders AD. Chronic cough in infants and children: an update. *Laryngoscope.* 1991;101:596–605, with permission from John Wiley & Sons.

■ Clinical Assessment of the Child With Chronic Cough

The etiologies of cough are diverse and numerous (Box 18-1). As a result, it is critical that the primary care practitioner develop a conceptual framework for clinical and laboratory assessment of the child with cough.

HISTORY

Age

Patient age is one of the most important factors in determining etiology of cough (Box 18-2). Among children from birth to 18 months of age, the most common causes of chronic cough are gastroesophageal reflux

Box 18-1. Etiologies of Cough

Cough-dominant asthma
Infections
Acute and chronic sinusitis
Adenoiditis
Pneumonia
Tuberculosis
Pertussis
Adenovirus
Influenza

Congenital
Laryngeal cleft
Tracheoesophageal fistula
Subglottic stenosis
Tracheomalacia
Vascular compression
Congenital heart disease
Vocal cord paralysis

Environmental
Cigarette smoke
Pollution

Genetic
Cystic fibrosis
Immotile cilia syndrome

Aspiration
Saliva
Gastroesophageal reflux disease
Foreign body

Psychogenic

Neoplastic
Neoplasms of the tracheobronchial tree
Laryngotracheal papillomatosis
Airway hemangioma
Mediastinal tumor

Box 18-2. Causes of Chronic Cough According to Age

Infants
GERD and feeding disorders
Airway anomalies
Pertussis

Toddlers and young children
Recurrent viral illness
GERD
Cough-dominant asthma
Allergy
Chronic sinusitis
Airway foreign body
Pertussis
Bronchitis/bronchiolitis
Pneumonia
Cystic fibrosis

Older children and adolescents
Recurrent viral illness
Cough-dominant asthma
Allergy
Chronic sinusitis
Psychogenic cough
Bronchitis/bronchiolitis
Pneumonia
Cystic fibrosis

Abbreviation: GERD, gastroesophageal reflux disease.

disease (GERD); congenital airway abnormalities such as tracheomalacia, laryngeal cleft, tracheoesophageal fistula (TEF) with direct aspiration, and long segment tracheal stenosis; and pertussis. In toddlers and young children, the most common cause of chronic cough is recurrent viral illness; in affected children, the illnesses are of typical duration, but the disease-free interval is very brief. Allergies, chronic sinusitis, cough-dominant asthma, cystic fibrosis, bronchitis, and pneumonia are also frequently encountered in this age group. This is also the age group in which bronchial or other airway foreign bodies most commonly present. In school-aged children, cough-dominant asthma, infections (sinus and lung), psychogenic cough (habit cough), and allergies predominate as the causes of cough.

Character of Cough

Cough can be characterized based on tonal qualities as well as the presence or absence of secretions. Barky cough is typical of subglottic disease (croup, subglottic stenosis, subglottic cyst, or hemangioma). Brassy cough is similar in tone but emanates more from the chest, suggesting tracheobronchial disorders (bronchitis, tracheomalacia, tracheal stenosis). In pertussis, a high-pitched "whoop" sound frequently follows the paroxysms of cough in the early stages of the disease. A wet or productive cough usually is present in pulmonary infections, bronchitis, chronic sinusitis, or any infection producing an abundance of mucous and secretions. A dry cough may be related to infections producing minimal secretions or to noninfectious processes such as airway anomalies, cough-dominant asthma, airway foreign body, or habit cough. Hemoptysis may suggest the presence of a neoplasm, vascular anomaly, or severe inflammation.

Frequency, Duration, and Timing of Cough

In the absence of upper respiratory illness (URI) or other pathology, children will experience 10 or 11 cough episodes per day. Cough considered pathologic should be substantially in excess of this number.

Although some infectious processes may last several weeks, it is critical that pathologies such as foreign bodies of the airway be discovered in a reasonable amount of time. As a result, cough persisting for more than 4 weeks should be considered chronic and merits more than clinical evaluation. Cough that recurs after appropriate therapy may warrant endoscopic evaluation for an underlying airway problem.

In newborns and infants, timing of the cough in relation to feeding may suggest a cause. Babies with laryngotracheal clefts or TEF typically cough *during* the swallow. Children with gastroesophageal reflux more commonly cough *after* feeding and when positioned supine.

As a rule, sleep generally suppresses cough. However, because night-time is the quietest time of day, the presence of any cough at night is often unsettling to parents. Wet cough due to postnasal drip may be exacerbated in the supine position. Conversely, habit cough will completely disappear during sleep.

Cough during URI may increase with exertion or exercise. However, cough present only during exercise is more typically associated with asthma or psychogenic etiology.

> **Pearl:** Habit cough disappears completely during sleep.

Additional History

Additional historical information may be useful in identifying the etiology of a chronic cough. A history of endotracheal intubation, especially in a young child with a history of prematurity, suggests the presence of an acquired airway lesion. Parents of toddlers should be asked about circumstances that might suggest ingestion or aspiration of a foreign body. Symptoms of wheezing in association with chronic cough are common in very young children because of the small caliber of their airways; however, wheezing should also alert the clinician to the possibility of asthma. The clinician should also inquire about environmental irritants that delay the resolution of cough, such as tobacco smoke, and about any recurrent infections that might suggest an immune deficiency.

PHYSICAL EXAMINATION

General appearance of the coughing child may provide some insight into the severity and cause of the problem. For example, the absence of cough during the office visit may prompt further inquiry into the actual frequency of cough and exacerbating factors. Children whose coughing ceases when asked to focus on other things during the examination are more likely to have habit cough. Tachypnea and stridor associated with cough are often immediately apparent on initial patient contact. Other patients may show obvious signs of allergy or URI.

Anterior rhinoscopy may be performed using an otoscope with a large-diameter speculum. Findings of swollen, edematous mucosa and clear, watery rhinorrhea may suggest the presence of allergy, while mucoid or purulent secretions are associated with viral URI or sinusitis. Postnasal drip may also be evident on oropharyngeal examination. Nasal polyps are pathognomonic of cystic fibrosis.

Auscultation of the neck and chest will yield important information about the condition of the lower airway and lungs. In cough caused by subglottic pathology, stridor can generally be appreciated over the neck. Decreased breath sounds over the chest may indicate an aspirated foreign body or consolidation due to infection. Wheezing is most suggestive of asthma, although foreign bodies and airway anomalies should be entertained as well.

■ Additional Investigation

The history and clinical examination are useful in establishing those diagnoses from Box 18-1 that are the most likely causes of chronic cough in a child. A clinical practice guideline from the American College of Chest Physicians proposes that these causes be further classified as *specific* or *nonspecific* causes of cough evaluated based on a set of indicators (Box 18-3). Specific cough is often wet and associated with underlying respiratory or systemic disease. The diagnosis is often made based on coexisting symptoms or laboratory findings suggestive of a particular disease. Nonspecific cough is defined as cough in the absence of these indicators; in such cases, the cough is the primary symptom and is usually dry. Such individuals may also have a higher level of cough sensitivity, which can occur following routine viral URI.

The causes of chronic cough vary in prevalence among epidemiologic studies depending on the population studied. The most common etiologies are persistent bacterial bronchitis, asthma, gastroesophageal reflux, and upper airway cough syndrome (UACS), the latter referring to disorders including URI, allergy, and sinusitis in which the cough clears secretions of nasal origin from the larynx. Based on these data, it is reasonable to begin empiric pharmacotherapy with antibiotics for possible bronchitis or sinusitis, or with a trial of inhaled corticosteroids to treat suspected asthma. Children who are unresponsive should undergo, at a minimum, a radiograph of the chest and spirometry.

Plain radiographs of the chest are useful for delineating infiltrates, radiopaque foreign bodies, and other types of infections. Inspiratory and expiratory views or lateral decubitus views may also show hyperinflation suggestive of a foreign aspiration with air trapping. Additional images of the neck may demonstrate subglottic pathology including stenosis, hemangiomas, or cysts.

Box 18-3. Indicators of Specific Cough in Children	
Daily, wet, or productive cough	Recurrent pneumonia
Auscultatory findings (wheeze or crackles)	Cardiac abnormalities (including murmurs)
Chronic dyspnea	Immune deficiency
Exertional dyspnea	Failure to thrive
Hemoptysis	Digital clubbing
Duration >6 months	Swallowing problems

After Chang AB, Glom WB. Guidelines for evaluating chronic cough in pediatrics: ACCP evidence based clinical practice guidelines. *Chest.* 2006;129:2605–2835

Spirometry is indicated to identify disorders of reversible airway obstruction associated with cough. Testing is limited, in many cases, by the age of the patient, but should be achievable in most children older than 3 years. When age or developmental status prohibits such testing, empirical treatment for asthma may be necessary.

> **Pearl:** Children with specific cough who are unresponsive to a trial of pharmacotherapy should undergo, at a minimum, a radiograph of the chest and spirometry.

EVALUATION OF SPECIFIC COUGH

Patients with signs and symptoms of respiratory disease, abnormalities on chest radiograph or spirometry, or cough characteristic of a particular disorder are considered to have specific cough and should undergo a directed evaluation. Diagnoses such as bronchiectasis, cystic fibrosis, and immune deficiency should be entertained in children with chronic purulent cough. Computed tomography (CT) of the chest may be performed to demonstrate bronchiectasis, interstitial lung disease, or foreign bodies. Computed tomography may also be useful in the diagnosis of chronic sinusitis but should be reserved for children with a consistent clinical picture who have failed empirical medical therapy. Patients with findings consistent with asthma should be treated empirically for 4 weeks and then reassessed. Diagnostic laboratory testing based on clinical indicators includes purified protein derivative (PPD), sweat chloride, and immunoglobulin titers.

Recommended testing for gastroesophageal reflux may vary among clinicians and may be delayed in favor of a trial of pharmacologic therapy including H_2 blockers or proton pump inhibitors. Such testing typically involves pH probes, impedance testing, or endoscopic evaluation. Upper gastrointestinal (GI) radiographic studies and nuclear scans are somewhat less useful, although swallow studies in infants who cough in association with feeding may demonstrate aspiration as a potential cause of the cough.

When diagnosis behind chronic cough remains uncertain, referral to a pulmonologist or otolaryngologist for endoscopy should be considered. In most cases, examination of the airway is performed under sedation using a flexible fiber-optic bronchoscope with side-port suction placed via face mask or laryngeal mask airway. Mobility of the vocal folds is best assessed at this time and any airway anomalies are noted. Bronchoalveolar lavage is performed to obtain cultures and stains for bacteria (including mycobacteria), fungi, and viruses. Specimens are also obtained for quantitation of lipid laden macrophages and to assay for pepsin, both of which are suggestive of aspiration due to reflux. Mucosal biopsies may be taken from the carina, bronchi, or nasal turbinates and sent for ultrastructural analysis of the cilia. Rigid airway endoscopy is less ideal for bronchial lavage but facilitates delivery of anesthesia and removal of foreign bodies when present while providing a superior view of the airway. Upper GI endoscopy is often performed under the same anesthetic to obtain biopsies of the esophagus that may suggest GERD or eosinophilic esophagitis, 2 common causes of cough. When recommended by the gastroenterologist, the procedure can be combined with impedance probes.

EVALUATION OF NONSPECIFIC COUGH

Children with no signs or symptoms of respiratory disease and normal chest radiographs and spirometry have nonspecific cough. Because most cases of nonspecific cough are post-infectious, a 1- to 2-week period of additional observation is recommended prior to consideration of additional intervention. During this time, it is important to avoid environmental irritants that may prolong the inflammation of the airway or maintain a higher level of cough sensitivity. If cough persists, additional empiric treatment with inhaled corticosteroids or antibiotics is recommended. In children who remain unresponsive, a diagnosis of habit cough should be entertained; however, this is usually a diagnosis of exclusion, and referral to a pulmonologist is prudent.

> **Pearl:** Nonspecific cough is usually
> postinfectious and self-limited.

■ Treatment

Successful treatment of cough depends on accurate diagnosis of the cause. Management of the myriad causes of cough is beyond the scope of this chapter; however, several disorders are worthy of brief discussion.

INFECTIONS OF THE LUNGS

Cough caused by lung infections may require prolonged courses of intravenous antibiotics as well as inhalational steroids and bronchodilators. *Streptococcus pneumoniae* and *Staphylococcus aureus* are common bacterial causes, although anaerobes may be present in cases of suspected aspiration. When sputum can be obtained, an accurate culture, Gram stain, and sensitivity may determine the optimal antimicrobial agent of choice. Often, the disease must be treated empirically with broad-spectrum antibiotics and may take weeks to eradicate.

Other infectious etiologies include viral infections, *Mycoplasma pneumoniae*, *Bordetella pertussis*, and mycobacteria. Diagnosis of mycoplasma may be made based on specific IgM and IgG antibody production and cold agglutinins. *Bordetella* outbreaks are not unusual despite required vaccination programs. In the early phase, rhinitis, conjunctivitis, low-grade fever, and mild cough are seen. However, as the airway mucosa is infiltrated with lymphocytes and polymorphonuclear leukocytes, it begins to slough, leading to violent coughing paroxysms associated with a characteristic whoop. The disease may progress to complete respiratory failure in infants and young children. Treatment involves isolation to prevent further spread, especially from low-risk hosts to higher-risk hosts, and erythromycin (40 to 50 mg/kg/day) for at least 14 days. In infections caused by mycobacteria tuberculosis, exposure results in few early symptoms and respiratory symptoms usually progress slowly. Chest radiographs will remain negative even as the PPD converts to positive. Several months later, patients may develop progressive cough, malaise, and night sweats. Chest radiographs ultimately demonstrate lobar infiltrates, cavitary lesions, or military pattern. Treatment includes multidrug antituberculosis therapy.

COUGH-DOMINANT ASTHMA

The diagnosis of cough-dominant asthma is often difficult to make. The methacholine challenge test for bronchoprovocation is still occasionally performed in pulmonology practices, but more commonly the diagnosis is establish based on the response to bronchodilators and inhaled steroids. Treatment failures may be due to noncompliance with medications or failure to recognize and treat a secondary problem.

CHRONIC SINONASAL ILLNESS

Recurrent viral URI, recurrent acute sinusitis, chronic sinusitis, and allergic rhinitis all may present with a moist, productive cough related to constant postnasal drip. In most children, chronic cough of sinonasal etiology results from frequent viral illness with only brief periods of improvement or recovery. As a result, in children with chronic cough and rhinorrhea, it is imperative to try to ascertain whether the disorder improves at all within the typical duration of viral illness, 10 to 14 days. Nasal saline irrigations may be useful in treating these self-limited cases. In recurrent acute or chronic sinusitis, a course of empiric antimicrobial therapy is usually indicated. Children who fail to improve should be considered for referral to an otolaryngologist for endoscopic examination with or without cultures. In most refractory cases, adenoidectomy will be considered prior to consideration of CT scanning of the sinuses or sinus surgery.

Symptoms of allergy should be distinguished from those of sinusitis based on systemic manifestations and quality of the rhinorrhea. Ultimately, affected children should undergo formal testing by an allergist or a trial of some combination of intranasal steroids, antihistamines, and leukotriene inhibitors.

GASTROESOPHAGEAL REFLUX AND FEEDING DISORDERS

Dietary modification, prokinetic agents, proton pump inhibitors, and H_2 blockers are used to treat GERD. Refractory cases may require surgery such as Nissen fundoplication or feeding assess for post-pyloric feeds.

Swallowing dysfunction may be a cause of cough with chronic aspiration. Treatment strategies are based on the results of radiologic or endoscopic swallow evaluations or operative endoscopy. Certain feeding strategies such as thickening or avoidance of certain textures may minimize cough. Surgery may be required if laryngeal cleft or TEF are present.

CONGENITAL AIRWAY DISORDERS

These disorders require endoscopic or open surgical repair and comprise the aberrant innominate artery with tracheal compression, laryngeal clefts, TEFs, subglottic stenosis, and tracheomalacia. Small laryngeal clefts (type 1) respond to endoscopic surgical closure; larger clefts and TEFs require open repair. The aberrant innominate artery requires aortopexy, which relieves the cough and lower airway symptoms. Subglottic stenosis requires intervention in severe cases.

HABIT COUGH AND PARADOXICAL VOCAL CORD DYSFUNCTION

Habit cough is usually related to stress and behavioral factors. The cough often begins with a viral syndrome but persists after improvement of the other symptoms. The cough is usually worse during the day and disappears at night. Biofeedback, breathing exercises, and psychologic counseling may help. Benzonatate may help in refractory cases. In most cases, habit cough will be self-limited.

Paradoxical vocal cord dysfunction is also typically stress-related. Presenting most commonly with stridor, obstructive and cough-like symptoms may be seen as well. Treatment is aimed at education through awareness, biofeedback, and stress relaxation. Specific breathing exercises with sniffing techniques can be performed with a speech/swallow specialist.

■ Selected References

Chang AB, Glomb WB. Guidelines for evaluating chronic cough in pediatrics: ACCP evidence-based clinical practice guidelines. *Chest.* 2006;129(1 Suppl):260S–283S

Denoyelle F, Leboulanger N, Enjolras O, Harris R, Roger G, Garabedian EN. Role of propanolol in the therapeutic strategy of infantile laryngotracheal hemangioma. *Int J Pediatric Otorhinolaryngol.* 2009;73(8):1168–1172

Goldsobel AB, Chipps BE. Cough in the pediatric population. *J Pediatr.* 2010;156(3):352–358

Holinger LD. In: Cotton RT, Myer III CM, eds. *Practical Pediatric Otolaryngology.* Philadelphia, PA: Lippincott-Raven Publishers; 1999:117–128

Holinger LD, Sanders AD. Chronic cough in infants and children: an update. *Laryngoscope.* 1991;101(6 Pt 1):596–605

Leigh MW, Zariwala MA, Knowles MR. Primary cilia dyskinesia: improving the diagnostic approach. *Curr Opin Pediatr.* 2009;21(3):320–325

Mayerhoff RM, Pitman MJ. Atypical and disparate presentations of laryngeal sarcodosis. *Ann Otol Rhino Laryngol.* 2010;119(10):667–671

Meyer AA, Aitken PV. Evaluation of persistent cough in children. *Prim Care.* 1996;23(4):883–892

Milgrom H, Corsello P, Freedman M, Blager FB, Wood RP. Differential diagnosis and management of chronic cough. *Compr Ther.* 1990;16(10):46–53

Shaikh N, Wald ER, Pi M. Decongestants, antihistamines and nasal irrigation for acute sinusitis in children. *Cochrane Database Syst Rev.* 2010;12:CD007909

CHAPTER 19

Aerodigestive Tract Foreign Bodies

Kristina W. Rosbe, MD

Introduction	Imaging
Epidemiology and Prevention	Treatment
Signs and Symptoms	Complications

■ Introduction

Foreign body ingestion and aspiration are an important cause of morbidity and mortality in the pediatric population. Foreign bodies remain a diagnostic challenge because their presentation can vary from life-threatening airway compromise to subtle respiratory symptoms that often are misdiagnosed. A high level of clinical suspicion can prevent delays in diagnosis and complications related to these delays.

■ Epidemiology and Prevention

Aerodigestive tract foreign bodies are the cause of approximately 150 pediatric deaths per year in the United States, and choking causes 40% of accidental deaths in children younger than 1 year. Most aerodigestive tract foreign bodies occur in children younger than 4 years. The high incidence of aerodigestive foreign bodies in children of this age is related to their increased mobility, introduction of adult food, high propensity for placing objects in their mouths, incomplete dentition, and immature swallowing coordination. Other populations at risk for esophageal foreign bodies include psychiatric patients, patients with underlying esophageal or neurologic disease, and edentulous adults. Coins are the most commonly swallowed foreign bodies in infants and toddlers (Figure 19-1); in older children and adults, fish or chicken

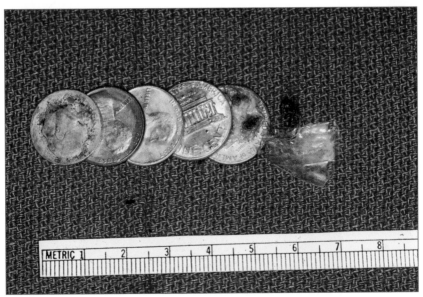

Figure 19-1. Coins are the most commonly swallowed foreign bodies in infants and children.

bones may lodge in the oropharynx. Nuts and seeds are the most commonly aspirated foreign bodies (Figure 19-2). Fortunately, mortality is rare in foreign body accidents; however the foreign bodies most commonly responsible in such cases are latex balloons.

The prevention of ingestion is the most important intervention for potential aerodigestive tract foreign body ingestions. The Consumer Products Safety Act was passed in 1979 and includes criteria for the minimum size of objects (>3.17 cm in diameter and >5.71 cm in length) allowable for children to play with, but these regulations are not uniformly enforced. The small parts test fixture (SPTF) is a cylinder simulating the mouth (diameter) and pharynx (depth) with these dimensions. If an object can fit within the SPTF, it is considered a small part. Small balls are held to an even stricter standard given their high-risk shape and must be 1.75 inches or greater for children younger than 3 years. The Consumer Product Safety Improvement Act of 2008 amended the Federal Hazardous Substances Act (FHSA) to include choking-hazard warnings in all media (eg, Web sites, catalogs) with direct means for purchase of objects for which a warning is required under the FHSA. Some suggest that even stricter dimensions should be adopted for the small part cylinder and could potentially prevent at least 20% of the injuries and fatalities resulting from foreign body ingestions and aspirations in children. Young children should remain under constant adult supervision and allowed to play only with age-appropriate toys. Small and hazardous objects should be safely stored so as not to be accessible to a newly mobile and curious child. Food should be age appropriate and presented only in an observed setting.

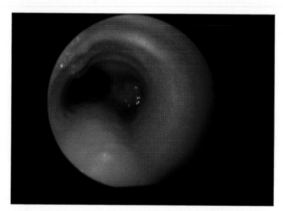

Figure 19-2. Peanut obstructing right main bronchus.

Children with esophageal motility disorders or neurologic disorders should be encouraged to chew food slowly and completely to avoid esophageal impactions or aspiration.

■ Signs and Symptoms

A witnessed ingestion or aspiration episode should be brought to the attention of a physician. Information that is important to elicit from parents includes the approximate time of ingestion, any history of esophageal dysfunction, and severity and duration of swallowing and respiratory symptoms since the time of ingestion. When an unusual foreign body is aspirated or ingested, it may also be helpful to have parents bring in a similar object from home.

Typical signs and symptoms of esophageal foreign body ingestion include drooling, dysphagia, emesis, food refusal, and chest pain. Esophageal foreign bodies may also cause respiratory symptoms in a young child due to swelling in the wall shared by the trachea and esophagus. Airway foreign bodies may initially present with an episode of choking, gagging, and cyanosis followed by coughing, wheezing, or stridor. Physical examination may reveal asymmetric breath sounds or unilateral wheezing. However, the patient may be asymptomatic if air can pass through or around the foreign body or when the reflexes fatigue after the foreign body has been present a long time. This can make diagnosis difficult, especially when the initial event is not witnessed.

> **Pearl:** A high index of suspicion should be maintained when evaluating children presenting with a sudden onset of respiratory symptoms or with recurrent croup, asthma, chronic cough, or pneumonia without the expected response to treatment.

■ Imaging

Posteroanterior and lateral plain films of the neck and chest are the imaging studies of choice. Radiopaque foreign bodies should be straightforward to diagnose, whereas organic and other radiolucent foreign bodies may be more difficult. Unilateral hyperinflation, localized atelectasis or infiltrates, mediastinal shift, and esophageal air trapping can all be clues to the presence of a foreign body, even when no foreign body is visualized (Figure 19-3). Posteroanterior (PA) and lateral views should be obtained because they can help differentiate between esophageal and tracheal foreign bodies and provide clues as to the type of foreign body. For example, the "halo" associated with button batteries on PA views is not always apparent. The clinician also should look for the characteristic "double contour" on lateral view in such cases (Figure 19-4).

Imaging studies should not be used to rule out the presence of a foreign body. High clinical suspicion or historical evidence (ie, witnessed

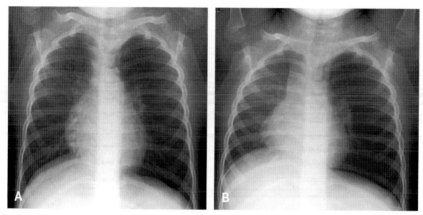

Figure 19-3. Inspiratory (A) and expiratory (B) radiographs of the chest demonstrating air trapping in the left lung.

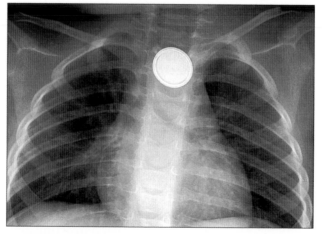

Figure 19-4. Button battery in esophagus. Note "halo" near rim, diagnostic of this foreign body. If not present, lateral radiograph may demonstrate "double contour."

ingestion or aspiration) warrants rigid endoscopy even if imaging studies are normal. If plain films are not diagnostic or the patient cannot cooperate for the imaging examination, airway fluoroscopy is sometimes used. This study has the added advantage of demonstrating a dynamic view of the airway; however, it is dependent on the expertise of the radiologist performing the examination. Barium swallow is generally not indicated, and the presence of barium can make esophageal foreign body extraction more difficult.

■ Treatment

Most surgeons agree that an airway foreign body should be addressed at the time of presentation. Rapid sequence anesthesia techniques may be preferred if aspiration of stomach contents is a concern. The timing of esophageal foreign body removal can be debated based on the type and location of the foreign body, the elapsed time since ingestion, and patient age. An asymptomatic older child with a distal or midesophageal coin present for less than 24 hours and no history of esophageal disorders may be observed for a period of 8 to 16 hours to see if the coin will pass. Spontaneous coin passage rates range widely from 9% to 77% in this patient population. Young children, foreign bodies present for longer than 24 hours, sharp metallic or caustic foreign bodies (eg, button batteries), and symptomatic patients (eg, respiratory symptoms, discomfort, pooling or intolerance of oral secretions) should not be observed for spontaneous passage. A child with suspected disc battery ingestion requires urgent removal in the operating room to avoid mucosal erosion or perforation.

The treatment of choice for most aerodigestive tract foreign bodies is rigid endoscopic removal under general anesthesia. This is carried out in the operating room with proper pediatric endoscopic equipment and pediatric anesthesiologists. Rarely, an oropharyngeal foreign body in an older, cooperative child, such as a fish bone impaling the tonsil, may be successfully extracted when the patient is awake. Alternate methods of removal (eg, Fogarty or Foley catheters, bougienage, flexible endoscopes) have been used successfully at some facilities but are generally not recommended because of the difficulty in protecting the airway and controlling the foreign body with these methods. Meat tenderizers, muscle relaxants, and promotility agents have been used in the past for esophageal foreign bodies in adults, but no evidence supports their use in pediatric patients.

Airway foreign bodies should be retrieved with the patient spontaneously breathing. This facilitates passage of a bronchoscope, prevents distal migration of the foreign body during positive-pressure ventilation, and takes advantage of the natural increase in tracheal and bronchial cross-sectional area during inspiration. It also lowers the risk of inability to ventilate should the foreign body strip off the extraction forceps during the procedure. After mask induction with an inhalational agent, topical lidocaine should be used to anesthetize the vocal folds. Direct laryngoscopy is performed and a rigid bronchoscope introduced under direct vision. Once the bronchoscope has been introduced, the anesthesiologist may connect to the ventilation port. The foreign body is identified, secured, and removed. Removal may require withdrawing, as a unit, the telescopic forceps and bronchoscope. Care should be taken to avoid premature release of the foreign body because this can result in an obstructing laryngotracheal foreign body. The surgeon should also communicate with the anesthesiologist to confirm the depth of anesthesia so as to avoid laryngospasm on withdrawal of the bronchoscope. Nuts and other foods may require multiple passes. Care should be taken to minimize mucosal trauma. Before completion, at least one more pass should be performed to evaluate for multiple foreign bodies and mucosal damage. Depending on the ease of extraction, the child may require a postoperative chest x-ray and close follow-up to rule out the development of pneumonia.

If the foreign body is removed easily without mucosal trauma, the child can be extubated and discharged from the recovery room if he is able to take adequate oral intake. If the foreign body has been present for an unknown length of time and there are signs of mucosal damage, the patient may require a longer period of observation postoperatively. Dexamethasone (ie, Decadron) at a dose of 0.5 to 1.0 mg/kg intravenous may be given in the operating room and continued postoperatively if significant edema is present. A chest x-ray should be performed if there is evidence of a traumatic extraction and any concern of significant mucosal damage to rule out perforation and mediastinal air.

Most children make a full recovery without permanent sequelae from aerodigestive tract foreign body ingestion. Delays in the diagnosis cause the most severe morbidity. Children who have a delayed or technically difficult extraction should be observed postoperatively in an inpatient setting until they no longer require airway support or can tolerate an age-appropriate diet.

■ Complications

Complications from aerodigestive tract foreign bodies result from the type of foreign body and duration of entrapment. Damage to the surrounding aerodigestive tract mucosa may result in granulation tissue formation, erosive lesions, and infection. Objects such as button batteries can cause mucosal erosion in as little as 6 hours from the time of ingestion (Figure 19-5). The risk of complications increases with duration of time the foreign body remains in place. The initial complications from a laryngeal or bronchial foreign body can be severe, including cyanosis, respiratory distress, and even respiratory arrest and death. A ball-valve effect can occur with a partially occluding bronchial foreign body causing hyperexpansion of the affected lung. If complete bronchial occlusion is present, total or partial lung collapse can occur. Late complications of bronchial foreign bodies include granulation tissue formation, pneumonia, empyema, bronchial fistula, and pneumothorax. In the case of esophageal foreign bodies, late complications include granulation tissue formation, mucosal erosions, esophageal perforation, tracheoesophageal fistula, esophageal-aortic fistula, and mediastinitis.

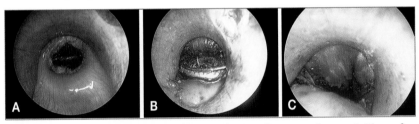

Figure 19-5. Endoscopic removal of button battery from esophagus. A, View of battery prior to instrumentation. Note eschar due to superficial necrosis; small bubbles at surface demonstrate ongoing electrolytic reaction. B, Battery after eschar removal and prior to extraction. C, Residual burns in esophageal wall where battery rim contacted mucosa.

■ Selected References

American Academy of Pediatrics Committee on Injury, Violence, and Poison Prevention. Prevention of choking among children. *Pediatrics.* 2010;125(3):601–607

Betalli P, Rossi A, Bini M, et al. Update on management of caustic and foreign body ingestion in children. *Diagn Ther Endosc.* 2009:969868

Crysdale WS, Sendi KS, Yoo J. Esophageal foreign bodies in children. 15-year review of 484 cases. *Ann Otol Rhinol Laryngol.* 1991;100(4 Pt 1):320–324

Digoy GP. Diagnosis and management of upper aerodigestive tract foreign bodies. *Otolaryngol Clin North Am.* 2008;41(3):485–496

Donnelly LF, Frush DP, Bissett GS 3rd. The multiple presentations of foreign bodies in children. *AJR Am J Roentgenol.* 1998;170(2):471–477

Lin V, Daniel SJ, Papsin BC. Button batteries in the ear, nose and upper aerodigestive tract. *Int J Pediatr Otorhinolaryngol.* 2004;68(4):473–479

Reilly JS. Prevention of aspiration in infants and young children: federal regulations. *Ann Otol Rhinol Laryngol.* 1990;99(4 Pt 1):273–276

Reilly JS, Walter MA, Beste D, et al. Size/shape analysis of aerodigestive foreign bodies in children: a multi-institutional study. *Am J Otolarngol.* 1995;16(3):190–193

Waltzman ML, Baskin M, Wypij D, Mooney D, Jones D, Fleisher G. A randomized clinical trial of the management of esophageal coins in children. *Pediatrics.* 2005;116(3):614–619

Zaytoun GM, Rouadi PW, Baki DH. Endoscopic management of foreign bodies in the tracheobronchial tree: predictive factors for complications. *Otolaryngol Head Neck Surg.* 2000;123(3):311–316

CHAPTER 20

Gastroesophageal Reflux

J. Paul Willging, MD

■ Introduction

Gastroesophageal reflux occurs when gastric contents pass from the stomach into the esophagus. Physiologic reflux occurs in normal individuals with episodes occurring infrequently and associated with rapid clearance of refluxed material from the esophagus. Physiologic reflux causes no irritation to esophageal mucosa. However, when esophageal mucosa is exposed to an increasing frequency of reflux events, or the duration of acid exposure within the esophagus increases with each reflux event, the mucosa becomes inflamed. Chronic inflammation of esophageal mucosa by reflux is a hallmark of gastroesophageal reflux disease (GERD). In children, GERD may manifest with irritability, failure to thrive, food refusal, cough, dysphagia, stridor, hoarseness, bronchospasm, recurrent pneumonia, and apnea. Episodes of regurgitation need not be present with GERD.

> **Pearl:** Gastroesophageal reflux occurs commonly in children. Gastroesophageal reflux disease only occurs when secondary problems develop, such as the development of esophagitis, failure to thrive, food refusal, and airway symptoms.

Several physiologic mechanisms protect against GERD. The lower esophageal sphincter (LES) is a tonic high-pressure zone at the level of the diaphragm that prevents reflux events. It is composed of involuntary smooth muscle fibers and must allow a bolus transiting the esophagus from above into the stomach. The LES also relaxes for belching and vomiting. The upper esophageal sphincter (UES) is another high-pressure zone at the level of the cricoid cartilage. It is composed of a combination of smooth and striated muscle fibers that limit the transfer of reflux material into the hypopharynx, where it may be aspirated.

When reflux events do occur, they are normally cleared from the esophagus. Saliva and secretions produced by mucus glands within the esophagus neutralize gastric acid. Peristaltic action within the esophagus clears gastric secretions from the esophagus, protecting the lining of the esophagus from inflammatory actions of the reflux material.

■ Diagnosis of Gastroesophageal Reflux Disease

No single symptom or symptom complex is diagnostic of GERD. Clinical suspicion may lead to specific tests to determine the presence and severity of gastroesophageal reflux.

ESOPHAGEAL pH MONITORING

Intraluminal pH is monitored and recorded continuously for 24 hours. The length of time the esophagus is exposed to a pH less than 4, number of episodes of acidic reflux, and number of reflux episodes lasting more than 5 minutes are determined. The probe is positioned within 3 cm of the LES for accurate recordings. To increase the sensitivity of the study, a second sensor can be positioned at the UES to assess the number of reflux events ascending to the level of the pharynx.

pH monitoring can detect only acidic events reaching the level of the sensor. Volume of reflux cannot be determined. Gastric contents that have been buffered to a neutral pH by foods, bile, or medications do not trigger the sensor as an event.

Esophageal pH monitoring is useful for evaluating the effectiveness of anti-acid and antisecretory therapies for gastroesophageal reflux.

> **Pearl:** Combined multiple intraluminal impedance with pH monitoring is the best method of evaluating gastroesophageal reflux. It provides the most complete assessment of reflux episodes.

COMBINED MULTIPLE INTRALUMINAL IMPEDANCE WITH pH MONITORING

A probe that measures a change in impedance between pairs of electrodes allows a determination of the presence of liquid, air, or solids in the esophagus passing the probe. Multiple pairs of electrodes allow a reflux event to be followed as it ascends the esophagus and again as it is cleared from the esophagus. A pH sensor is incorporated into the sleeve of the sensor to allow a determination of the acidic or neutral nature of the reflux event.

Impedance monitoring provides significantly more information on reflux events than does a pH probe study. Anterograde and retrograde flow through the esophagus can be measured. Acidic and neutral events can be identified. The height of a single event can be followed and the rate of clearance from the esophagus defined.

CONTRAST STUDIES

The upper gastrointestinal study (barium contrast study) is useful in determining anatomic abnormalities of the upper gastrointestinal tract, but it is not a useful study for the diagnosis of GERD. Reflux may be seen during the study, but the lack of identified reflux events does not rule out the diagnosis of GERD. Conversely, reflux events may be seen in normal individuals without disease.

SCINTIGRAPHY

Food materials labeled with radio nucleotides are ingested and prolonged imaging is obtained to provide a means of determining the rate of gastric emptying and identifying reflux events. Pulmonary aspiration of a reflux event may be recorded by presence of label within the lung fields. A negative test result does not rule out the possibility of pulmonary aspiration of reflux materials because of the episodic nature of the events. These nuclear medicine scans are not recommended for routine evaluation of patients suspected of gastroesophageal reflux.

ENDOSCOPY WITH BIOPSY

Esophagogastroduodenoscopy allows visualization of esophageal mucosa and permits biopsy specimens to be obtained from the proximal and distal esophagus. The stomach and duodenum are also examined. Breaks in the distal esophageal mucosa are the most reliable sign of reflux esophagitis. Mucosal erythema, pallor, and altered vascular patterns are suggestive but not specific findings of reflux.

Histologic findings suggestive of gastroesophageal reflux are eosinophilia, elongation of the rete pegs, vascular hyperplasia, and dilation of intercellar spaces. Correlation between impedance monitoring and esophageal biopsies are only moderate in pediatric populations.

MOTILITY STUDIES

Although rarely indicated in evaluation of gastroesophageal reflux, esophageal manometry may be abnormal in patients with GERD. Manometry is best suited to confirm the diagnosis of achalasia, but it is not sufficiently sensitive nor specific to diagnose GERD.

■ Gastroesophageal Reflux and Airway

Reflux contributes to development of a variety of symptoms associated with the upper airway digestive tract. Gastric acid or activated digestive enzyme-containing fluid may ascend up the esophagus from the stomach and enter the hypopharynx. Reflux may then bathe the laryngeal structures, causing edema, erythema, and pain. It may penetrate into the larynx through the interarytenoid notch and irritate the vocal folds, causing hoarseness or trigging a cough response. Reflux may be aspirated, causing tracheal or bronchial irritation. In such cases, tracheal washings taken via bronchoscopy may reveal the presence of pepsin in the airway. In cases of chronic aspiration, areas of consolidation in lung fields may develop.

> **Pearl:** Extra-esophageal reflux episodes can irritate the airway. Symptoms related to the airway may be the only outward sign of gastroesophageal reflux.

Chronic exposure of the supraglottic larynx to refluxed materials induces chronic throat clearing and cough behaviors. Bronchospasm has been linked to gastroesophageal reflux. Aspiration of gastric contents or stimulation of vagally mediated reflexes from the irritation of receptors in the esophageal mucosa may be responsible for this phenomenon.

Globus pharyngeus (sensation of a mass in the throat) is often linked to gastroesophageal reflux. Chronic pharyngitis may be caused by reflux. Pharyngeal pain, worse in the morning, may be caused by increased frequency of reflux events occurring when in a supine or recumbent position.

Patients with recurrent croup may have a component of their symptoms related to gastroesophageal reflux. Baseline edema found in the airway of reflux patients may predispose to airway compromise. When the patient is exposed to a concomitant viral infection, chronic inflammation of the airway caused by reflux may also be an etiology for development of subglottic stenosis.

Extra-esophageal reflux may also worsen symptoms of laryngomalacia. Edema of the supraglottic structures worsens symptoms of laryngomalacia, increasing the degree of airway collapse and increasing work associated with breathing. This increased work of breathing increases negative pressure within the thoracic cavity. The pressure differential across the LES is thus raised, increasing the incompetence of the LES, producing more reflux events of increasing volume.

■ Treatment of Gastroesophageal Reflux

Treatment of gastroesophageal reflux is approached in stages. Infants given thickened formula (1 tablespoon of rice cereal per ounce of formula) see a reduction in incidence of reflux events reaching the hypopharynx. Overall nutrition is enhanced and the number of reflux events reaching the hypopharynx is diminished.

Alteration in positioning affects reflux. Upright positioning and the prone position reduce reflux events. Conversely, infants in a seated or semi-recumbent position tend to increase pressure on the abdomen and promote reflux events.

Medical treatment of reflux is reserved for individuals with excessive emesis episodes, irritability related to gastroesophageal reflux, failure to thrive, or recurrent respiratory symptoms. Antacids neutralize gastric acid. High doses of aluminum medications may reach toxic levels in children, causing neutropenia, anemia, and neurotoxicity. Only occasional use of aluminum-containing antacids is recommended in children.

Prokinetic agents increase resting tone of the LES, increasing esophageal peristalsis and accelerating gastric emptying. All of these mechanisms reduce gastroesophageal reflux events. Cisapride provides the greatest prokinetic affect and is least likely to induce bronchospasm. Cases of prolonged QT interval and fatal arrhythmias have been associated with cisapride when used concurrently with macrolide antibiotics and antifungal medications. Use of cisapride should be limited to select infants failing lifestyle changes and antisecretory therapy. Careful monitoring is required for the duration of its use, limiting the utility of this medication.

Metoclopramide facilitates gastric emptying; it is associated with lethargy and irritability and may cause irreversible tardive dyskinesia.

Sucralfate adheres to the surface of gastric ulcers and protects esophageal mucosa from the corrosive effects of gastric acid. Because it contains aluminum, care must be taken in children.

Histamine receptor antagonists (H_2 blockers) ranitidine and cimetidine suppress gastric acid production. They reduce symptoms of gastroesophageal reflux and promote healing of the histologic changes associated with esophagitis.

Proton pump inhibitors are the most affective acid suppressants. There is concern about safety of prolonged proton inhibitor use. Increased rates of community-acquired pneumonia, gastroenteritis, and *Candida* infections have been associated with prolonged use of proton pump inhibitors.

> **Pearl:** Proton pump inhibitors are the most effective medication used for the treatment of gastroesophageal reflux disease.

Surgical treatment of gastroesophageal reflux is reserved for patients with severe, medically unmanageable gastroesophageal reflux. A fundoplication procedure, of which there are many types, attempts to recreate a functional LES by wrapping a portion of the greater curvature of the stomach around the esophagus. The primary complication associated with this procedure is gas bloat, gas-bloat syndrome, retching, gagging, dumping syndrome, and recurrent reflux symptoms.

■ Selected References

Ali T, Roberts DN, Tierney WM. Long-term safety concerns with proton pump inhibitors. *Am J Med.* 2009;122(10):896–903

Dalby K, Nielsen RG, Markoew S, Kruse-Andersen S, Husby S. Reproducibility of 24-hour combined multiple intraluminal impedance (MII) and pH measurements in infants and children. Evaluation of a diagnostic procedure for gastroesophageal reflux disease. *Dig Dis Sci.* 2007;52(9):2159–2165

Euler AR, Byrne WJ. Twenty-four-hour esophageal intraluminal pH probe testing: a comparative analysis. *Gastroenterology.* 1981;80(5 pt 1):957–961

Kaul A, Rudolph CD. Gastrointestinal manometry studies in children. *J Clin Gastroenterol.* 1998;27(3):187–191

McMurray JS, Gerber M, Stern Y, et al. Role of laryngoscopy, dual pH probe monitoring, and laryngeal mucosal biopsy in the diagnosis of pharyngoesophageal reflux. *Ann Otol Rhinol Laryngol.* 2001;110(4):299–304

Piquette RK. Torsade de pointes induced by cisapride/clarithromycin interaction. *Ann Pharmacother.* 1999;33(1):22–26

Putnam PE. Gastroesophageal reflux disease and dysphagia in children. *Semin Speech Lang.* 1997;18(1):25–38

Rosbe KW, Kenna MA, Auerbach AD. Extraesophageal reflux in pediatric patients with upper respiratory symptoms. *Arch Otolaryngol Head Neck Surg.* 2003;129(11):1213–1220

Sondheimer JM. Continuous monitoring of distal esophageal pH: a diagnostic test for gastroesophageal reflux in infants. *J Pediatr.* 1980;96(5):804–807

Tsou VM, Young RM, Hart MH, Vanderhoof JA. Elevated plasma aluminum levels in normal infants receiving antacids containing aluminum. *Pediatrics.* 1991;87(2):148–151

Tutuian R, Vela MF, Shay SS, Castell DO. Multichannel intraluminal impedance in esophageal function testing and gastroesophageal reflux monitoring. *J Clin Gastroenterol.* 2003;37(3):206–215

SECTION 6

General

CHAPTER 21

Otolaryngologic Disorders in Down Syndrome

Sally R. Shott, MD; Dorsey Heithaus, MA; and Anthony Sheyn, BS

■ Introduction

Disorders of the ears, nose, and throat are common among children with Down syndrome (DS). The otologic problems observed include conductive hearing loss caused by the presence of chronic middle ear fluid, as well as sensorineural hearing loss. Management of these problems in children with DS may be further complicated by congenital ear canal stenosis. Obstructive sleep apnea and sleep-disturbed breathing are also very common, occurring in as many as 60% of children as young as 3 to 4 years; this incidence increases as children grow older. The subglottic and tracheal airways of children with DS are smaller than in other children of the same age. This is of particular importance if surgery requires endotracheal intubation of the airway for general anesthesia. Tracheomalacia, with stridor due to partial collapse of the trachea with respiration, is not uncommon. Because of delay in development of the immune system and the midfacial hypoplasia with smaller nasal passages and smaller paranasal sinuses, young children are more prone to upper respiratory tract infections and rhinorrhea.

■ Chronic Otitis Media

EPIDEMIOLOGY

Chronic ear infections are common in children with DS, occurring in up to 95%. Etiologic factors include midface hypoplasia with a contracted nasopharynx, an abnormally configured eustachian tube, a higher incidence of upper respiratory infections due to immaturity and delay in the immune system, and poor function of the tensor veli palatini muscle of the soft palate, the muscle responsible for opening and closing the eustachian tube.

The duration of eustachian tube dysfunction in DS is unknown, but it appears that chronic middle ear disease continues much longer and to an age older than that in the general population. Studies demonstrate that aggressive medical and surgical management of chronic otitis media results in better hearing levels and a lower occurrence of tympanic membrane (TM) perforations and cholesteatoma.

PRESENTING SIGNS AND SYMPTOMS

Symptoms associated with acute otitis media are no different in children with DS than other children and include fever, pulling on ears, irritability, poor sleep, poor feeding, and otorrhea in the event of an acute perforation. However, establishing a diagnosis of otitis media on physical examination can be more difficult in children with DS. Up to 50% of newborns with DS will have stenosis of the external auditory canals, often making visualization of the ear drum difficult or impossible. In addition, many affected children have developmental delay that complicates the office examination. As a result, there is a high incidence of under-diagnosis and under-treatment of middle ear disease in DS.

For children with DS in whom the TM can be seen with an otoscope, the primary care practitioner should monitor both ears for recurrent otitis media and chronic middle ear fluid. Patients with eustachian tube dysfunction resulting in severe retraction or retraction pockets, or chronic middle ear fluid causing potential hearing loss, should be referred to an otolaryngologist for evaluation.

The examiner's inability to adequately visualize the eardrum should not be trivialized if the child does not have classic symptoms of otitis media. Although the canals slowly grow during the first 3 years of life, many children will need to have their ear examinations and cerumen removal performed under a microscope to adequately rule out otitis media until routine office examination of the TMs is possible. Chronic middle fluid or negative middle ear pressure can present insidiously in DS, and affected children may have difficulty expressing the associated symptoms. Left untreated, these middle ear disorders may result in erosion of the ossicles and cholesteatoma that requires extensive and aggressive surgical management.

Tympanometry may be a useful tool for screening children with DS for middle ear disease. However, it is suggested that such children be examined by an otolaryngologist every 3 to 4 months, under sedation if necessary, to avoid lengthy delays in diagnosis.

TREATMENT OPTIONS

Similar to other children, initial treatment is medical management with antibiotics for acute otitis media. In addition, environmental risk factors such as exposure to cigarette smoke and appropriately sized child care environments need to be discussed with the child's family and eliminated. It is important to stress that because of the delay in maturity of the immune system for children with DS, these risk factors place the child at an even higher risk of recurrent ear infections.

Children with DS fall outside of the published guidelines for management of otitis media. Insertion of pressure equalization (PE) tubes should generally be considered when fluid associated with hearing loss has not resolved within 3 months or if the child has had 3 to 4 ear infections in 6 months or 5 to 6 in 12 months. It has been shown that children with DS with tubes in place have a 3.6 times higher chance of having normal hearing compared with audiograms done when tubes were not in place.

NATURAL HISTORY AND PROGNOSIS

Due to more prolonged eustachian tube dysfunction, continued problems with ear infections and development of chronic TM changes associated with chronic otitis media occur more frequently in children with DS. Multiple sets of PE tubes may be needed for an individual child. Children should continue to have their ears monitored at least every 6 months as long as chronic retraction of the eardrums, ear effusions, or recurrent infections persist. Audiometric testing is recommended after clearance of middle ear disease to ensure hearing is otherwise normal. For children with minimal ear problems and normal hearing, hearing should be tested periodically to rule out hearing loss that may develop from middle ear fluid or otitis infection. A recent study by Lee et al showed that with aggressive medical surveillance and proactive surgical treatment of chronic ear disease, the need for more extensive otologic surgery can be minimized.

> **Pearl:** Children with Down syndrome who have ear canal stenosis should have regular visits to an otolaryngologist at intervals no greater than 6 months for debridement, microscopic examination, and audiometric testing.

■ Hearing Loss: Audiologic Testing

Although most hearing loss in DS can be attributed to conductive pathology, data suggest that 4% to 20% of DS patients may have sensorineural or mixed hearing loss. As a result, children with DS should have an initial audiologic evaluation in the first month of life following universal newborn screening and American Academy of Pediatrics (AAP) recommendations. Initial audiologic evaluations during the newborn period are done by a screening auditory brain stem response (ABR) or otoacoustic emissions (OAE) hearing test. Otoacoustic emissions are generated at the level of the cochlea and thus will miss more central dysfunction. They are also inaccurate in the presence of middle ear fluid. Auditory brain stem response testing evaluates the hearing via neural pathways and can be done without the child's cooperative participation. Auditory brain stem response testing is felt to be a superior test, as it can differentiate between sensorineural and moderate conductive hearing loss and can also be used for the detection of auditory neuropathy. However, the standard screening ABR uses broadband click stimuli set at a fixed intensity (eg, 20 dB) to determine a pass/fail level. A child with mild otitis media with effusion might pass a screening ABR, and a low-frequency hearing loss could be missed.

Following an initial *abnormal* OAE, a more comprehensive diagnostic ABR should be done by age 3 months. For those children who *passed* the screening ABR, a diagnostic ABR should be done by age 6 months. Diagnostic ABRs better capture the full spectrum of frequencies and can help to determine whether the hearing loss present is conductive or sensorineural.

Once normal hearing is confirmed bilaterally, behavioral testing is initiated. Behavioral testing may be performed in an open-room setting (sound field testing) or with headphones. Unfortunately, children younger than 3 years can rarely be tested with headphones, and sound field testing does not provide audiometric information that is ear specific; as a result, a unilateral hearing loss could be missed. Therefore, behavioral testing should continue every 6 months until the child is found to have normal hearing by ear-specific testing using insert/TDH earphones for at least 3 frequencies (500 Hz, 1,000 Hz, and 4,000 Hz) and normal speech awareness or speech reception threshold. Once this is achieved, annual audiologic testing can be initiated.

If a child fails screening and diagnostic ABRs, the child should be seen by an otolaryngologist who has experience working with children with DS. The otolaryngologist can then determine if medical or surgical interventions are indicated to treat or minimize hearing loss. After successful treatment, the child should undergo a repeat diagnostic ABR. Behavioral audiometry would be acceptable at this time if ear-specific information can be obtained.

Once the ear examination is normal, abnormal audiometric testing usually indicates a sensorineural loss. Such patients should be fitted with hearing aids as early as possible. These children are then followed according to standards established for children with sensorineural hearing loss. The otolaryngologist should participate in long-term monitoring and management of the child's hearing loss and provide information and recommendations with regard to amplification, hearing-assistive devices, and surgical intervention. Amplification with hearing aids should be considered even if there is only mild hearing loss.

Children with DS have a 3-times higher incidence of hearing loss secondary to chronic ear infections than other children with developmental delays. Blaser et al have shown through evaluations of computed tomography scans and magnetic resonance imaging (MRI) a high incidence of inner ear abnormalities in children with DS. Multiple studies have shown a relationship between mild hearing loss and educational, language, and emotional development. Mild hearing loss can also affect a child's articulation skills. Initial studies evaluating the incidence of hearing loss in children with DS reported rates as high as 78%. However, with more fastidious monitoring and more aggressive medical and surgical management, this incidence can be much lower.

A policy statement regarding management of children with DS published in 2011 by the AAP Committee on Genetics recommends audiologic testing at birth and then every 6 months until ear-specific testing is achieved. A study by Maurizi et al shows that reliable, ear-specific results by behavioral audiometry could not be achieved in children with DS younger than 3½ years of age. Ear-specific testing was achieved only rarely in this study. This was further confirmed by Shott et al, who found that only 12% of the children with DS were able to do ear-specific testing at 3 years of age, and only 41% could be tested at 4 years. Testing protocols should therefore be determined by the child's developmental levels and not by chronologic age. The goal is to have ear-specific measurements of pure tones as well as speech awareness levels, and eventually speech reception levels and a determination of speech discrimination abilities. Therefore, hearing levels should be established by objective hearing testing such as ABR, and evaluations should continue every 6 months until ear-specific behavioral testing is achieved. If hearing is normal, annual follow-up hearing tests would be adequate. More frequent audiologic evaluations are necessary in the presence of hearing loss.

Amplification with hearing aids should be considered even if there is only mild hearing loss, especially in view of data linking mild hearing loss with delays in educational, emotional, and language development. This is of particular importance for children with DS, in whom expressive language skills are delayed compared with cognitive abilities. Statistically significant differences in IQ levels were demonstrated among children with mild hearing loss caused by otitis media and matched controls. These studies, however, were all done on otherwise healthy children with hearing loss. It is possible that developmental problems associated with hearing loss may have greater effect in children with the mental and physical handicaps associated with DS.

■ Obstructive Sleep Apnea Syndrome

Studies report a 50% to 100% incidence of obstructive sleep apnea syndrome in individuals with DS, with almost 60% of children with DS having abnormal sleep studies by age 3½ to 4 years. Further evidence shows that these numbers increase as children grow older. Fitzgerald et al showed a 97% incidence of obstructive sleep apnea in children with DS aged 0.2 to 19 years who snored (mean age, 4.9 years). Predisposing factors include midface hypoplasia, mandibular hypoplasia, a relative macroglossia, medially displaced tonsils, adenoid sitting in a contracted nasopharynx and thus causing more obstruction, and hypotonia of the upper airway with resultant collapse at multiple levels of the airway during sleep. Increased upper airway infections and nasal secretions, obesity, and hypotonia further contribute to oropharyngeal and hypopharyngeal collapse and obstruction with sleep.

Sleep-disordered breathing has been shown to affect cognitive abilities, behavior, growth rate, and more serious consequences of pulmonary hypertension and cor pulmonale. Because of the high incidence of underlying congenital cardiac anomalies in individuals with DS, there is a higher risk of development of more severe complications. Abnormalities in the pulmonary vasculature also increase risk of development of pulmonary hypertension.

Unfortunately, the ability of parents to predict sleep abnormalities in their children with DS has been shown to be poor. A sleep study or polysomnogram continues to be the gold standard test from which to evaluate sleep-disordered breathing and sleep apnea. Because of the poor correlation between parental reporting and sleep study results, the AAP recommends a baseline sleep study or polysomnogram for all children with DS by 4 years of age.

PRESENTING SYMPTOMS

Starting at birth, primary care physicians should actively inquire about restless sleep, snoring, heavy breathing, uncommon sleep positions, frequent waking during the night, daytime sleepiness, apneic pauses, and behavior problems associated with poor sleeping. Sleep positions should also be discussed, such as sleeping sitting up, sleeping with the neck hyperextended, or sleeping bent forward at the waist in a sitting position.

Although the focus of sleep-disturbed breathing tends to center around the tonsils and adenoid (T/A), other causes of obstruction, such as chronic rhinorrhea and congestion, nasal septal deviation, and nasal turbinate enlargement, need to be assessed and treated. If the oral examination shows edema of the posterior pharyngeal wall, thus decreasing the size of the posterior pharyngeal airway, gastroesophageal reflux (GER) or chronic postnasal drainage should be considered as the cause of these findings. Treatment with anti-reflux medications or decongestants, nasal steroid sprays, or antihistamines should be considered. Families should be counseled on the risk of sleep apnea due to obesity and the importance of weight control and need for continued exercise.

If there is any question of airway disturbances during sleep, a referral to an otolaryngologist should be done to determine if a sleep study or surgical intervention is needed. In most cases, a sleep study is appropriate to evaluate the severity of the obstruction and to aid in preoperative planning, particularly if the T/A do not appear enlarged. Similar to all children, removal of enlarged T/A is the first-line surgical treatment. In children with DS, because of their midface hypoplasia and contracted nasopharynx, even mildly enlarged T/A may have a greater than expected effect with regard to airway obstruction. If the T/A do not appear enlarged, it has been suggested that a sleep study be done to confirm that the child does *not have* sleep apnea.

MANAGEMENT

Although T/A is the most common initial surgical intervention, studies have shown that residual airway obstruction after this surgery is possible, and further surgical and medical interventions may be needed. This has recently been shown to be more common than previously believed in typical children with preoperative sleep apnea. Mitchell in 2007 showed a 10% to 20% incidence of persistent sleep apnea in a group of 79 typical children after T/A. Tauman et al, using a much more strict definition of surgical cure, showed complete normalization of all components evaluated in a sleep study in only 25% of the test population of "typical" children. This compares with the 5% total success rate seen in the paper by Shott et al in which a similarly strict definition of *cure* was used in a group of children with DS. If cure is more akin to the definitions used in the study by Mitchell, almost 50% to 70% of the children with DS in this study continued to have obstructive sleep apnea after T/A.

All of these studies illustrate the need for postoperative evaluation of children with DS for residual sleep apnea after T/A surgery with a sleep study or polysomnogram. Because of the higher rate of respiratory complications after removal of the T/A in children with DS, overnight observation in the hospital after this surgery is also recommended.

If residual obstruction is present despite T/A surgery, medical treatments with continuous positive-pressure ventilation, weight loss, and oxygen use with sleep are still an option. Evaluations to determine the site(s) of residual airway obstruction include flexible nasopharyngoscopy and laryngoscopy examination in the office to rule out enlarged lingual tonsils, residual or regrowth of adenoid tissue, and possible glossoptosis. Radiographic studies using cine-MRI studies have shown that the base of tongue obstruction from a combination of relative macroglossia and glossoptosis, enlarged lingual tonsils, and adenoid regrowth are some of the most common sites of residual obstruction in individuals with DS despite previous T/A.

Surgical options for persistent obstructive sleep apnea in children with DS need to be tailored to each patient's individual pattern of obstruction. Surgical approaches currently used include lingual tonsillectomy, uvulopalatopharyngoplasty, midline posterior glossectomy, genioglossus advancement, and craniofacial surgery, including mandibular and midface advancements. Dental appliances to promote mandibular stabilization have also been shown to be helpful in cases of mild residual sleep apnea. However, in cases of severe sleep apnea with associated pulmonary hypertension, severe hypoxemia, or cardiac complications, tracheostomy may also need to be considered.

■ Airway Abnormalities: Laryngeal and Tracheal

In comparison to the general pediatric population, children with DS have smaller subglottic and tracheal airways than typical children. An association between DS, stridor, and subglottic stenosis is commonly discussed in the anesthesia literature. It has been shown that children with DS, when compared with other children matched for age and weight with otherwise healthy controls, require an endotracheal tube that is 2 sizes smaller when intubated appropriately, such that there is an air leak around the tube. The hypotonia seen in DS also affects the larynx and trachea, and laryngomalacia and tracheomalacia with associated stridor is not uncommon. Postoperative airway complications are higher in children with DS than typical children, usually caused by airway issues. The combination of the smaller airway, hypotonia, a high incidence of GER, and a high percentage of procedures for children with DS done under general anesthesia places them at higher risk for development of subglottic stenosis.

Although no ongoing monitoring is required, primary care physicians need to be aware of potential airway problems when their patient is scheduled for surgery, especially when intubation is expected to take place and if the child undergoes surgery in a center not accustomed to caring for children with DS. Recurrent croup should be treated aggressively, especially because it is most likely that the child is starting off with a subglottic airway smaller than usual. Treatment of GER should be considered, especially in cases of recurrent croup or if significant edema is seen in the posterior oropharynx. Mitchell found a high incidence of GER in his review of a cohort of children with DS, and GER has been linked as a risk factor for recurrent croup. There is also a higher incidence of GER in children who have laryngomalacia. Although initial reports suggested a lower success rate in surgical treatment of subglottic stenosis in children with DS, more recent reports have shown similar success rates as other children.

Because of the higher potential for postoperative airway problems after general anesthesia, especially if intubation of the airway occurs, overnight hospitalization, following even after a short procedure, should be considered in children with DS and is strongly advocated after adenotonsillectomy.

Due to the higher incidence of airway anomalies such as laryngomalacia, tracheomalacia, and smaller subglottic airways, an otolaryngology consultation should be included when children with DS have recurrent croup, noisy breathing, or stridor.

■ Chronic Rhinitis and Sinusitis

The chronic rhinitis frequently seen in young children with DS in the past has traditionally been dismissed as something that was "just part of DS" and was noted to improve as the child got older. However, chronic rhinitis in DS should not be accepted as an inevitable and untreatable condition, and specialty evaluation of refractory chronic rhinitis should be considered.

Radiographic studies have shown abnormal development of the frontal, maxillary, and sphenoid sinuses, including hypoplasia or lack of pneumatization of the paranasal sinuses. Similarly, midface hypoplasia in DS results in smaller than usual nasal and nasopharyngeal airway and predisposes to stasis of secretions and poor ventilation. Delay in development of the immune system also contributes to response to infectious rhinitis in children with DS. Saline nasal drops, sprays, and irrigations have long been used for treatment of chronic rhinitis and have recently been further confirmed as effective treatment in adults. For children with midface hypoplasia and thus smaller than usual nasal passages, this is an invaluable and effective treatment. Further evaluation and treatment of chronic sinusitis should follow similar pathways of treatment as would be used in typical children.

EVALUATION AND EXAMINATION

In the newborn with DS, or if not done previously in the older child, patency of the nasal choanae should be confirmed by passing a size 8F suction catheters through each naris. If this is not possible, referral to an otolaryngologist to rule out an anatomic or congenital cause of the obstruction may be needed. Examination of the nose will usually rule out foreign bodies, enlarged nasal turbinates, blockage from significant nasal crusting, or purulent rhinitis.

Education of parents should also include discussions on the need to eliminate any cigarette exposure, especially in view of the delay in immune system development and higher incidence of upper respiratory infections in children with DS.

Other causes of nasal obstruction, such as adenoid hypertrophy and nasal turbinate enlargement, should be considered. Symptoms consistent with environmental allergies should be discussed and allergy testing be considered. This should include an assessment of the immune system, including IgG (total and subclass levels), IgA, IgM, IgE, titers to diphtheria, tetanus, and pneumococcus. High-risk exposures such as child care, cigarette smoke, and common environmental allergens should be addressed.

TREATMENT OPTIONS

Successful medical management of rhinitis and sinusitis in DS depends significantly on establishing the correct diagnosis. Although antibiotics, nasal steroid sprays, topical nasal saline, and antihistamines or decongestants may be useful, the indiscriminate use of any of these agents will make further management even more difficult, particularly in lower functioning children. If nasal crusting and clear rhinitis is a problem, a trial of saline nose drops or spray used on a regular basis may be result in improvement. In older children, empiric trials of decongestants or antihistamines may be considered; use of antihistamines that do not cross the blood-brain barrier and thus are less sedative are suggested. If rhinitis is chronically purulent, treatment with antibiotics may be indicated.

If rhinitis continues despite medical management, referral to the allergist or otolaryngologist may be needed to refine medical management including immunotherapy, topical therapies, intravenous immunoglobulin, and surgical intervention. Adenoidectomy with or without turbinate reduction may reduce nasal obstruction and rhinorrhea by improving nasal ventilation and reducing bacterial colonization of the nasopharynx. Studies have shown that adenoid regrowth after adenoidectomy is not uncommon in DS; as a result, persistence or recurrence of nasal obstruction after adenoidectomy should prompt a follow-up lateral neck radiograph to rule out adenoid recurrence.

■ Selected References

American Academy of Family Physicians, American Academy of Otolaryngology–Head and Neck Surgery, American Academy of Pediatrics Subcommittee on Otitis Media With Effusion. Otitis media with effusion. *Pediatrics.* 2004;113(5):1412–1429

Balkany TJ, Downs MP, Jafek BW, Krajicek MJ. Hearing loss in Down's syndrome. A treatable handicap more common than generally recognized. *Clin Pediatr (Phila).* 1979;18(2):116–118

Balkany TJ, Mischke RE, Downs MP, Jafek BW. Ossicular abnormalities in Down's syndrome. *Otolaryngol Head Neck Surg.* 1979;87(3):372–384

Bess FH. The minimally hearing-impaired child. *Ear Hear.* 1985;6(1):43–47

Blaser S, Propst EJ, Martin D, et al. Inner ear dysplasia is common in children with Down syndrome (trisomy 21). *Laryngoscope.* 2006;116(12):2113–2119

Bonnet MH. The effect of sleep fragmentation on sleep and performance in younger and older subjects. *Neurobiol Aging.* 1989;10(1):21–25

Borland LM, Colligan J, Brandom BW. Frequency of anesthesia-related complications in children with Down syndrome under general anesthesia for noncardiac procedures. *Pediatr Anaesth.* 2004;14(9):733–738

Boseley ME, Link DT, Shott SR, Fitton CM, Myer CM, Cotton RT. Laryngotracheoplasty for subglottic stenosis in Down syndrome children: the Cincinnati experience. *Int J Pediatr Otorhinolaryngol.* 2001;57(1):11–15

Bower CM, Richmond D. Tonsillectomy and adenoidectomy in patients with Down syndrome. *Int J Pediatr Otorhinolaryngol.* 1995;33(2):141–148

Brooks DN, Wooley H, Kanjilal GC. Hearing loss and middle ear disorders in patients with Down's syndrome (mongolism). *J Ment Defic Res.* 1972;16(1):21–29

Bull MJ, American Academy of Pediatrics Committee on Genetics. Health supervision for children with Down syndrome. *Pediatrics.* 2011;128(2):393–406

Cone-Wesson B, Vohr BR, Sininger YS, et al. Identification of neonatal hearing impairment: infants with hearing loss. *Ear Hear.* 2000;21(5):488–507

Dahle AJ, McCollister FP. Hearing and otologic disorders in children with Down syndrome. *Am J Ment Defic.* 1986;90(6):636–642

Davies B. Auditory disorders in Down's syndrome. *Scand Audiol Suppl.* 1988;30:65–68

Dobie RA, Berlin CI. Influence of otitis media on hearing and development. *Ann Otol Rhinol Laryngol Suppl.* 1979;88(5 Pt 2 Suppl 60):48–53

Donaldson JD, Redmond WM. Surgical management of obstructive sleep apnea in children with Down syndrome. *J Otolaryngol.* 1988;17(7):398–403

Donnelly LF, Shott SR, LaRose CR, Chini BA, Amin RS. Causes of persistent obstructive sleep apnea despite previous tonsillectomy and adenoidectomy in children with Down syndrome as depicted on static and cine MRI. *AJR Am J Roentgenol.* 2004;183(1):175–181

Dyken ME, Lin-Dyken DC, Poulton S, Zimmerman MB, Sedars E. Prospective polysomnographic analysis of obstructive sleep apnea in Down syndrome. *Arch Pediatr Adolesc Med.* 2003;157(7):655–660

Fitzgerald DA, Paul A, Richmond C. Severity of obstructive apnoea in children with Down syndrome who snore. *Arch Dis Child.* 2007;92(5):423–425

Gershwin ME, Crinella FM, Castles JJ, Trent JK. Immunologic characteristics of Down's syndrome. *J Ment Defic Res.* 1977;21(4):237–249

Halstead LA. Role of gastroesophageal reflux in pediatric airway disorders. *Otolaryngol Head Neck Surg.* 1999;120(2):208–214

Harada T, Sando I. Temporal bone histopathologic findings in Down's syndrome. *Arch Otolaryngol.* 1981;107(2):96–103

Harley EH, Collins MD. Neurologic sequelae secondary to atlantoaxial instability in Down syndrome. Implications in otolaryngologic surgery. *Arch Otolaryngol Head Neck Surg.* 1994;120(2):159–165

Holm VA, Kunze LH. Effect of chronic otitis media on language and speech development. *Pediatrics.* 1969;43(5):833–839

Jacobs IN, Gray RF, Todd NW. Upper airway obstruction in children with Down syndrome. *Arch Orolaryngol Head Neck Surg.* 1996;122(9):945–950

Jacobs IN, Teague WG, Bland JW Jr. Pulmonary vascular complications of chronic airway obstruction in children. *Arch Otolaryngol Head Neck Surg.* 1997;123(7):700–704

Johnson JL, White KR, Widen JE, et al. A multicenter evaluation of how many infants with permanent hearing loss pass a two-stage otoacoustic emissions/automated auditory brainstem response newborn hearing screening protocol. *Pediatrics.* 2005;116(3):663–672

Joint Committee on Infant Hearing. Year 2007 position statement: principles and guidelines for early hearing detection and intervention programs. *Pediatrics.* 2007;120(4):898–921

Lee K, Richter G, Shott S, Hall, Choo D. Surgical management of otologic disease in Down syndrome patients. Abstract presented at American Society of Pediatric Otolaryngology, May 2008

Levanon A, Tarasiuk A, Tal A. Sleep characteristics in children with Down syndrome. *J Pediatr.* 1999;134(6):755–760

Levine OR, Simpser M. Alveolar hypoventilation and cor pulmonale associated with chronic airway obstruction in infants with Down syndrome. *Clin Pediatr (Phila).* 1982;21(1):25–29

Marcus CL, Keens TG, Bautista DB, von Pechmann WS, Ward SL. Obstructive sleep apnea in children with Down syndrome. *Pediatrics.* 1991;88(1):132–139

Marcus CL, Lutz J, Carroll JL, Bamford O. Arousal and ventilatory responses during sleep in children with obstructive sleep apnea. *J Appl Physiol.* 1998;84(6):1926–1936

Maurizi M, Ottaviani F, Paludetti G, Lungarotti S. Audiologic findings in Down's children. *Int J Pediatr Otorhinolaryngol.* 1985;9(3):227–232

Merrell JA, Shott SR. OSAS in Down syndrome: T&A versus T&A plus lateral pharyngoplasty. *Int J Pediatr Otorhinolaryngol.* 2007;71(8):1197–1203

Miller JD, Capusten BM, Lampard R. Changes at the base of skull and cervical spine in Down syndrome. *Can Assoc Radiol J.* 1986;37(2):85–89

Mitchell RB. Adenotonsillectomy for obstructive sleep apnea in children: outcome evaluated by pre- and postoperative polysomnography. *Laryngoscope.* 2007;117(10):1844–1854

Mitchell RB, Call E, Kelly J. Ear, nose and throat disorders in children with Down syndrome. *Laryngoscope.* 2003;113(2):259–263

Mitchell V, Howard R, Facer E. Down's syndrome and anaesthesia. *Paediatr Anaesth.* 1995;5(6):379–384

Moos DD, Prasch M, Cantral DE, Huls B, Cuddeford JD. Are patients with obstructive sleep apnea syndrome appropriate candidates for the ambulatory surgical center? *AANA J.* 2005;73(3):197–205

Ng DK, Chan CH, Cheung JM. Children with Down syndrome and OSA do not necessarily snore. *Arch Dis Child.* 2007;92(11):1047–1048

Ng DK, Hui HN, Chan Ch, et al. Obstructive sleep apnoea in children with Down syndrome. *Singapore Med J.* 2006;47(9):774–779

Pynnonen MA, Mukerji SS, Kim HM, Adams ME, Terrell JE. Nasal saline for chronic sinonasal symptoms: a randomized controlled trial. *Arch Otolaryngol Head Neck Surg.* 2007;133(11):1115–1120

Roizen NJ, Ben-Ami MV, Shalowitx DK, Yousefzadeh. Sclerosis of the mastoid air cells as an indicator of undiagnosed otitis media in children with Down syndrome. *Clin Pediatr (Phila).* 1994;33:439–443

Rowland TW, Nordstrom LG, Bean MS, Burkhardt H. Chronic upper airway obstruction and pulmonary hypertension in Down's syndrome. *Am J Dis Child.* 1981;135(11):1050–1052

Sherry KM. Post-extubation stridor in Down's syndrome. *Br J Anaesth.* 1983;55(1):53–55

Shibahara Y, Sando I. Congenital anomalies of the eustachian tube in Down syndrome. Histopathologic case report. *Ann Otol Rhinol Laryngol.* 1989;98(7 Pt 1):543–547

Shott SR. Down syndrome: analysis of airway size and a guide for appropriate intubation. *Laryngoscope.* 2000;110(4):585–592

Shott SR. Down syndrome: common ear, nose and throat problems. *Down Syndrome Quarterly.* 2000;5:1–6

Shott SR. Down syndrome: common otolaryngologic manifestations. *Am J Med Genet C Semin Med Genet.* 2006;142C(3):131–140

Shott SR, Amin R, Chini B, Heubi C, Hotze S, Akers R. Obstructive sleep apnea: should all children with Down syndrome be tested? *Arch Otolaryngol Head Neck Surg.* 2006;132(4):432–436

Shott SR, Donnelly LF. Cine magnetic resonance imaging: evaluation of persistent airway obstruction after tonsil and adenoidectomy in children with Down syndrome. *Laryngoscope.* 2004;114(10):1724–1729

Shott SR, Heithaus D, Sheyn A. Audiologic testing in children with Down syndrome. Abstract presented at Society for Ear, Nose and Throat Advances in Children Annual Meeting

Shott SR, Heubi C, Akers R. Hearing loss in Down syndrome—do PETs help? Abstract presented at Society for Ear, Nose and Throat Advances in Children, 2003.

Shott SR, Joseph A, Heithaus D. Hearing loss in children with Down syndrome. *Int J Pediatr Otorhinolaryngol.* 2001;61(3):199–205

Southall DP, Stebbens VA, Mirza R, Lang MH, Croft CB, Shinebourne EA. Upper airway obstruction with hypoxaemia and sleep disruption in Down syndrome. *Dev Med Child Neuro.* 1987;29(6):734–742

Spina CA, Smith D, Korn E, Fahey JL, Grossman HJ. Altered cellular immune functions in patients with Down's syndrome. *Am J Dis Child.* 1981;135(3):251–255

Strome M. Down's syndrome: a modern otorhinolaryngological perspective. *Laryngoscope.* 1981;91(10):1581–1594

Tauman R, Gulliver TE, Krishna J, et al. Persistence of obstructive sleep apnea syndrome in children after adenotonsillectomy. *J Pediatr.* 2006;149(6):803–808

Vernail F, Gardiner Q, Mondain M. ENT and speech disorders in children with Down's syndrome: an overview of pathophysiology, clinical features, treatments, and current management. *Clin Pediatr (Phila).* 2004;43(9):783–791

Yamaguchi N, Sando I, Hashida Y, Takahashi H, Matsune S. Histologic study of eustachian tube cartilage with and without congenital anomalies: a preliminary study. *Ann Otol Rhinol Laryngol.* 1990;99(12):984–987

CHAPTER 22

Vascular Birthmarks

John Gavin, MD

■ Introduction

The evaluation and management of vascular birthmarks can be difficult because terminology used to describe these lesions may be vague or confusing. One term may be used to describe multiple types of lesions, or different authors may use different terms to describe the same lesion. Inconsistent use of terminology or including multiple entities under one heading can lead to errors in diagnosis and inappropriate treatment recommendations. In 1982, Mulliken and Glowacki suggested a classification system based on endothelial characteristics of these lesions and their biological behavior. Using this classification system as a framework for evaluating these lesions can improve diagnostic accuracy, which in turn should lead to use of logical treatment algorithms.

Vascular anomalies, both tumors and malformations, involve the head and neck 70% to 80% of the time; can affect vision, hearing, and breathing; and may be severely disfiguring with significant psychosocial sequelae for patient and family.

■ Classification

Mulliken and Glowacki used information from clinical history of vascular lesions, their histology, and their radiographic appearance to separate vascular birthmarks into 2 large categories, tumors and vascular malformations. They found that the terms *cavernous hemangioma, lymphangiohemangioma, strawberry nevus,* and *capillary hemangioma* were used inconsistently and for multiple types of lesions. More than 25 years after Mulliken and Glowacki clarified classification of these lesions, the term *cavernous hemangioma* is still used to describe venous and capillary-venous malformations. Within their system, tumors consist primarily of hemangiomas and malformations and include capillary, venous, arterial, and lymphatic malformations. The International Society for the Study of Vascular Anomalies established a formal classification system in 1996.

■ Vascular Tumors

Vascular tumors are true neoplasms that result from disordered angiogenesis. Hemangiomas are by far the most common vascular tumor in newborns and infants, and in fact are the most common soft tissue tumor of infancy. Other vascular tumors include tufted angiomas and kaposiform hemangioendothelioma (KHE).

EPIDEMIOLOGY

In term babies of normal weight, incidence of hemangioma is between 1.1% and 2.6% during the first 3 days of life and may be as high as 12.6% or as low as 3.5% during the first year of life. Inconsistent nomenclature historically associated with these lesions as well as a lack of prospective studies make knowing true incidence of hemangiomas difficult. It is probably closer to 4% or 5% rather than the 10% or more often cited. Among babies weighing less than 1,000 g, incidence is 22.9%. Babies born to mothers of advanced maternal age or with a history of chorionic villus sampling between weeks 9 and 12 of gestation are 21% more likely to have a hemangioma. Girls are affected twice as often as boys. Caucasians are affected more often than other races. The estimated incidence in African Americans is 1.4%; in Asians, 0.8%.

Hemangiomas are typically single and sporadic. Only 3% of patients present with multifocal (more than 8) lesions. A few families show an autosomal-dominant inheritance pattern. The responsible gene is located on chromosome 5q31-33. Four of 5 children with a hemangioma will have a single lesion.

ETIOLOGY

Although pathogenesis of hemangiomas is uncertain, they likely arise from vessels whose growth is hormonally driven. It has been suggested that they may be the result of transfer of placental cells to the fetus. The presence of glucose transporter 1 (GLUT1), which is also found in placenta but not other vascular lesions, supports this, as does increased risk of hemangiomas after chorionic villus sampling. However, absence of villous architecture and trophoblastic elements makes ectopic placental tissue an unlikely explanation. Proliferating hemangiomas express human chorionic gonadotrophin and human placental lactogen, indicating they may originate from the placental chorionic villous mesenchymal core. Proliferating hemangiomas also demonstrate embryonic stem cell–associated proteins. Infantile hemangiomas may result from new blood vessels originating from circulating stem cells rather than disordered angiogenesis. Immunophenotype of hemangiomas resembles the cardinal vein during early embryogenesis, suggesting that hemangiomas may be arrested in an early developmental stage of vascular differentiation.

NATURAL HISTORY

Hemangiomas are not typically present at birth but appear during the first year of life. They have a proliferating phase followed by an involuting phase. During both phases, levels of basic fibroblast growth factor, urokinase, and von Willebrand factor are elevated.

Proliferating phase begins shortly after the hemangioma appears. A period of rapid growth is seen within the first 3 to 6 months of life. Eventually, growth rate slows and parallels the patient's growth, and the lesion achieves maximum size by 1 year of age. Proliferating phase is driven by endothelial cells. These cells demonstrate high levels of alkaline phosphatase. Factor 8 antigen is elevated and toward the end of proliferation, mast cells are present at 30 times their normal numbers. Pro-angiogenic factors include proliferating cell nuclear antigen, vascular endothelial growth factor, basic fibroblast growth factor, and type 4 collagenase. In hemangiomas, endostatin, an angiogenesis inhibitor, stimulates migration of endothelial cells. In normal endothelial cells, migration is inhibited by endostatin.

Mature lesions are made up of lobules separated by fibrous septa and demonstrate large feeding and draining vessels. A multi-laminated basement membrane is seen on electron microscopy.

Involuting phase usually begins by 18 months of age but can occur significantly later, especially in lesions of the lip. Involution is completed by age 5 years in 50% of patients but may last until age 12. During involution, the lesion is noted to be lighter, softer, and smaller. Histologically, vascular channels decrease in number and perivascular spaces demonstrate fibrous deposition. Antiangiogenic effects during involution are a function of tissue inhibitor of metalloproteinase, mast cells, and scavenger macrophages. Involution is apoptotic and likely immune mediated, with cytotoxic T cells playing an important role. Proliferating lesions show high levels of indoleamine 2,3-dioxygenase, which decrease significantly during involution. Indoleamine 2,3-dioxygenase inhibits T-cell function. It is also present in the placenta and may protect the placenta and fetus from the mother's immune response.

At least half of hemangiomas completing involution will heal without permanent changes in skin color or texture. The vascular network is replaced with fibrofatty tissue and dense collagen. Midface hemangiomas have an involution that is less predictable than lesions in other locations and may be more likely to leave cosmetic deformity. Hemangiomas that leave a residuum may be appropriate for treatment at the end of involution. The residuum may appear as epidermal atrophy, telangiectasia, fibrofatty tissue, or excess skin.

Congential hemangiomas are present at birth but similar in appearance to infantile hemangiomas. They can be divided into rapidly involuting congenital hemangioma (RICH) and non-involuting congenital hemangioma (NICH) types. Neither shows rapid proliferation, but they are both similar to infantile hemangiomas histologically and radiographically. The only histologic difference that distinguishes these lesions from hemangiomas of infancy is the absence of GLUT1 staining. Rapidly involuting congenital hemangiomas are present at birth, raised with a blue or violet color, and often surrounded by a hypopigmented halo. Regression begins early and is usually complete between 6 and 14 months of age. Non-involuting congenital hemangiomas are well-circumscribed, solitary lesions with a reddish pink plaque, central telangiectasia, and hypopigmentation around the rim. They behave like vascular malformations, growing with the child and persisting into adulthood.

DIAGNOSIS

History

An accurate and thorough history is the key to diagnosing vascular birthmarks. With regard to hemangiomas, the age at which the lesion first appeared and changes in the lesion over time will usually lead the clinician to the correct diagnosis.

Physical Examination

The appearance and tactile qualities of the lesion can also aid in diagnosis. Hemangiomas typically have a fleshy quality and will not completely empty with compression. This helps distinguish them from many vascular malformations.

Hemangiomas can be described based on appearance and location. Lesions can be superficial, deep, or compound. Superficial lesions are usually red in color and do not involve deeper tissues (Figure 22-1). Deep lesions create a mass effect in soft tissues, and overlying skin typically has a bluish discoloration. Care must be taken in diagnosing deep lesions as hemangiomas because some of these deep vascular lesions without a skin component may represent other vascular tumors or vascular malformations, especially venous malformations Compound hemangiomas (Figure 22-2) have deep and superficial components. Lesions may be further characterized as focal or segmental. Segmental lesions (Figure 22-3) are more often superficial and are more likely to have associated morbidity than focal lesions. Segmental lesions

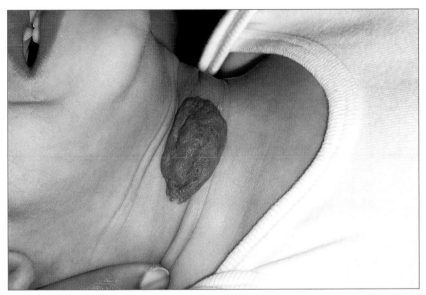

Figure 22-1. Superficial hemangioma. Such lesions may be raised and focal as seen, or flat and diffuse (segmental).

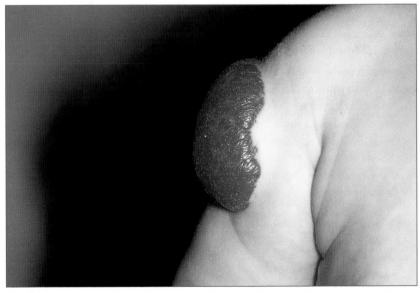

Figure 22-2. Compound hemangioma, with superficial and deep components.

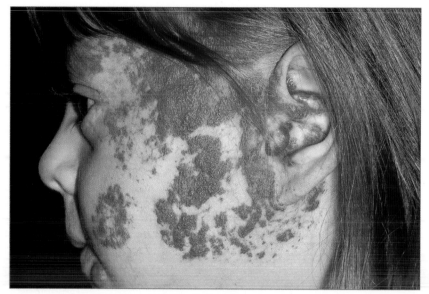

Figure 22-3. Segmental hemangioma of the face.

in the lower face are associated with a hemangioma involving the airway more than half the time.

Airway Evaluation

When an airway lesion is suspected, fiber-optic laryngoscopy, operative endoscopy, computed tomography (CT) or magnetic resonance imaging (MRI) scanning, and/or hospital admission may be warranted. Computed tomography scanning helps determine whether an airway lesion is focal or segmental. This information can be critical to developing a treatment plan. If presence of an airway hemangioma is in question, especially in a patient with a cutaneous hemangioma, a trial of corticosteroids that relieves stridor strongly suggests the diagnosis.

> **Pearl:** Late-onset progressive stridor in a patient with a cutaneous hemangioma should prompt an airway evaluation.

Imaging

Imaging is often not required to diagnose hemangiomas, but lesions with uncommon features or unusual histories may make imaging necessary. Plain films are not useful in evaluating vascular lesions. Doppler ultrasound is cost-effective and easily performed in infants without the need for sedation and without the radiation risk associated with other imaging modalities. This modality is 84% sensitive and 98% specific in diagnosing hemangiomas when lesions demonstrate high vessel density ($>5/cm^2$) and high Doppler shift (>2 kHz).

Computed tomography scans with intravenous (IV) contrast demonstrate a homogenous lesion with uniform enhancement. As lesions begin to involute, associated fibrofatty tissue gives lesions a heterogenous appearance. As compared with ultrasound, CT has increased risk because of radiation exposure, need for IV contrast, and possible need for sedation.

Magnetic resonance imaging is an excellent imaging study for evaluating hemangiomas. On MRI lesions appear as soft tissue masses that are typically lobulated and clearly separated from surrounding muscle. During involution, fibrofatty tissue is seen as increased areas of high-intensity foci. Unfortunately, MRI in infants typically requires general anesthetic. Fortunately, most lesions do not require imaging. Imaging usually is reserved for operative planning or in rare cases when the diagnosis is in question.

Deep hemangiomas may be difficult to distinguish from venous malformations. Magnetic resonance imaging, CT, and ultrasound may not always be able to distinguish these lesions from one another. In patients in whom diagnosis is in question, especially if treatment is indicated, 3-D CT angiography may be a valuable tool for confirming diagnosis.

Patients with 4 or more cutaneous hemangiomas should be imaged to rule out visceral lesions, especially hepatic lesions. This can be achieved with abdominal ultrasound.

> **Pearl:** While patients with multiple hemangiomas are at increased risk of visceral lesions, many visceral lesions can be followed with serial imaging and do not require intervention.

Histologic Evaluation

Lesions that require excision or biopsy may provide immunohisto-
chemical markers on the surface of the endothelium for diagnosis.
Hemangiomas of infancy show GLUT1 on the endothelium. This
marker is not present in vascular malformations or congenital hemangiomas. Hemangiomas also demonstrate multi-laminated basement
membranes not found in malformations.

Proliferating lesions show compact capillaries lined with plump
endothelial cells with high mitotic rates. Stromal components include
fibroblasts, pericytes, and mast cells.

While many vascular lesions are lobular, infantile hemangiomas
differ from other lesions in that lobules are separated by normal stroma
as opposed to fibrotic bands seen separating lobules in other lesions.

DIFFERENTIAL DIAGNOSIS

Other lesions that may be mistaken for hemangiomas include pyogenic
granulomas, tufted angiomas, infantile hemangiopericytomas, fibro-
sarcomas, KHEs, neuroblastomas, and embryonic rhabdomyosarcomas.
Biopsy is warranted if the presumed hemangioma cannot be distinguished from these lesions.

Congenital Hemangiomas

Rapidly involuting congenital hemangiomas and NICH are similar to
one another histologically, but their etiologies are not well understood.
These lesions are present at birth and distinct from infantile hemangiomas. Both lack the placenta-associated phenotype of infantile hemangiomas. They occur with equal frequency in males and females.

Rapidly involuting congenital hemangiomas and NICH have a
peripheral rim of pallor, and RICH typically demonstrate a central
depression or ulcer. Histologically, lobules of these lesions are separated by dense fibrous tissue, not the normal stroma seen in infantile
hemangiomas. Rapidly involuting congenital hemangiomas show a
central core containing large, central draining channels correspond-
ing to the region of central depression. Non-involuting congenital
hemangiomas sometimes demonstrate large capillary lobules and
arteriovenous fistulae.

Kaposiform Hemangioendothelioma

Kaposiform hemangioendotheliomas are rare in the head and neck.
They occur anywhere on the body and are benign lesions with a significant lymphatic component. They are usually cutaneous nodules with

a purple color extending into deeper tissues. Most appear before age 2 years and may be present at birth. They occur with equal frequency in boys and girls. Biopsy may be required to make diagnosis.

The lesion is associated with Kasabach-Merritt phenomenon, a life-threatening condition related to platelet trapping within the lesion. More deeply seated lesions are at greater risk.

Magnetic resonance imaging demonstrates a tumor involving multiple tissue layers with poorly defined margins. Lesions may be multifocal.

Tufted Angioma

Tufted angiomas (TAs) tend to be more localized than KHEs and appear as pink or red macules with papules. They occur with equal frequency in boys and girls. More than half appear before age 5 years, and 15% are congenital. Like KHE, biopsy is often required for diagnosis.

These lesions can also produce the Kasabach-Merritt phenomenon, which has only been seen with congenital TA.

Pyogenic Granuloma

A pyogenic granuloma may be easily mistaken for an infantile hemangioma. While common during childhood, pyogenic granulomas are very uncommon during the first year of life. Pathogenesis of pyogenic granuloma is not well understood. They are often associated with minor trauma and may represent an exaggerated vascular proliferation in response to local irritation. They are usually raised but may be sessile or pedunculated (Figure 22-4). They bleed easily with even mild trauma and are prone to ulceration. Histologically, there is endothelial proliferation and vascular spaces are present. This accounts for the term *lobular capillary hemangioma*. Many lesions demonstrate a lymphocytic infiltrate. Conservative local excision is usually curative.

COMPLICATIONS

At least 80% of all hemangiomas resolve without sequelae. In some anatomic locations, complications will be more likely. Lesions near the eye may cause visual deficits, and lesions involving the airway may threaten breathing.

Complications are most commonly seen in early to mid-proliferating phase when growth is most rapid. Ulceration, obstruction, bleeding, infection, congestive heart failure, and physical deformity can be seen.

Ulceration occurs in 5% of hemangiomas (Figure 22-5). Hemangiomas of the lips, neck skin folds, and diaper area are most at risk for

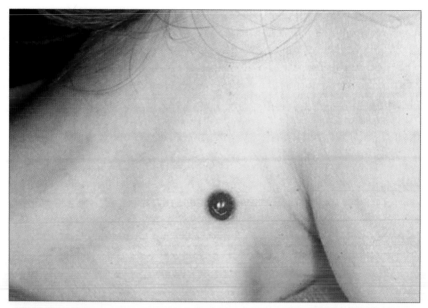

Figure 22-4. Pyogenic granuloma of the neck.

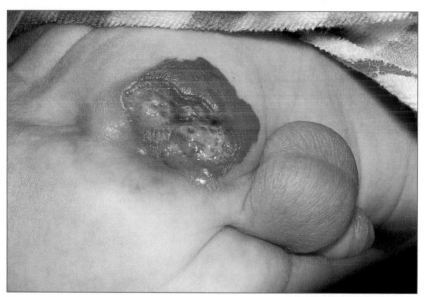

Figure 22-5. Ulcerated hemangioma. Ulceration occurs most commonly in hemangiomas that are segmental and those occurring around the lips or diaper area.

ulceration. Segmental lesions ulcerate 8 times more than focal lesions. Bleeding may occur with ulceration but is easily controlled with pressure. Ulcers in the diaper area may be chronically soiled and are at increased risk of infection.

Obstruction of the visual axis or auditory canal can lead to changes in vision and hearing. Periorbital lesions produce complications 54% to 80% of the time. Because of this, periocular lesions warrant close evaluation, including serial cycloplegic refractions, and early treatment. Patients with periorbital hemangiomas are at risk for amblyopia, refractive errors secondary to pressure on the cornea, proptosis, blepharoptosis, and optic atrophy. Lesions obstructing the visual axis may lead to deprivation amblyopia. Compressive lesions may deform the eye, leading to astigmatic amblyopia. Left unchecked, some of these changes may be irreversible, especially if there is compression of the optic nerve.

Periorbital hemangiomas often require imaging and must be distinguished from lymphatic malformations, neurofibroma, rhabdomyosarcoma, and neuroblastoma. Ultrasound and CT can provide information about the size of the lesion and involved structures but are not as useful as MRI in distinguishing hemangiomas from other lesions.

Bilateral lesions affecting the external auditory canal may produce conductive hearing loss severe enough to hinder speech and language development.

Airway obstruction is one of the most feared complications of hemangiomas. Lesions occurring anywhere from the nasal passage to the subglottic airway may produce life-threatening airway obstruction. Because babies are obligate nasal breathers, lesions involving the nasal airway should be closely monitored for impending airway obstruction. Lesions of the subglottis are often detected late because stridor may not occur for several weeks or months. Patients with cutaneous hemangiomas in the beard distribution have airway lesions creating some degree of obstruction more than 60% of the time.

Skeletal deformity can occur as a result of pressure effects from locally expanding deep hemangiomas.

Congestive heart failure may be seen with large cutaneous or hepatic hemangiomas. Patients with more than 4 cutaneous lesions are at increased risk for hepatic lesions.

After age 3 years, as body image begins to develop, significant psychosocial sequelae may be seen. Children aged 3 to 5 years with head and neck hemangiomas feel that others do not value them as highly as children of the same age without hemangiomas. Negative psychosocial effects have also been demonstrated in family members of children with head and neck hemangiomas. Family members are frequently subjected to questions or comments from friends and other family members, or even from complete strangers. They may have to field questions about child abuse. Families notice that other people tend to stare at, ignore, or avoid children with hemangiomas. School-yard bullying or cruelty can lead to withdrawal, anger, or aggression in patients with vascular birthmarks.

> **Pearl:** Early treatment of head and neck hemangiomas may be warranted to minimize psychosocial sequelae associated with disfiguring lesions.

Kasabach-Merritt Phenomenon

Thrombocytopenia secondary to sequestration and destruction of platelets within a large vascular tumor are known as Kasabach-Merritt syndrome or phenomenon. This complication is seen with KHE and TA and not with infantile hemangiomas as was originally believed. This phenomenon occurs in infancy. Chemotherapy is often required to minimize the bleeding risk.

SYNDROMES

Posterior Fossa Malformations, Hemangiomas, Arterial Anomalies, Coarctation or Cardiac Defects, Eye Abnormalities, Sternal Cleft (PHACES)

This collection of abnormalities noted to occur together is abbreviated PHACES. Dandy-Walker syndrome is the most commonly seen brain lesion. In general, hemangiomas associated with posterior fossa lesions are more likely to occur in the airway or on the face and lead to complications. Associated ocular defects include optic nerve hypoplasia, increased retinal vascularity, exophthalmos, choroidal hemangiomas, strabismus, colobomas, cataracts, glaucoma, and microphthalmia. One of these findings is present in 20% of patients with the PHACES syndrome and may be contralateral to the facial hemangioma. Central nervous system sequelae include developmental delay, seizure, and stroke. Any baby with a large, segmental facial hemangioma in a dermatome distribution should have neurologic evaluation and imaging as part of the workup for PHACES.

Other Associated Anomalies

Lumbar hemangiomas may be associated with intraspinal lipomas, tethered spinal cord, or tight fila terminalia. Sacral lesions are seen with imperforate anus, renal anomalies, lipomeningoceles, and fistulas. When encountering lesions in these locations, a high degree of suspicion is needed so as not to overlook potentially severe associated deformities.

TREATMENT

Observation

Most hemangiomas will resolve without intervention. For this reason, these lesions can frequently be observed. It must be kept in mind that observation is an active process, and the clinician must be on alert for impending complications. In deciding to treat a hemangioma, the clinician must consider indications for treatment and goals of the clinician and the patient's family. Indications for treatment include location and size of the lesion, possibility of complications, and psychosocial factors associated with the lesion. Any treatment plan should be directed at minimizing morbidity associated with the lesion, ameliorating psychosocial effects of the lesion, and avoiding toxic side effects or undue scarring.

Children younger than 3 years do not have a well-developed body image, but as they approach school age they begin to be aware of differences between themselves and other children. Of course the patients are not the only ones who suffer psychosocial effects of hemangiomas. Their families are also affected, and maladaptive behavior patterns among families of children with cosmetically significant hemangiomas are not uncommon.

Hemangiomas that show significant improvement by 18 to 24 months of age are considered early involuters and are likely to resolve by age 5 years. Lesions that show little or no change by 2 years of age are late involuters and will often benefit from intervention.

When considering airway lesions, avoiding tracheostomy is an important goal of any treatment strategy. However, in some patients, especially those with segmental airway lesions, tracheostomy may be unavoidable

> **Pearl:** Early referral to a specialist is always appropriate when risk of visual loss is suspected.

Medical Therapy

The ability of corticosteroids to arrest growth or accelerate regression of hemangiomas has been recognized for more than 50 years. Corticosteroids are anti-inflammatory and antiangiogenic. They may be used locally or systemically. They are most useful during the proliferative phase because they have no significant effect on involution.

Corticosteroids may be injected to treat small, localized lesions. Injecting periorbital lesions is controversial given the risk of blindness. Eyelid lesions may be injected under general anesthesia while visualizing the retina. Periorbital injections carry risks of retinal artery occlusion, eyelid necrosis, depigmentation, and subcutaneous fat atrophy. To decrease these risks, clobetasol may be applied topically, although it works more slowly and likely is not as effective as injected corticosteroids.

Systemic corticosteroids are used to treat large lesions that pose a threat to normal function or are life-threatening. Segmental lesions are more likely to require therapy. Side effects of steroid treatment include cushingoid facies, gastrointestinal complaints, changes in mood, weight gain, insomnia, and growth retardation. Throughout the course of systemic corticosteroid therapy, effectiveness of the therapy should be followed, live vaccines should be avoided, and blood pressure should be monitored. A recent study of immunosuppressive effects in children with hemangiomas treated with corticosteroids showed decreases in B and T lymphocytes as well as loss of protective titers in patients previously immunized against diphtheria and tetanus. Corticosteroids have been considered a first-line therapy for hemangiomas for many years, but propanolol may soon replace corticosteroids in that role.

Propanolol was serendipitously found to be an effective treatment for hemangiomas at Bordeaux Children's Hospital. Two patients with large hemangiomas were admitted for systemic corticosteroid therapy. Neither lesion regressed with therapy, but one child developed an obstructive hypertrophic myocardiopathy and the other demonstrated increased cardiac output on ultrasonography. Both children were treated with propanolol and subsequently showed regression of their hemangiomas. Subsequently, 9 more children were treated with propanolol, all with good outcomes. Propanolol has now replaced corticosteroids as the primary medical therapy for hemangiomas at most institutions (Figure 22-6). Mechanisms of action to explain the effect of propanolol on hemangiomas include vasoconstriction, decreased expression of basic fibroblast growth factor and vascular endothelial growth factor, and triggering apoptosis of capillary endothelial cells. Protocols for starting and maintaining propanolol therapy are not yet established. The medication should be started and the patient monitored by specialists with experience using the drug for hemangioma management.

Interferon 2α and 2β have been used as a second-line medical therapy. Interferon is not considered first-line therapy because of the risk of severe side effects. It is typically reserved for severely disabling or life-threatening lesions when corticosteroids are ineffective, contraindicated, or not tolerated by the patient. Interferon is more effective the earlier it is started and should be continued for 9 to 14 months. Interferon therapy carries the risk of spastic diplegia, especially before age 1 year.

Laser Therapy

Laser therapy may be useful in reducing the surface color of hemangiomas. Argon and neodymium:yttrium-aluminum-garnet (Nd:YAG) lasers have been use to treat hemangiomas but are limited because of their relatively nonselective tissue destruction. The pulsed dye laser (PDL) with a wavelength of 595 nm (oxyhemoglobin has its absorption peak at 577 nm) is much more selective and has become the preferred laser for treatment of hemangiomas. It is not particularly effective in treating

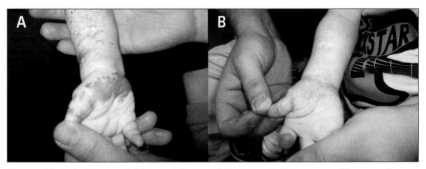

Figure 22-6. A, Segmental hemangioma of the arm. B, Response of hemangioma to propranolol.

the deeper component of lesions, as its penetration is only 1 mm. Laser therapy is useful early in the course of the lesion, for hemangiomas with a high risk of complication, and for treating residual defects after involution. When used before 6 months of age, there may be some risk of epithelial disruption, ulceration, and scarring.

Chemotherapy

Vincristine, cyclophosphamide, and bleomycin have all been used to treat hemangiomas, but associated toxicity and side effects make these a second- or third-line therapy. Vincristine is used most commonly and is probably more useful in treating other vascular lesions, including KHE.

Surgical Treatment

Early surgical therapy (within the first year of life) is reserved for lesions with severe acute complications not responding to medical therapy. The most common complications requiring early surgical intervention are obstructive, affecting vision, hearing, and respiration. Disfiguring lesions of the face may benefit from early surgical intervention to avoid deposition of fibrofatty tissue requiring more extensive surgery later.

Late surgical intervention, when involution is complete, is aimed at correcting abnormal contouring and distortion related to fibrofatty tissue.

Other Treatment Options

Embolization is useful in treating lesions that pose a risk of hyperdynamic heart failure, especially liver lesions. Radiation is no longer considered appropriate treatment for hemangiomas given associated risks, including secondary neoplasm.

■ Vascular Malformations

Vascular malformations are present at birth and can contain arterial, venous, and lymphatic vessels. These lesions result from errors in vasculogenesis. Lesions are often associated with local soft-tissue or bony overgrowth. Malformations are one-tenth as common as hemangiomas.

VENOUS MALFORMATIONS

Etiology

Venous malformations can be inherited and are linked to a mutation in the tyrosine kinase protein receptor. Mutations in this receptor lead to defects in the smooth muscle layer of the vessels, which in turn lead to development of venous malformation.

Natural History

Lesions are seen at birth. They may become painful due to nerve irritation or consumptive coagulopathy, which can be detected by an elevated D dimer with a low fibrinogen. During puberty they may enlarge or become painful.

Diagnosis

Venous malformations are present at birth and enlarge over time. They are compressible and frequently found in muscle tissue. Overlying skin has a bluish discoloration (Figure 22-7). On Valsalva maneuver, the lesions enlarge. Often presentation alone is enough to make the diagnosis.

Plain films may demonstrate phleboliths within the involved soft tissues. On MRI, these will appear as flow voids (Figure 22-8). Computed tomography often is not diagnostic, and MRI may be

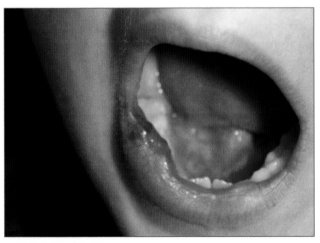

Figure 22-7. Venous malformation of right lower lip. Purple color is typical of these lesions.

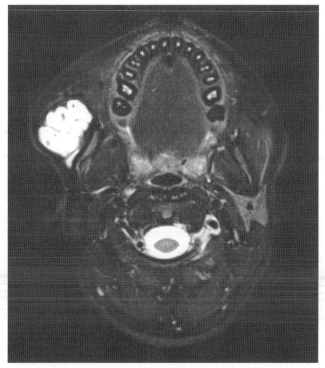

Figure 22-8. Magnetic resonance imaging scan demonstrating venous malformation of right buccal fat space. Flow voids in mass are due to phlebolith formation.

required to confirm the diagnosis. Magnetic resonance imaging also helps define the extent of the lesion to plan treatment.

Usually, biopsy is not required to make the diagnosis. If biopsy is performed, histologic evaluation shows venous and lymphatic elements. On ultrasound they demonstrate slow blood flow. Magnetic resonance imaging reveals a bright signal on T2-weighted signals. Calcified phleboliths may be seen on CT.

Treatment

Pain associated with these lesions can be controlled with anti-inflammatory agents. For severe consumptive coagulopathy, low-dose heparin may be used. Discrete lesions may be amenable to complete surgical excision. Sclerotherapy can be used alone or in combination with surgery. Sclerotherapy alone may be considered first-line treatment for some venous malformations.

ARTERIOVENOUS MALFORMATIONS

Etiology

Arteriovenous malformations (AVMs) contain an abnormal precapillary connection between arteries and veins. Lesions associated with cutaneous capillary malformations may be secondary to gene abnormalities. Arteriovenous malformations are caused by errors in vascular development between the fourth and sixth weeks of gestation. They may be caused by a failure of apoptosis in primitive arteriovenous connections. The possibility that these lesions occur as a result of a failure of apoptosis is supported by the fact that AVMs appear in the central nervous system 20 times as often as they appear elsewhere. Less apoptosis occurs in the central nervous system, especially with regard to neurons.

Epidemiology

Arteriovenous malformations occur 1½ times more often in females than males. Lesions appearing at birth or during childhood are equal among males and females, but lesions occurring after puberty are seen 4 times as often in females.

Natural History

Arteriovenous malformations are present at birth 59% of the time. Ten percent appear in childhood, 10% in adolescence, and 20% in adulthood. They frequently involve the midface. The lesions tend to go through 4 stages. The first is dormancy; during this stage, the lesion may be mistaken for other vascular lesions. These malformations demonstrate cutaneous blush and warmth. Expansion, the second stage, often occurs during adolescence. During expansion, lesions demonstrate bruit or audible pulsation. Intraluminal hydrostatic pressure associated with the arterial component seems to predispose these lesions to expansion at a much greater rate than other vascular malformations. It has been suggested that arteriovenous communications dilate surrounding veins. This may lead to dilation of normal arteriovenous shunts, which then lose their ability to contract, becoming part of the malformation. Destruction and heart failure are the final 2 stages. During destruction, lesions are painful and ulcerative. They may bleed or become infected. Ischemia secondary to arterial steal can cause pain and skin breakdown. High-output cardiac failure may occur early, even in infancy. These lesions may undergo rapid change during puberty, after trauma or surgery, and with pregnancy. Once symptoms present, they persist or worsen until the lesion is treated. Lesions can involve bone, especially the mandible and maxilla, and can create significant deformity.

Diagnosis

Lesions demonstrate high flow, enlarge over time, and can occur anywhere in the head and neck. Often, they involve the cheek or auricle. Lesions are often pulsatile and a bruit may be present.

On arteriography, early venous filling is diagnostic of these lesions. Magnetic resonance imaging demonstrates extent of the lesion and allows for treatment planning. Computed tomographic angiography gives excellent detail of vascular architecture and can guide treatment as well. These lesions may progress rapidly, so diagnostic workup should be completed in a timely fashion.

Physical examination and imaging usually provide diagnosis. Biopsy of an AVM can produce significant blood loss and should be avoided.

Treatment

Treatment typically consists of embolization followed by surgery. Lesions are prone to recurrence, so the treatment plan must be carefully considered. Arteriovenous malformations undergoing biopsy, subtotal excision, or proximal ligation often demonstrate sudden expansion. Extensive lesions may require free tissue transfer for reconstruction.

No other treatment modality has been show to be effective. Laser treatments, corticosteroids, and radiation have all failed to improve or cure AVMs.

Deciding which lesions to treat and timing of treatment remain controversial for some lesions. Discrete stage 1 lesions can be removed relatively easily. Treating these lesions early may eliminate the need for riskier or more urgent treatment later. Treatment success has been shown to be higher in stage 1 lesions. Stage 2 and 3 lesions, which may be painful, rapidly enlarging, or ulcerating, warrant timely treatment because they may progress to cause more serious and potentially life-threatening complications. Deciding when or if to treat extensive stage 1 lesions is more difficult because surgery may be disfiguring and have significant effect on normal function. Complete resection may not be possible, leading to high rates of recurrence, and there is no way to predict which lesions will ultimately progress to stage 2 or 3.

CAPILLARY MALFORMATIONS

Natural History

Capillary malformations (malformations of postcapillary venules) are commonly referred to as port-wine stains (PWSs). Port-wine stains are seen in 0.3% to 0.5% of children and occur equally in boys and girls. They are frequently found on the face or neck (Figure 22-9) and can have significant psychosocial effect. Lesions are present at birth and become darker, thicker, and more nodular over time.

Diagnosis

Port-wine stains are frequently seen on the mid- and upper face. Lesions with V1 or V2 distribution are seen in Sturge-Weber syndrome. Lesions with significant eyelid involvement should raise suspicion for this syndrome, and imaging to rule out leptomeningeal involvement is warranted. Magnetic resonance imaging is the modality of choice to evaluate for leptomeningeal involvement. If the eyelids are significantly involved, evaluation by an ophthalmologist to rule out glaucoma is appropriate.

Histologic evaluation of a PWS shows a plexus of dilated blood vessels at a depth of 100 to 1,000 µm (in the upper dermis). Overlying epidermis is histologically normal.

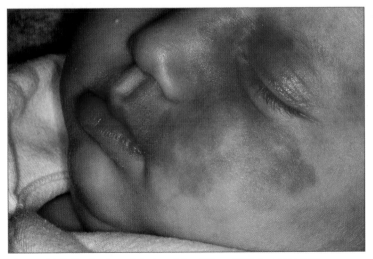

Figure 22-9. Port-wine stain involving V1 and V2 dermatomes.

Treatment

Historically, skin grafting, radiation, dermabrasion, cryosurgery, tattooing, and electrotherapy have been used to treat PWS. However, because of poor cosmetic outcomes and associated risks, none of these modalities is currently considered appropriate therapy for PWS.

The argon laser has been used to treat PWS. It achieves blanching of lesions, but hypertrophic scarring was seen up to 40% of the time.

While there is no curative therapy, current treatment consists of serial PDL treatments. Using light at a wave length of 585 to 595 nm allows selective treatment of abnormal blood vessels seen in PWS by targeting oxyhemoglobin and deoxyhemoglobin. Because melanin is a barrier to PDL, patients with darker skin may benefit from the use of bleaching creams in the weeks leading up to treatment. Lesions that do not respond to PDL can be treated with potassium titanyl phosphate laser at a wavelength of 532 nm or with an Nd:YAG at 1,064 nm. Potassium titanyl phosphate lasers have a higher thermal risk in patients with darker skin because they also target melanin.

LYMPHATIC MALFORMATIONS

Epidemiology

Lymphatic malformations are the most common vascular malformation affecting children. They occur in 1 out of 2,000 to 4,000 live births. Three-quarters of these lesions are found in the head and neck (Figure 22-10). Lesions occur sporadically, likely as a result of de novo somatic mutations.

Natural History

Lesions tend to have recurring episodes of swelling, usually in association with infection or trauma. These episodes are particularly common in suprahyoid microcystic lesions. Large lesions may be associated with lymphocytopenia affecting T, B, and natural killer cells. Facial lesions may involve and distort the facial skeleton. Most commonly, bony overgrowth is seen, but in some cases bone loss occurs. Severe bone loss is seen in Gorham disease as lymphatic vessels replace bony structures.

Diagnosis

Lesions are usually present at birth and in more than half of cases are detected in utero. Some may not be recognized until later in life when they enlarge following infection or trauma. They are usually seen as

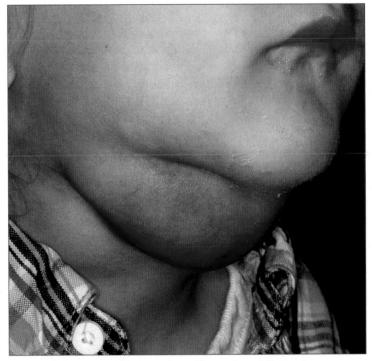

Figure 22-10. Inflamed lymphatic malformation of the neck.

easily compressible soft tissue swelling without involvement of over-lying skin.

T1-weighted MRI shows non-enhancing muscle signal intensity, and T2-weighted images show a high signal intensity lesion without feeding or draining vessels. Computed tomography shows a fluid density lesion that does not enhance. Both MRI and CT allow distinction between microcystic and macrocystic lesions. Macrocystic lesions have cystic spaces measuring 2 cm or more. Imaging both confirms diagnosis and delineates relationship of the lesion to surrounding structures.

Physical examination and imaging alone are usually adequate for diagnosis. Biopsy is not ordinarily required.

Staging

Staging is based on relationship to the hyoid and laterality. Stage 1 is unilateral and infrahyoid. Stage 2 is unilateral and suprahyoid. Stage 3 is unilateral suprahyoid and infrahyoid. Stage 4 is bilateral suprahyoid. Stage 5 is bilateral suprahyoid and infrahyoid.

Complications

Lymphatic malformations are particularly prone to infection, especially suprahyoid microcystic lesions. Swelling associated with infection may compromise feeding and respiration. Infections are treated with broad-spectrum antibiotics. Systemic corticosteroids may help resolve compressive or obstructive sequelae associated with infection.

Bony involvement, especially of the mandible, can lead to significant cosmetic deformity and functional deficits, including malocclusion, excessive drooling, and articulation difficulties. Excising soft tissue component of a lymphatic malformation does not change incidence of bony involvement.

Airway compromise can occur via extrinsic compression or intrinsic involvement of the tongue, larynx, or other structures in the airway. Airway compromise is most likely to present in infancy or following infection or trauma. Patients may require early intervention or placement of a surgical airway.

Treatment

The goal in treating lymphatic malformations should be preservation or, when necessary, restoration of functional and aesthetic integrity. Severe or life-threatening functional impairment requires prompt treatment. If there is no significant functional deficit, treatment may be delayed to allow the patient to grow.

Observation is appropriate for some lesions. Macrocystic lesions, especially those in the posterior neck, may be observed and even spontaneously regress. Small lesions without functional deficit may also be observed. However, trauma or infection may lead to rapid enlargement.

Sclerotherapy is most useful in treating macrocystic lesions. Sclerosing agents include doxycycline, bleomycin, OK-432 (picibanil), and ethanol. Erythema, pain, fever, and skin blistering are sometimes seen. Bleomycin has been associated with pulmonary fibrosis and interstitial pneumonia. Microcystic lesions can be treated with sclerosing agents with a complete response rate of 14% and partial response rate of 50%.

Surgery continues to be the most common treatment modality. Complication rates for some lesions, including large mixed suprahyoid lesions, are high. Complications include cranial nerve injury, bleeding due to great vessel injury, infection, and airway compromise. Complete excision should be performed whenever possible, but extensive lesions may require subtotal excision to protect vital structures.

Macrocystic lesions, whether suprahyoid or infrahyoid, are often amenable to resection. Infiltrative microcystic lesions are much less easily resected, especially if they are bilateral or suprahyoid, or compromise the aerodigestive tract. These lesions are more likely to require tracheostomy and gastrostomy.

COMBINED VASCULAR ANOMALIES

Klippel-Trenaunay Syndrome

Klippel-Trenaunay syndrome (KTS) is defined by a low-flow lesion affecting a lower extremity. Lesions in KTS are capillary-lymphatic-venous malformations that produce overgrowth of the affected limb. Superficial PWS and venous varicosities are hallmarks (Figure 22-11).

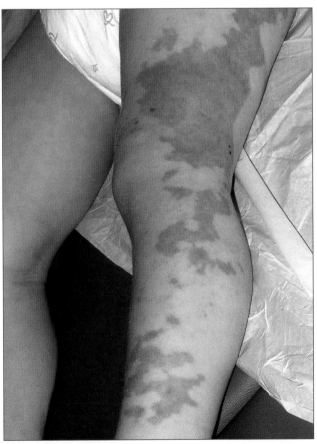

Figure 22-11. Diffuse port-wine stain and venous varicosities are typical of patients with Klippel-Trenaunay syndrome.

Enlargement of the lower extremity associated with this malformation provides a typical clinical presentation. Patients should undergo MRI before treatment is initiated to evaluate extent of the lesion and ensure that the deep venous system is patent. Magnetic resonance imaging can also rule out Parkes-Weber syndrome. Klippel-Trenaunay syndrome is usually treated with sclerotherapy, surgery, or a combination of the two.

Parkes-Weber Syndrome

Parkes-Weber syndrome is a high-flow lesion that consists of a capillary-arterial-venous malformation. It affects extremities, with overgrowth of the involved limb. Evaluation consists of physical examination and MRI. Treatment is often with embolization of the arterial component.

■ Selected References

Beck DO, Gosain AK. The presentation and management of hemangiomas. *Plast Reconstr Surg.* 2009;123(6):181e–191e

Boscolo E, Bischoff J. Vasculogenesis in infantile hemangioma. *Angiogenesis.* 2009;12:197–207

Ceisler EJ, Santos L, Blei F. Periocular hemangiomas: what every physician should know. *Pediatr Dermatol.* 2004;21(1):1–9

Chen H, Lin X, Jin Y, et al. Deep infantile hemangiomas and early venous malformations: differential diagnosis by 3D CT angiography. *Ann Plast Surg.* 2010;64(6):755–758

de Serres LM, Sie KC, Richardson MA. Lymphatic malformations of the head and neck. A proposal for staging. *Arch Otolaryngol Head Neck Surg.* 1995;121(5):577–582

Dubois J, Patriquin HB, Garel L, et al. Soft-tissue hemangiomas in infants and children: diagnosis using Doppler sonography, *AJR Am J Roentgenol.* 1998;171(1):247–252

Gampper TJ, Morgan RF. Vascular anomalies: hemangiomas. *Plast Reconstr Surg.* 2002;110(2):572–588

Itinteang T, Tan ST, Guthrie S, et al. A placental chorionic villous mesenchymal core cellular origin for infantile haemangioma. *J Clin Pathol.* 2011;64(10):870–874

Kelly KM, Choi B, McFarlane S, et al. Description and analysis of treatments of port-wine stain birthmarks. *Arch Facial Plast Surg.* 2005;7(5):287–294

Kelly ME, Juern AM, Grossman WJ, Schauer DW, Drolet BA. Immunosuppressive effects in infants treated with corticosteroids for infantile hemangiomas. *Arch Dermatol.* 2010;146(7):767–774

Kilcline C, Frieden IJ. Infantile hemangiomas: how common are they? A systematic review of the medical literature. *Pediatr Dermatol.* 2008;25(2):168–173

Kohout MP, Hansen M, Pribaz JJ, Mulliken JB. Arteriovenous malformations of the head and neck: natural history and management. *Plast Reconstr Surg.* 1998;102(3):643–654

Konez O, Burrows PE. An appropriate diagnostic workup for suspected vascular birthmarks. *Cleve Clin J Med.* 2004;71(6):505–510

Léauté-Labrèze C, Dumas de la Roque E, Hubiche T, Boralevi F, Thambo JB, Taïeb A. Propanolol for severe hemangiomas of infancy. *N Engl J Med.* 2008;358(24):2649–2651

Lee SJ, Shin DJ, Kim HY, et al. A fraction of deep vascular birthmarks are true deep hemangiomas of infancy. *Int J Dermatol.* 2009;48(8):817–821

Mulliken JB, Glowacki J. Hemangiomas and vascular malformations in infants and children: a classification based on endothelial characteristics. *Plast Recontr Surg.* 1982;69(3):412–422

North PE, Waner M, Buckmiller L, James CA, Mihm MC Jr. Vascular tumors of infancy and childhood: beyond capillary hemangioma. *Cardiovasc Pathol.* 2006;15(6):303–317

Perkins JA, Chen EY. Vascular anomalies of the head and neck. In: *Otolaryngology Head & Neck Surgery.* 5th ed. Philadelphia, PA: Mosby; 2010

Perkins JA, Manning SC, Tempero RM, et al. Lymphatic malformations: review of current treatment. *Otolaryngol Head Neck Surg.* 2010;142(6):795–803

Phung TL, Hochman M, Mihm MC. Current knowledge of the pathogenesis of infantile hemangiomas. *Arch Facial Plast Surg.* 2005;7(5):319–321

Railan D, Parlette EC, Uebelhoer NS, Rohrer TE. Laser treatment of vascular lesions. *Clin Dermatol.* 2006;24(1):8–15

Sandler G, Adams S, Taylor C. Paediatric vascular birthmarks—the psychological impact and the role of the GP. *Aust Fam Physician.* 2009;38(3):169–171

Sheth SN, Gomez C, Josephson GD. Pathological case of the month. Diagnosis and discussion: pyogenic granuloma of the tongue. *Arch Pediatr Adolesc Med.* 2001;155(9):1065–1066

Smith SP Jr, Buckingham ED, Williams EF 3rd. Management of cutaneous juvenile hemangiomas. *Facial Plast Surg.* 2008;24(1):50–64

Williams EF 3rd, Stanislaw P, Dupree M, Mourtzikos K, Mihm M, Shannon L. Hemangiomas in infants and children. An algorithm for intervention. *Arch Facial Plast Surg.* 2000;2(2):103–111

Index